TOTAL GUT BALANCE

TOTAL GUT BALANCE

Fix Your Mycobiome Fast for Complete Digestive Wellness

With 50 Recipes to Lose Weight and Feel Great

Mahmoud Ghannoum, PhD
with Eve Adamson

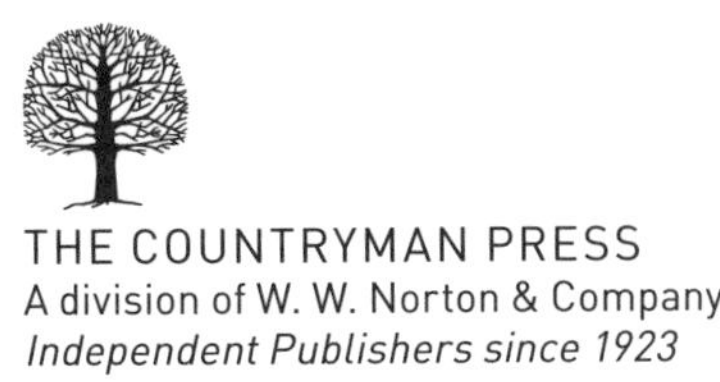

THE COUNTRYMAN PRESS
A division of W. W. Norton & Company
Independent Publishers since 1923

DISCLAIMER: This volume is intended as a general information resource. It is not a substitute for professional advice and no recommendation in this book to eat or drink anything is intended to substitute for any prescribed medication. Consult your healthcare provider before changing your diet in any significant way and before eating any new foods in significant quantities, especially if you are diabetic or suffer from any other health condition, if you are pregnant or nursing, or if you have food or other allergies. Also consult your doctor before you *start* to take any vitamin or other dietary supplement and before you *stop* taking any antibiotic, antifungal, or other prescribed medication.

As of press time, the URLs displayed in this book link or refer to existing websites. The publisher is not responsible for, and should not be deemed to endorse or recommend, any website other than its own or any content not created by it. The author, also, is not responsible for third-party material.

Printed in the United States of America

For information about permission to reproduce selections from this book, write to Permissions, The Countryman Press, 500 Fifth Avenue, New York, NY 10110

For information about special discounts for bulk purchases, please contact W. W. Norton Special Sales at specialsales@wwnorton.com or 800-233-4830

Manufacturing by Versa Press
Book design by Anna Reich
Production manager: Devon Zahn

The Countryman Press
www.countrymanpress.com

A division of W. W. Norton & Company, Inc.
500 Fifth Avenue, New York, NY 10110
www.wwnorton.com

978-1-68268-368-2

10 9 8 7 6 5 4 3 2 1

To my wife, Marie, and children, Afif, Emma, and Adam.
Your love always inspires me to keep going.

CONTENTS

INTRODUCTION

In all the discussions about the community of microorganisms living in the human gut (the microbiome) and its "good" and "bad" bacteria; in all the science about how to manipulate bacterial populations to increase gut health; and in all the media urging greater awareness of the microbiome's influence on us all, there has been a missing link. The science of the microbiome has, until recently, largely neglected an active and potentially virulent community within: It is fungus, and it is among us.

The fungi in your microbiome may not outnumber the bacteria, but it can compromise your health, contributing to weight gain, digestive problems, inflammatory bowel disorders, and even mood disorders and mental illness. As a research scientist specializing in fungus, I have dedicated my life to the study of the fungi that live in our guts, as well as in and on other parts of our bodies. I've witnessed firsthand what kind of trouble fungi can cause. Infections and systemic inflammation are a couple of obvious ways fungi can cause trouble, but they are devious in other ways—fungi can work in an insidious partnership with "bad" bacteria to foil even the most aggressive medications and render useless our most vigorous efforts at dietary control.

Intestinal fungi in particular can work with disease-causing gut bacteria, forming sticky biofilms that are a lot like the plaque on your teeth. These biofilms coat the lining of your digestive tract, protecting harmful fungal and bacterial microbes from the body's immune system, and even from antibiotic and antifungal treatment.

But we can outsmart them. *Total Gut Balance* is the first general-audience health book to explain how fungi work in the human gut, in ways that are beneficial, neutral, and detrimental to human health. If you have recently gained a lot of weight, or are having trouble losing weight; if you have digestive disorders such as irritable bowel syndrome (IBS), stomach pain, bloating after eating, flatulence, belching, nausea, vomiting, acid reflux or heartburn, chronic constipation or diarrhea (or both); if you have a diagnosed chronic disease such as Crohn's disease (CD), inflammatory bowel disease (IBD), or colitis; or even if you just have a general feeling of poor health and low energy, then you need to know how to manage your total gut balance. It could be a root cause of your health and weight issues.

The good news is that gut fungi change *rapidly.* Gut bacteria, by contrast, is largely established at birth and while it can shift gradually with dietary changes, it can never completely be remade. Not so with fungus. The community of fungi inside and on the surface of a human host (that's you) is called the **mycobiome**—a term I coined in 2010 that is now in widespread use in both the scientific community and in popular culture. The mycobiome is dynamic, shifting significantly with every meal.

We know that what you eat and do directly influence your gut fungi, and that your gut fungi, in turn, can directly influence what you weigh, how you feel, how well your immune system works, how much inflammation you have, and more. Within 24 hours, you can remake your mycobiome for better or for worse based on what you decide to eat and other factors within your control. When you make gut-friendly choices, you can set yourself on the fast track to total gut balance, which translates to weight loss, better digestion, improved health, and more energy. If you want results and you want them now, fungi are your inroad to a short-term as well as a long-term gut makeover.

In this book, you will learn a new way of eating for gut health that specifically targets fungi and takes advantage of its changeable nature. You'll also learn how to target the beneficial bacteria whose job it is to keep fungi under control. This can help you get the specific and dramatic results you've been hoping for, in record time.

The Mycobiome Diet is my potent and fast-acting solution to achieve total gut balance through direct intervention with gut fungi. This diet takes the best elements from many current popular research-based diets, but combines them for maximum total gut balance effect as follows:

Microbiome diets not only primarily target bacteria exclusively, but are often very low in carbs and sugars, which can help to decrease harmful bacteria but may leave beneficial microbes without sufficient fuel. To resolve this problem, the Mycobiome Diet addresses both bacteria and fungi, for a more encompassing approach to total gut balance. Another key difference is that the Mycobiome Diet contains more beneficial microbe-feeding fiber and resistant starch than typical microbiome diets, but avoids the potential problems associated with these dietary elements through a precise balancing and timing, so you will never eat too much of them at one time. This controls sugar-loving bacteria and fungi while at the same time sufficiently feeding microbes. Unlike other microbiome diets, the Mycobiome Diet also targets harmful biofilms with specific foods proven to break them down; offers detailed, evidence-based explanations for why it contains these specific foods and limits or eliminates other foods; and offers a much wider range of foods for maximum microbial diversity. Finally, the Mycobiome Diet addresses lifestyle elements proven to impact microbiome balance, in addition to dietary elements, making it truly unique and comprehensive.

The Paleo diet is similar to the Mycobiome Diet in its liberal use of natural whole foods. But the Mycobiome Diet does not prohibit foods that provide important fuel for beneficial fungi and bacteria, such as legumes and whole grains. It also limits inflammatory fats and animal proteins more than a typical paleo diet does.

The Mycobiome Diet can be (but need not be) **vegetarian, plant-based, or vegan,** but it specifically limits pathogenic fungi-enhancing foods (like sugar and refined grains) that are not typically prohibited on a plant-based diet. Moreover, the Mycobiome Diet has a more organized way of doling out healthy carbohydrate-rich foods throughout the day.

The Mycobiome Diet is a relatively **low-carb diet,** which helps to control sugar-loving pathogenic fungi, but unlike low-carb diets, it limits or eliminates certain types of animal products that we know are inflammatory and specifically linked to a less favorable, more disease-promoting microbiome balance.

Although the Mycobiome Diet contains plenty of healthy fats, the fats are primarily plant-based, unlike the typically animal-based fats in a standard ketogenic diet. Plant-based fats contain more gut-friendly monounsaturated and polyunsaturated fats and fewer saturated fats that we know contribute to microbial imbalance.

The Mediterranean diet is similar to the Mycobiome Diet in that it is made up primarily of natural whole plant foods. But, in order to keep pathogenic fungi under control, the Mycobiome Diet does not overuse carbohydrate-rich foods. (Recent findings[1] showed an increased prevalence of harmful fungi in subjects who ate a Mediterranean diet.) The Mycobiome Diet also limits (although does not completely prohibit) alcohol, which some versions of the Mediterranean diet do not specifically limit. The Mycobiome Diet sets these limits because we know that the combination of alcohol and certain fungi are linked to several health issues, including excessive inflammation and liver damage.

For all these reasons and more, the Mycobiome Diet is not just a best-of-all-diets approach but is also a specifically formulated diet for optimizing fungal populations and beneficial bacteria. It is designed to balance your total gut ecosystem, facilitate weight loss, inhibit cravings, strengthen immunity, boost energy, elevate mood, and promote robust health. In this book, you'll also learn which fungi (and supporting bacteria) are most likely to occupy your internal territory based on your current diet and lifestyle; what fungi could be doing to your weight, health, and well-being right now; and most important, how to get the upper hand in managing all those microbes interacting inside of you and influencing your life.

Armed with my effective, simple, proven, and delicious four-week plan, you will be able to improve your fungal balance as well as the health and abundance of your good bacteria. The improvements start on day one, and you will learn how to sustain those positive changes and better manage your mycobiome.

The strategies in this book are tested (I'll share my human test results with you), research-backed (consult the endnotes whenever you want to know more), and evidence-based. Prepare to learn more than you ever thought you needed to know about what's going on inside your gut, and how you can manipulate your intestinal microbes for your own benefit, rather than allowing them to manipulate you. Specifically, the Mycobiome Diet will help you to:

- **Limit the growth of pathogenic fungi,** especially *Candida*, with a diet specifically designed to stifle its proliferation.
- **Foster and nourish beneficial fungi** (like *Saccharomyces boulardii)* to crowd out *Candida* and solve uncomfortable gastrointestinal (GI) symptoms.
- **Enhance the growth of certain beneficial bacteria** that are particularly good at keeping fungi from overgrowing (like *Bifidobacteria* and *Lacto-*

bacilli) by providing plenty of prebiotic food for them to grow, flourish, and multiply.

- **Break down dangerous intestinal biofilms** you may already have with targeted foods that are proven to have biofilm-dissolving properties.
- **Reduce overall inflammation that weakens the immune system** with potent anti-inflammatory and antioxidant foods.

You'll also learn everything I know about how lifestyle influences the mycobiome specifically and total gut balance in general. My recommendations for exercise, sleep, and stress management are based on this knowledge. I want you to enjoy the same benefits our test subjects have enjoyed. I want you to feel better, lose weight more easily (if that is your desire), and demolish the chronic health issues that plague you.

Let's work together to balance your gut by increasing its diversity, optimizing the good fungi and bacteria, and putting the bad guys in their place to strengthen your immunity, regulate your weight, improve your mood, and make you feel better and better every day. There may be fungus among us, but what kind of impact it has is in your hands and on your plate.

PART ONE

THE SECRET SOCIETY IN YOUR GUT

The Mycobiome in Your Microbiome

Fungus. It's a funny word, perhaps calling to mind mushrooms on a pizza, mold under a basement carpet, or the yeast that makes bread rise (or the kind that causes athlete's foot). Fungus, or its plural, fungi (don't get me started on the "fun guy" jokes), doesn't necessarily sound like something you would care about or want or need . . . except maybe on that pizza. What's so interesting about fungi? How does it affect you? And what is it, anyway? Are mushrooms, yeast, and mold really all fungi?

Yes they are, but the scope of fungi encompasses more than just the culinary and the occasional household nuisance. Fungi affect you more than you may have ever guessed. *Penicillium* is a fungus, and it has saved many lives. *Candida, Aspergillus,* and *Fusarium* are fungi that have taken many lives. Humankind has had a strange and enigmatic relationship with fungi. It was first described in 1588 by an eccentric Italian Renaissance man named Giambattista della Porta, who noted the little black "seeds" he found embedded on fungi that, when planted, produced more fungi. He could not have known that these "seeds" were actually spores. He also could not have known that fungi exist not just in the crevices of rotting logs or on that orange on your kitchen counter that you forgot about, but that it lives inside all of us, where it may behave itself or proliferate out of control and cause all kinds of trouble.

We've come a long way in our knowledge of fungi since the 16th century, when many scientists thought fungi were plants (they aren't) that generated spontaneously out of nothing (they don't). Many others believed they were not alive at all. This is because they look and behave in a manner almost alien. The idea that fungi could exist inside us was even more alien. Although Hippocrates first described the white plaque-like ulcerations that can grow in the mouth and on the tongue (what we now call thrush) in 400 BC, mycologists

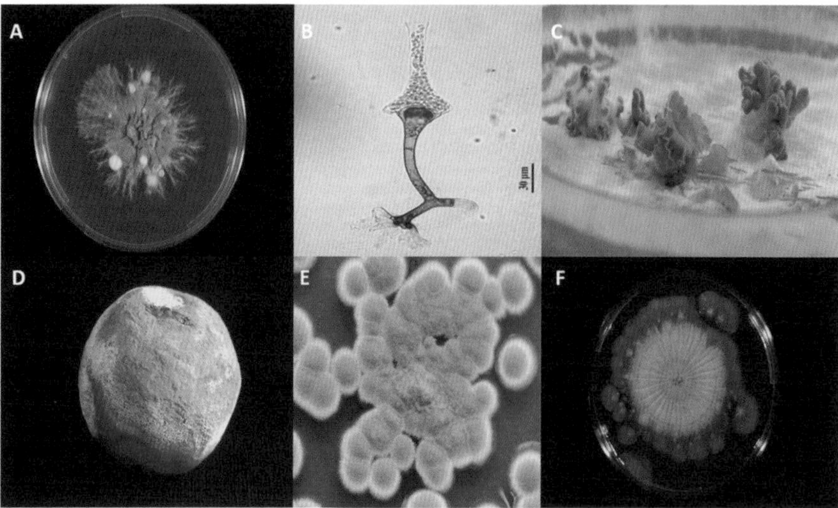

Fungi have a double personality. For example, *Penicillium* gave us penicillin, the first antibiotic discovered. However, this same fungus spoils our produce before we get around to eating it. Similarly, mushrooms can be delicious or poisonous. (A) *Epidermophyton floccosum,* a fungus that causes nail infections; (B) sporangium of *Saksenaea vasiformis,* a fungus that can cause superficial fungal infections following a trauma but which could lead to systemic infections (mild to severe) when it enters the bloodstream; (C) basidiocarps of *Schizophyllum commune* mushroom, which grows on hard wood—this fungus has a beautiful structure that resembles corals or Chinese fans, and can be edible or poisonous; (D) *Penicillium* species on an orange—these species of fungus play an important role in the natural environment as well as in their better known action as an antibiotic (used to produce penicillin) and food (used in cheesemaking). Although they are beneficial, they can cause allergic reactions in some humans; (E) *Penicillium* species growing in culture; and (F) *Basidiobolus ranarum,* a filamentous fungus that lives in the guts of reptiles and on decaying fruits and soil. It can cause subcutaneous infections, although this is rare and mostly affects children—these infections usually resolve without treatment. *Credit:* Dr. David Ellis and Dr. Sarah Kidd of the National Mycology Reference Centre, University of Adelaide.

have only recently agreed that this affliction was fungal in nature and not some strange emanation oozing from the oral tissue of a sick person.

By the 18th century, scientists had shown that fungal spores could reproduce (asexually, another curiosity). But even into the early 19th century, some die-hard, old-school botanists still insisted that fungi were inanimate objects. One "imaginative German . . . proposed, in 1804, that fungi were birthed by shooting stars."[2] Looking at a particularly weird mushroom or puffball, that theory is almost believable.

And yet, fungi are not just of this earth, but in many ways, have influenced what our earth is today. Fungi are the main microbes that break down plant debris, as we see in compost. Without fungi "processing" leaves, wood, and other plant products, we would be wading around in a world covered in layer upon layer of dead plant matter. Yet, fungi are also capable of causing plant diseases such as mildews, smuts, and rusts. Plants are even more susceptible to fungal infections than animals are—you need only observe how quickly fungus grows on strawberries just a couple of days after you buy them at the grocery store. But fungi may also work symbiotically with plants to sustain them.[3]

Animals are not immune, of course. Recently in the United States, bats were being decimated by a fungus that caused a disease called white-nose syndrome. The US Fish and Wildlife Service asked for my help, and I tested a number of antifungal agents to see if they could be used to treat the bats. Eventually, as it turned out, UV light was the most effective treatment. In an earlier time, these bats might have become extinct from this fungus.

In fact, fungi have wiped out entire species of amphibians, reptiles, and algae, epidemic-style, upending ecosystems and directing the course of evolution.[4] There is an interesting theory—unprovable, but convincing—that fungi may even have been responsible for the death of the dinosaurs and the rise of mammals as the dominant class on earth, since reptiles and the plants they eat are particularly susceptible to fungal disease.[5] We may very well owe our place as masters of the planet to fungi, and fungi will likely continue to influence life on earth for as long as it continues to spin around the sun.

But what's most relevant for our current focus, as you will soon see, is that fungi are not just all around us, but inhabit us, change us, influence us, and in many ways, determine how healthy we are, how much we weigh, how we feel, and even whether we will live or die. They work together with bacteria to outsmart us, or to help us, depending on their fungal agenda. They are an influential minority within the human microbiome and they act (like most living things) in their own best interest. To me, as a mycologist who has spent a lifetime studying them, they are utterly enthralling.

WHAT'S IN A MICROBIOME?

To understand how influential fungi can be for human health, we must first understand the microbiome as a whole. The microbiome, to put it simply, is a collection of microbes that live inside and on the human body. They are in us but not of us, and each microbe has its own DNA and will to survive. In a sense, these microbes are the aliens within, because they are not technically human and do not come from our bodies. They have been "invading" us since before our birth, and that invasion has had many beneficial effects, as well as some harmful ones. For the most part, our relationship with our microbiome is symbiotic—we depend on those microbes and they depend on us for health and survival. Our microbiomes have about as many cells as we have human cells, so while their cells are a lot smaller and make up only a little bit of our mass (maybe a pound or two), you could say that cell-for-cell, we are only about half human.[6]

Also, the microbiome is fraught with mystery. Honestly, there are a lot of microbes inside you that science has not identified yet, and others that we know exist but cannot grow or culture in a lab (many fungi fall into this category), which makes them more difficult to study.

When most people think about the microbiome, they think about bacteria. Bacteria are a large part of the microbiome, it's true. They are the majority. Bacteria are also relatively easy to culture and study, so we know a lot about them compared to what we know about fungi. Interest in bacteria is also a current fad—many books, articles, and blogs have been written about the "bacteria in your gut" and how to manage it. "Gut bacteria," "microbiome," "gut garden," and other similar terms have become buzzwords in the health community. Most of the research on the human microbiome right now focuses on bacteria, and only bacteria. There is no doubt that the study of bacteria in the microbiome is an exciting new avenue of research that shows a lot of promise for addressing health issues.

But many people believe that "microbiome" and "bacteria" are synonymous. They are not. Your population of inner bacteria is called your bacteriome. The microbiome is much bigger, encompassing *all* the microbes that live in you and on you—not just bacteria but fungi, parasites, protozoa, amoebae, archaea (single-celled bacteria-like microorganisms that can survive under extreme conditions), viruses, and bacteriophages (which are essentially viruses that infect bacteria). Each of these microbial categories has its own community, but they are all mingled together inside you.

Fungi are a little like the black sheep of the microbiome. They are a part of the microbiome—a subcommunity—but they can cause big trouble by going against the current of what is most beneficial for the microbiome's human host (that's you). But fungi aren't all bad. Some are helpful, contributing to the complex workings of your body, and some are helpful in small amounts but harmful if they become too numerous or abundant.

As a whole, your microbiome directly or indirectly influences your weight, digestion, skin health, immunity, and chances for developing autoimmune disease, digestive cancers (such as colon cancer), kidney disease, HIV, liver disease, Parkinson's disease, Alzheimer's disease, type 2 diabetes, cystic fibrosis, neurodevelopmental disorders such as autism spectrum disorder and attention-deficit/hyperactivity disorder (ADHD), and more.[7] Your microbiome configurations can even influence your moods, due to something called the gut-brain axis (GBA). (I'll talk more about this in Chapter 7.)

Of all the systems in your body influenced by your microbiome, your digestive tract may be the most dramatically affected. We know from much scientific research that having a healthy gastrointestinal system depends upon having a healthy, well-balanced microbiome with a wide variety of species and a good balance of beneficial microbes to potentially harmful ones. When your microbiome is diverse and robust, it benefits you in many ways, such as:

- **Increasing nutrient absorption.** The microbiome is responsible for much of the biosynthesis of vitamins and essential amino acids.
- **Producing important metabolic by-products with useful properties that make you healthier.** These by-products, such as butyrate and short-chain fatty acids (SCFAs), come from your microbes digesting the foods you eat that you can't easily digest (like fiber and resistant starch). These by-products have many beneficial properties, such as being anti-inflammatory.
- **Improving immune function.** Many components of your immune system are manufactured or stimulated by the activity in your microbiome.
- **Preventing health problems.** Microbiomes have many mechanisms that help to prevent malnutrition, allergies, and infections.
- **Sealing the gut.** Microbiomes help to maintain your gastrointestinal (GI) barrier, so food particles and microbes don't "leak" out of the GI tract, and toxins don't get in.

Your microbiome is a crowded place, and its composition shifts constantly, depending on the conditions in you and on you—microbes reproduce, or die off, at different rates depending on what you feed them and how you live. They also interact with each other, sometimes helping each other, sometimes vying for power and influence. It is survival of the fittest in there . . . but *you* get to determine who is the fittest. You have more control than you may realize. Through diet and lifestyle, you can manipulate the environment in which those microbes exist, optimizing conditions for the good guys and stifling the bad guys so they don't take over and cause you problems.

Here are some other interesting things we know about the human microbiome:[8]

- **It contains the good, the bad, and the neutral.** The microbes (including fungi and bacteria) within you can be commensal (neutral), symbiotic (beneficial), or pathogenic (potentially harmful). Some microbes can fall under more than one of these categories, depending on how many there are. They may be neutral or beneficial in small numbers, but pathogenic in abundance.
- **It's not just in our guts.** Most of our microbes are in our gastrointestinal tracts, reproductive systems, mouths, and on our skin—they tend to accumulate nearest the portals of entry to our bodies.
- **Your diet influences who lives in there.** People with different diets have distinctly different microbiome configurations—for example, the typical vegetarian has a much different gut than people who eat a lot of meat.
- **Diversity is a good thing.** People with the most microbial diversity—in other words, those with a higher than average number of different species—tend to be the healthiest. Those with the lowest diversity, or the fewest species, tend to have more health issues such as allergies, obesity, arthritis, inflammatory bowel diseases, diabetes, high blood pressure, and neuropsychiatric disorders.
- **Most of your viruses won't harm you.** Most of the viruses in your gut are bacteriophages, or viruses that only infect your bacteria, not you. Many viruses that could affect you are easily wiped out by your immune system.
- **It started before birth.** Although scientists once believed babies were born with no microbiome, we now know that they do have a few microbes

within, which they get before birth. However, most of an infant's initial microbiome is established during the birthing process. (This is why infants born "naturally" have different microbiomes than those born by C-section—they are exposed to different kinds of tissues.)

- **It influences your weight.** Many studies show a consistent link between microbiome configuration and weight, with certain microbes consistently associated with people who are of normal weight, and other microbes, including fungi, associated with people who have obesity.
- **It influences your mood.** The microbiome produces the bulk of serotonin (a neurotransmitter that contributes to feelings of happiness and well-being) in your digestive tract, which directly impacts mood and health issues like depression and anxiety. Also, the gut-brain axis is a connection between the brain and the enteric nervous system in the gut that can deliver messages back and forth. Problems in the gut can impact the brain, and vice versa.
- **It can make you sick.** Imbalances in the microbiome (dysbiosis) can cause or contribute to many health problems. The most obvious ones are gut-related, such as inflammatory bowel diseases like Crohn's disease and ulcerative colitis (UC), as well as other digestive problems like irritable bowel syndrome and diarrhea that occurs while traveling or after antibiotic use. However, other health problems that are less obvious can also have a microbiome component, including cancer, autoimmune diseases, and mood disorders like depression.
- **Aging changes it—if you let it.** As humans age, their microbiomes often become less diverse and different species tend to predominate. Research has linked these changes to increased frailty, GI problems like colitis, certain cancers, and hardening of the arteries in older people. However, those who maintain a more robust microbiome through diet and lifestyle are likely to age more easily and with fewer health problems.

As you can see, your microbiome is incredibly influential at every stage of life, so it's no wonder the scientific and health communities are obsessed with discovering how to manipulate it for human benefit. There are a lot of ways to do this, but let's take a closer look at a shortcut that will help you optimize your microbiome efficiently, effectively, and quickly: by targeting fungus.

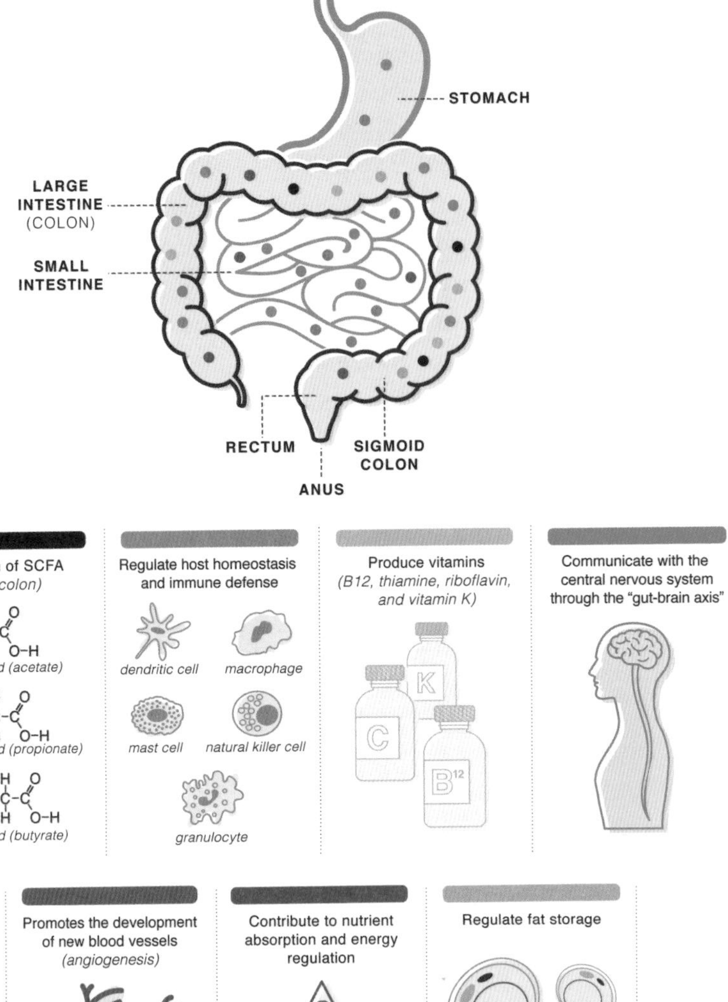

Schematic representation of how the microbiome influences our health. Microbes have a range of functions that support our well-being, including: (1) producing short-chain fatty acids (SCFAs) that have diverse physiological functions in our body (for example, they are a primary energy source for colonic cells), (2) regulating homeostasis, (3) producing vitamins, (4) communicating with our central nervous system, (5) promoting the development of blood vessels, (6) contributing to nutrient absorption and energy regulation, and (7) regulating fat storage.

Your Microbiome Fingerprint

Not only are human (and animal) microbiomes complex, but each one is different, like a fingerprint or a snowflake. Some of those differences are species-specific. Others are specific to diet, lifestyle, or location. Within subgroups, microbiomes often share certain characteristics. Particular bacteria and fungi are likely to be present or established in the microbiomes of most humans (but not in other animals), or in most mammals (but not in bugs or birds). For example, dogs can have similar microbiomes to humans, but honeybees have microbiomes that look much different (although not entirely different) than ours.

Also, some microbes are most likely to be established in people with particular diets and lifestyles, such as vegetarians versus those who eat a standard Western diet high in fat and sugar. There are similarities in the microbiomes of people who live in one country (such as people in France), and differences among the microbiomes of people who live in different countries. People who live in Ohio, where I live, have very different microbiomes than people who live in Lebanon, where I grew up. People who live in Korea and eat a lot of kimchi have different microbiomes than people who live in England and eat a lot of sausage. There are differences between the microbiomes of those who live in one environment (such as a big city) and those who live in a different kind of environment (such as on a dairy farm in a rural area).

To a large extent, we can predict many aspects of a microbiome's configuration by knowing how someone eats and lives, as well as where they live, and in what kind of immediate environment. (I'll tell you more about that in Chapter 7.) However, these consistencies are more likely to apply to bacteria than to fungi. Fungal populations are much less predictable and change easily and frequently. If you live in England and move to Korea, your bacteria will change slowly based on your changing diet and environment, but your fungi will likely change within hours.

The dominant fungi in any given group of humans, or in any individual human, is a wild card. We can't say that any one fungus is the prevalent one in all Americans, for example, because there are so many different ones that could potentially predominate. There is no known "normal." Nearly half of all the fungi we have identified so far in humans have only been reported to appear in one person, or in one study.[9] These fungi (mostly yeasts) may colonize the human body (they are resident fungi, also called autochthonous fungi), or they may be just passing through (nonresident or transient fungi). Either way, if you were to have your microbiome tested, you might very well have a yeast nobody else you know has ever had.

THE FUNGUS AMONG US

Now that we have the lay of the land, let's zoom in and give your mycobiome a closer look. While bacteria may be the "majority microbe," fungi are vying for the spotlight. They represent just 0.1% of your microbial species,[10] but they compensate by being larger in size. As you can see from an electron microscopy photo we recently published, one fungal cell is larger than 12 bacterial cells.

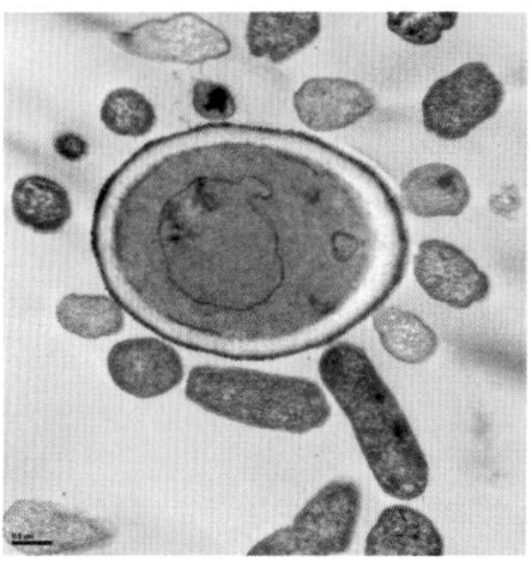

Transmission electron microscopy image showing a cross section of the fungus *Candida tropicalis* (large cell in the middle) surrounded by multiple bacteria. These organisms cooperate together to cause gastrointestinal issues in Crohn's disease patients.

Fungi are all over you. They exist in your mouth, in your gastrointestinal tract, on your skin, and sometimes in your lungs. Fungi can develop between your toes, under your fingernails and toenails, in and around your genitals. When it overgrows it can cause infections in all these places—superficial skin infections such as tinea pedis (athlete's foot), tinea corporis (ringworm, which is not caused by a worm but rather by fungus), tinea cruris (jock itch), and tinea versicolor (small pale, dark tan, or pink patches of skin), as well as thrush in the mouth (mostly in babies and the elderly), and vaginal yeast infections. Inhaling fungus can cause lung infections, and fungi can even get into your bloodstream.

Fungi have also been implicated in all sorts of gut disorders, from irritable bowel syndrome (IBS) to inflammatory bowel diseases (IBDs) like Crohn's disease (CD) and ulcerative colitis (UC). It causes many serious infections in hospitals and in people with compromised immune systems. It can also cause plenty of trouble for healthy people, like digestive problems, blood sugar imbalance, and excessive weight gain or weight loss resistance. For example, studies have linked obesity to higher levels of certain fungi, such as Eurotiomycetes, while weight loss is associated with higher levels of *Mucor.*[11] Fungi have been associated with increased inflammation,[12] and at least one study clearly demonstrated that a high-sugar diet leads to excessive growth of *Candida* species and related infections, but that decreasing sugar and artificial sweetener intake helped to decrease this growth and re-establish balance.[13] Studies have discovered higher numbers of *Candida* species in the gastrointestinal tracts of malnourished children, and theorize that vitamin and iron deficiencies may be risk factors for *Candida* infections.[14] These are just a few examples of the many ways in which fungi can influence human health, and how what you eat is closely linked to the fungus that lives inside you.

Fortunately, you can completely refurbish your fungi in 24 hours, just by changing your diet, which can help improve your health in numerous tangible ways. We call this the short-term diet effect, and it means that changing your diet can create swift and meaningful shifts in your mycobiome within hours, while your bacteriome slowly works to catch up.

Once you begin the Mycobiome Diet, you are likely to begin noticing positive changes in your energy level and gastrointestinal symptoms within the first 24 hours. As you shift your diet to modify your microbiome, you will continue to experience improvements in your energy and feelings of good health. After four weeks of eating to control your mycobiome and balance your gut, you are likely to notice significant changes in weight (if you have excess weight to lose) as well as even more profound differences in the way you feel. The longer you sustain these changes, the more lasting your microbiome shifts will be, resulting in longer-term effects like a strengthened immune system, enhanced weight regulation, rejuvenated skin, fewer allergies, less inflammation, and in many cases, the complete disappearance of gastrointestinal problems such as IBS and heartburn or acid reflux.

Rebalancing fungi is step one—as beneficial species like *Saccharomyces boulardii* increase and pathogenic fungi like *Candida* decrease, the beneficial bacteria (such as *Lactobacillus* and *Bifidobacterium*) that regulate fungal balance and do so much to improve health have more room and a better environment for growth and reproduction. Fungal control is the door that can lead to a whole new world of better microbiome balance for optimal health. You'll enjoy bolstered immunity, reduced inflammation, fewer digestive problems, easier weight loss, more energy, less fatigue, and a brightened mood.

THE **HUMAN** MYCOBIOME

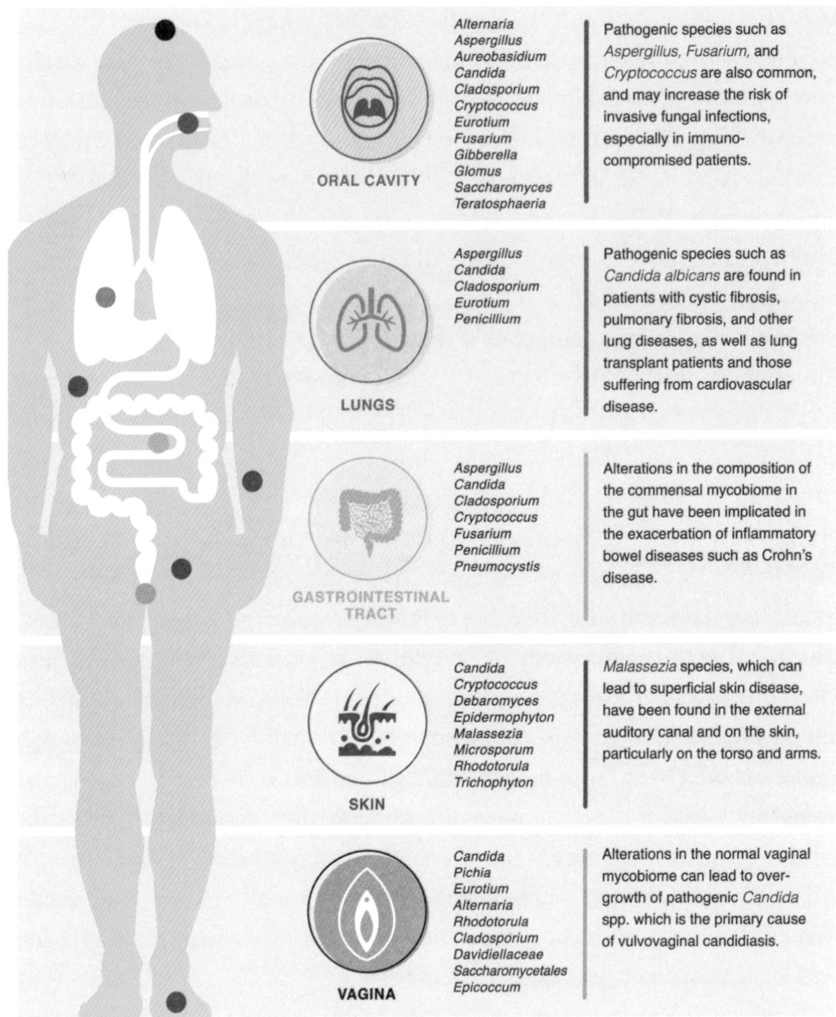

Fungal community members found in different compartments of the body.

Science Finally Focuses on Fungi

It has taken some time for the scientific community to recognize the importance and influence of fungi, and interest in the microbiome's fungal element has only begun to trickle down into the scientific research and the mainstream health media. Fortunately, researchers have started to use state-of-the-art sequencing technology, which allows us to study fungi without culturing it in a lab,[15] and we are now beginning to identify which fungi live where in our bodies.

When I first came to the United States, the idea that fungi such as yeasts could be harmful for human health was out there but considered to be a "fringe" idea that was often inaccurately portrayed in alternative health circles. In 2010, my team was the first to demonstrate the importance of fungal communities in the human body. That's not so long ago, in scientific terms. While those of us studying fungi still fight for recognition in a field that remains preoccupied with bacteria, we are making headway.

YOUR FUNGI LINEUP: GOOD GUYS AND BAD GUYS

When it comes to fungi, there are "good guys" and "bad guys." A great example of a good fungus is *Penicillium chrysogenum,* which is used to make the medicine we call penicillin (discovered in 1928). This fungus actually takes down pathogenic bacteria, such as when you get strep throat, or when your child gets an ear infection. In 1987, lovastatin (a drug used to reduce cardiovascular disease by lowering cholesterol) was produced using the fungus *Aspergillus terreus.* Fungi keep giving! In the gut, fungi called *Saccharomyces* are beneficial for human health in multiple ways—people who are healthy tend to have more of these fungi, and those with certain gut-related health conditions like Crohn's disease tend to have fewer. Other fungi are neutral—they don't seem to impact us directly, or we haven't yet discovered how they do.

Then there are those that are notorious troublemakers. *Candida albicans* can contribute to severe health issues, from irritable bowel syndrome to weight loss resistance to systemic infection. When their numbers are kept down, they don't do any harm and may even be useful. Problems occur when they get too numerous or transform shape and become more virulent and harmful to you, their human host.

Before we start targeting the bad guys and nurturing the good ones, let's get an idea of exactly who's who. While there are millions of fungal species on the planet, and we still haven't fully identified all of those inside the human microbiome, we do know there are some key players:

***Candida* yeasts:** Most of the fungi in your colon are probably from the *Candida* genus. Even perfectly healthy people host various species of *Candida,* and when it is kept in check and there isn't too much of it, *Candida* yeast won't cause a problem. People who tend to eat a lot of sugar also tend to have a larger population of *Candida* yeast, and so do people with inflammatory bowel disease and cystic fibrosis. The most prevalent *Candida* yeast in your digestive tract is *Candida albicans,* a pathogenic yeast that grows and spreads more quickly in people who eat high-sugar diets and who drink a lot of yeast-fermented beverages (like wine and beer). Another *Candida* yeast that tends to be more prevalent in the microbiomes of people with Crohn's disease is *Candida tropicalis.* Interestingly (or alarmingly), the population of *Candida* in your gut will multiply significantly within just 24 hours of a high-carbohydrate meal. *Candida*'s potential for harm results in a thumbs-down vote. **Verdict: Bad guys.**

***Saccharomyces* yeasts:** These are the yeasts that turn sugar into carbon dioxide, so they are used to bake bread, brew beer and wine, and distill spirits. The yeast called baker's yeast or brewer's yeast is *Saccharomyces cerevisiae,* and this is also the species used to make nutritional yeast. People with Crohn's disease and ulcerative colitis tend to have a low level of these yeasts, while healthy people have more of them, suggesting that having them is protective.

Some *Saccharomyces* species are especially beneficial, such as *Saccharomyces boulardii,* which helps control diarrhea caused by antibiotics; viral and bacterial infections, including the dangerous *Clostridium difficile* (*C. diff.*); and so-called traveler's diarrhea. These yeasts reduce inflammation, make it more difficult for bacteria and fungi to adhere to the intestinal wall, form biofilms, and break them down. They also inhibit the ability of pathogens to produce toxins, and on top of all that, they antagonize *Candida.* This yeast is a fungus superstar. Because of all these beneficial properties, *Saccharomyces boulardii* is sometimes used in probiotic supplements. **Verdict: Good guys.**

Pichia kluyveri: At least inside the human mouth, this yeast has been shown to be antagonistic against *Candida* in people with HIV-AIDS. *Pichia* also tends to be more abundant in people of normal weight than in people who are overweight. While we can't yet give *Pichia* to people in the United States to see if it helps with weight loss and digestive issues (the approval process is complex), this may be a treatment available in the future, so stay tuned.

Meanwhile, farmers in Europe spray their produce (for example, apples) with *Pichia* to prevent spoilage by molds. **Verdict: Good guys.**

Galactomyces geotrichum: This species is associated with a healthy gut. This fungus cooperates with beneficial bacteria to improve microbiome balance and to produce metabolites that can benefit you in many ways. **Verdict: Good guys.**

***Aspergillus* molds:** These fungi are all over the environment, in the food we eat and the air we breathe. One of the worst is *Aspergillus fumigatus,* which can lead to allergic reactions and life-threatening infections, especially in people who are immune-compromised. It's not as common as *Candida,* but it can do a lot of harm. **Verdict: Bad guys (although some species are neutral).**

***Fusarium* molds:** These molds are even less common than *Aspergillus* molds, but when they do get a foothold, they can cause serious opportunistic infections, especially in people with compromised immune systems, such as people with diabetes, transplant patients, or the very young and very old. **Verdict: Bad guys.**

***Zygomycetes* fungi:** Zygomycetes fungi generally aren't very abundant in the human gut, but some types, such as *Rhizopus* and *Mucor,* respond most vigorously to proteins and simple sugars like glucose. In the environment, you can find these fungi in spoiled fruit, soil, and dung. In humans, they can be pathogenic or beneficial. *Mucor* has been shown to contribute to pneumonia and other respiratory infections as well as skin infections, usually in immune-compromised people. However, one study showed that obese subjects had far fewer *Mucor* than normal-weight subjects, so it could also have a favorable effect on weight regulation. We have a lot more to learn about this group. **Verdict: Hung jury.**

Penicillium: This fungus is one of the most scientifically important types of fungus. When used therapeutically, it is well known for its ability to kill and control the growth of certain types of bacteria in the body. When it occurs in the gut, it seems to be present in larger numbers in vegetarians, which may be at least partially attributable to consumption of greater amounts of fruits, vegetables, and grains. **Verdict: Good guys.**

These are just a few of the fungal microbes that may be influencing your mycobiome right now. Later in this book, you will learn their needs and vulnerabilities: What feeds them, what starves them, and how to balance their populations for your benefit.

What You Need to Know About Taxonomy

Even though I have studied fungi for many years, I still have difficulty following the names of all the microbes and knowing exactly how to differentiate among them, due to their sometimes bewildering diversity. Taxonomy is the classification of organisms based on similarities, and its purpose is to organize the confusion. The Linnaean system of taxonomy divides all life into eight levels: domain, kingdom, phylum, class, order, family, genus, and species. This system has been continually modernized since the 1700s and made more complicated with subgroups and other variations, but the point is to make the relationships among organisms easier to comprehend.

For the purpose of this book and for best understanding the names of the various fungi and bacteria I will mention throughout, I will mainly be referring to phylum, genus, and species. I like to use the analogy of a family. The family includes everyone that is related. At the top, you have the parents. Then the children, then the grandchildren. It works like this:

Phylum: The phylum is like the parents. Ascomycota is an example of a fungal phylum, and Proteobacteria is a bacterial phylum. Note that phylum names are not written in italics, but their first letter is capitalized.

Genus: Next is the genus, which is like the children. *Candida* is a fungal genus, and *Escherichia* is a bacterial genus. Note that the genus is written in italics, and the first letter is also capitalized.

Species: The species is like the grandchildren. *Saccharomyces cerevisiae* is a fungal species and *Escherichia coli* (the dreaded *E. coli)* is a bacterial species. The species name is written in italics and the first letter is not capitalized. Species names always have two parts—the genus and then the species. The genus part of the name is capitalized, the species part of the name is not.

If we look at the two kingdoms of fungi and bacteria in this way, we can see how they separate out and how they are related. In some cases, we can pretty much dub all members of a phylum as "bad guys" (such as Proteobacteria), but more often, at the genus and species level, there are both good and bad guys, although one or the other might make up the majority.

YOUR BACTERIA LINEUP: THE KEY PLAYERS IN THE MYCOBIOME GAME

Next, let's look at just a few of the most influential bacteria that interact with fungi for good and for bad, so that when I talk about them throughout this book, you'll know who to cheer for, and when to yell "Boo!" These are the bacteria that are most influential in either wrangling troublemaking fungi like *Candida* into submission or teaming up with pathogenic fungi to make them even more harmful and virulent:

Proteobacteria: High levels of bacteria in this phylum are a red flag for systemic inflammation. **Verdict: Bad guys.**

Bacteroidetes: These are one of the most common organisms in the human gut microbiota. High levels of bacteria in this phylum are associated with a healthy gut. **Verdict: Mostly good guys, but a few bad guys.**

Firmicutes: Moderate levels of bacteria in this phylum are also associated with gut health, but very elevated levels are associated with obesity. **Verdict: Some good guys, many bad guys.**

Now let's look at some of the genus-level bacteria. These are key players in your gut that can influence or interact with fungi and bacteria:

Bifidobacterium: These bacteria produce short-chain fatty acids (SCFAs), which lower inflammation. They improve the gastrointestinal barrier and lower lipopolysaccharide levels, which also decrease inflammation. **Verdict: Good guys.**

Lactobacillus: These bacteria, part of the Firmicutes phylum, also produce SCFAs, reduce inflammation, and are particularly good at keeping *Candida* under control. **Verdict: Good guys.**

Bilophila: These bacteria promote pro-inflammatory activity. **Verdict: Bad guys.**

Clostridium: These bacteria are part of the Firmicutes phylum, but unlike *Lactobacillus,* they promote inflammation. Several different *Clostridium* species are highly pathogenic. **Verdict: Bad guys.**

Roseburia: Yet another member of the Firmicutes phylum, these bacteria produce SCFAs and are anti-inflammatory. **Verdict: Good guys.**

The following are some species that are particularly relevant for our mycobiome focus:

Faecalibacterium prausnitzii: This is the only known species in the *Faecalibacterium* genus, but it is one of the most common bacteria in the human gut microbiome. It boosts immunity and has many benefits, including the production of SCFAs and anti-inflammatory activity. **Verdict: Good guys.**

Akkermansia muciniphila: This bacterium is one of the few that doesn't get its food from you. It gets its food from mucin, which lines your gastrointestinal tract. When you don't eat, this puts other bacteria at a disadvantage but gives this one an advantage—and because it feeds on the degraded mucin, it helps restore strength and integrity to your gut lining. People with low levels of this species tend to have a thinner, less healthy gut lining. Use of this bacteria as a supplement improves several metabolic parameters. **Verdict: Good guys.**

Bacteroides fragilis: These drive the expansion of pro-inflammatory cytokines. **Verdict: Bad guys.**

Escherichia coli: You've probably heard of the notorious *E. coli* in food poisoning cases. This bacterium is elevated in people with Crohn's disease. It is particularly good at working in cahoots with *Candida tropicalis* to form detrimental biofilms. **Verdict: Bad guys.**

An important take-home message about the classification of organisms as being "bad" or "good" (in other words, beneficial to you or pathogenic to you) is that it's complicated. It's not just about whether an organism is present or absent. It depends on the relative levels of each. For example, take Firmicutes and Bacteroidetes. Even though these large groups of bacteria are present in the gut, whether or not they represent a good or bad influence depends on the ratio of one to the other. This is expressed as the Firmicutes/Bacteroidetes ratio (F/B). People with obesity tend to have high levels of Firmicutes compared to Bacteroidetes, meaning they have a high F/B ratio. In contrast, individuals falling within the normal weight range tend to have a lesser amount of Firmicutes compared to Bacteroidetes, resulting in a low F/B ratio. Are Firmicutes "bad"? Not necessarily. In proportion, they are just fine and contribute to human health. It is only when they grow too numerous that they can have a bad influence.

Also, within any phylum or genus, even if most of the species have a good influence, there may be a few that are more harmful, especially in greater abundance. In other words, don't take this "good guy" and "bad guy" list as set in stone. There are always exceptions. That being said, here's a table to give you a summary of the key players in the world of your mycobiome. The abbreviation "spp." is Latin for "multiple species," and it indicates when I'm referring to different types of bacteria within one genus. Refer back to this table as you read this book if you need to remember who's who.

The "Good Guys" (beneficial microbes)	The "Bad Guys" (pathogenic microbes)
FUNGI	
Saccharomyces cerevisiae	*Candida* spp.
Saccharomyces boulardii	*Candida albicans*
Pichia kluyveri	*Candida tropicalis*
Galactomyces geotrichum	*Fusarium* spp.
Penicillium spp.	*Aspergillus* spp.
Neutral or undetermined: *Zygomycetes* spp., including *Mucor*	
BACTERIA	
Lactobacillus spp.	Proteobacteria
Bifidobacterium spp.	*Clostridium* spp.
Faecalibacterium prausnitzii	*Bilophila* spp.
Akkermansia muciniphila	*Bacteroides fragilis*
Roseburia spp.	*Escherichia coli*
Contains both good and bad guys: Bacteroidetes, Firmicutes	

WHAT THE MYCOBIOME DIET CAN DO

When people learn about the fungi within them and how their own behavior (diet and lifestyle) directly affects the overgrowth or tight control of fungal species that impact health, I've seen them conquer health issues that they had never been able to control before. Over the years, I have seen many people suffering from gastrointestinal disorders, low energy, overall poor health, and unhappiness. By implementing dietary and lifestyle changes that address fungi, I've seen these same people become more energetic, with massive improvements in digestive health and a revitalized mood. This is my goal for you in creating the Mycobiome Diet.

I developed this diet based on my extensive research, the research of others in my field, and a massive database of information collected from thousands of people living in different parts of the United States. This data shed light on what microbiome configurations tended to coincide with various lifestyles and health issues. Importantly, this powerful data helped me understand the clinical impact of microbiome imbalance and gave me the information I needed to devise the Mycobiome Diet (as well as some other therapies—see the Appendix for more information).

Once the Mycobiome Diet was created, I went on to conduct a clinical trial with my team to evaluate the effectiveness of the Mycobiome Diet on the microbiome in general and on the mycobiome in particular for outcomes of improved health, reduced symptoms of gastrointestinal distress, weight loss, and subjective reports of changes in energy and mood.

Our subjects were healthy volunteers between the ages of 30 and 70 who agreed to follow the Mycobiome Diet for 28 days, and have their microbiomes tested periodically before, during, and after the study. The participants completed daily food logs, checking off the foods required for daily and weekly consumption, while noting various health measures such as weight and aspects of digestion and symptoms. The results of the study were exciting. The Mycobiome Diet was highly successful at reducing *Candida* species in general—the most troublesome and problematic of the gut fungi. Within just two weeks on the Mycobiome Diet, *Candida* species overall decreased by 72.4%; *Candida albicans* in particular decreased 1.42-fold, an impressive reduction; and *Candida tropicalis* disappeared completely after 4 weeks. (*Candida albicans* is among the most common and virulent pathogenic microbes, and *Candida tropicalis* tends to worsen symptoms and increase inflammation.)

Several beneficial fungal species increased over the course of the four-week trial. *Galactomyces geotrichum* increased by 58.4%, and *Pichia kluyveri* increased by 45.1%. *Galactomyces geotrichum* is one of the "good guys" typically associated with healthy gut function. It binds to lactic acid bacteria in a symbiotic positive relationship with *Lactobacillus,*[16] and it also produces peptides that can lead to better blood pressure control. My own lab has demonstrated how *Pichia* is particularly good at antagonizing the pathogenic *Candida* species.[17] More *Pichia* often means less *Candida,* including the inhibition of *Candida*-formed biofilms, and we have also shown that it can inhibit pathogenic *Fusarium* and *Aspergillus.*

Like the majority of the population in the United States, our study subjects came into the trial with high levels of pro-inflammatory Proteobacteria. After the 28-day trial, Proteobacteria was reduced from an unhealthy 38.6% to a much healthier 23.3%. Many studies support the concept that a high abundance of Proteobacteria is a sign of dysbiosis, or an unstable microbiome.

Subjects also significantly increased their levels of beneficial bacteria—specifically *Faecalibacterium prausnitzii* (up 35.8%), *Bifidobacterium adolescentis* (up 61.6%), *Roseburia* (up 57.5%), *Lactobacillus* (up 77.6%), and *Bacteroides* (up 22%). Pathogenic bacteria decreased significantly, including *Escherichia coli* (down 74%), *Bacteroides fragilis* (down 45.3%), and *Clostridium* (down 55.7%). One study showed that people who consume more junk food have increased *E. coli* in their guts, with less beneficial bacteria like *Lactobacillus* and *Faecalibacterium prausnitzii,* while a diet high in antioxidants inhibited the growth of *E. coli.*[18] Species of *Clostridium* have been associated with many GI issues, especially diarrhea but also constipation, vomiting, nausea, and irritable bowel syndrome.[19]

Many subjective improvements took place as well. Before starting the study, 60% of the participants reported health issues, especially symptoms of gastrointestinal distress. Thirty percent had SIBO (small intestinal bacterial overgrowth—see an explanation of this condition on page 29). Ten percent had celiac disease. Many reported problems with gas, bloating, constipation, heartburn, and diarrhea. Other reported issues included fatigue; low energy; cravings for sugar, bread, or salty carbs; and sleep disturbances, especially waking in the middle of the night.

After the study, all participants with GI symptoms reported moderate or dramatic improvements. Two-thirds of the participants who chose to track their weight lost a significant amount (between 2 and 10 pounds) over the testing period. (Note that all those participants who did not lose weight were at a normal BMI and did not need or want to lose weight, meaning all participants who wanted to lose weight did lose weight.) Thirty percent of the participants reported moderate or dramatically higher energy levels and reductions in fatigue. These were the participants who reported problems with fatigue and energy prior to the study. Thirty percent reported better sleep, less waking at night, and even reduced hot flashes—these were the same participants who complained of having these issues before the study began. Sixty percent of the participants decided to stay on the Mycobiome Diet after the trial.

Forty percent returned to their old diets at the end of the trial, and all of them experienced worsening of their symptoms except one subject, whose diet was already quite similar to the Mycobiome Diet. After symptom recurrence, some decided to go back on the Mycobiome Diet again or return to certain aspects of the diet that they believed were helpful.

Overall, we determined that adhering to the Mycobiome Diet does indeed lead to positive shifts in fungal and bacterial communities in the guts of participants, and that these shifts typically resulted in reduced GI distress symptoms, healthy weight loss, decreased fatigue, increased energy, more restful sleep, and fewer cravings for empty-calorie foods, in those people who had these particular issues.

In the second part of this book, you will get all the details about how to follow the Mycobiome Diet that our study subjects did. But first, let's look more deeply into the microbiome to see what's going on in there, and what you can start to do about it right away.

2

Prognosis: Dysbiosis

Balance is a beautiful thing. It brings calmness to life and calmness to the gut, too. The human body works very hard to achieve and maintain balance in all its systems, and this balanced state, especially when it comes to the internal workings of the human body, is sometimes called *homeostasis.* Homeostasis is a state of physiological stability within a system, and it is a marker of good health. When homeostasis is disrupted, problems can take root and ripple throughout the whole system. When uncorrected, the eventual result will be disease, dysfunction, even death.

There are many examples of homeostasis in the human body. Take, for example, body temperature. Your body should stay at around 98.6 degrees Fahrenheit. If you get hotter or colder than that, your internal systems go into high gear to regulate that temperature, by sweating to cool off or shivering to generate heat. To keep your blood sugar within a safe and healthy range, your body releases insulin after you eat, moving sugar out of the blood and into the liver or the fat cells. Similarly, your blood must stay within a very narrow pH range and your body must also regulate the amount of salt in your bloodstream to keep your blood pressure within the normal range.

Science continues to discover more ways the body attempts to compensate for imbalanced conditions. The immune system works tirelessly in your body's defense, shooting down potential disruptors like cancer cells, bacteria, fungi, or viruses, and rushing to surround and heal wounds. There is a theory that arterial plaque is meant to protect the arteries from inflammation, and another theory that the plaques and tangles (abnormal accumulation of a protein that collects inside neurons) of Alzheimer's disease are the body's attempt to protect the brain from inflammation and/or viruses.

These examples barely scratch the surface of what your body can do as it regulates and balances your water content, your breathing and oxygen intake, and many other processes far too complex to explain in this book. But in my world, there is no more interesting example of balance than the microbiome, which isn't exactly *your* body balancing and regulating its own processes, but *other bodies* (those microbes) existing in a community with each other as well as in symbiosis with you. The composition of the microbiome is the result of constant microbial attempts to balance their environment for maximum survival—theirs and (in the case of your more numerous and beneficial microbes) yours, because if you expire, so do they. As these microbes that live within you attempt to get along, complex dynamics are going on every second. Beneficial microbes (microbes that benefit you) constantly work to keep pathogenic microbes (microbes that could harm you) under control. Your health state coincides with the health state of your microbes, so it is in their best interest to keep you healthy. When they are successful, this is homeostasis, or more specifically, microbiome balance.

The opposite of total gut balance, or homeostasis in the gut, is gut imbalance, or dysbiosis. Your beneficial microbes aren't always able to maintain that balance. Sometimes, the odds against them are overwhelming. Maybe this is due to your dietary choices or stress or illness or injury or a course of antibiotics or antifungals. Anything you do that impacts your microbiome can potentially disrupt homeostasis. When that happens, you will feel it. Dysbiosis puts your beneficial microbes at risk and gives the pathogenic microbes a foothold, often causing uncomfortable symptoms for you and even potentially serious disease or infection.

Dysbiosis (diagnosed or not) can seriously interfere with your life, causing everything from bad breath to bloating, constipation to concentration problems, diarrhea to depression. And when fungi are involved—such as *Candida* overgrowing—you've got something akin to gastrointestinal anarchy.

When people talk about dysbiosis, they tend to talk about bacteria. But fungi are often behind the scenes, causing or worsening the trouble by growing excessively, by contributing to biofilms (see Chapter 4), or by exerting their own pathogenic effects when fungi-stifling bacteria are decimated, fungi can sweep in and cause problems swiftly.

Germ Warfare

Ever since Robert Koch and Louis Pasteur each showed that germs from the environment cause infectious diseases, society has been at war with microbes. When Alexander Fleming accidentally exposed a Petri dish containing bacteria to fungal contamination (the mold stopped the bacteria from growing), the concept that led to the development of life-saving antibiotics was born. Building on Pasteur's early work with chicken cholera, rabies, and anthrax, scientists developed vaccines to prevent many common childhood diseases, including polio and smallpox. More germ eradication! As the technology of microscopes advanced, we could see smaller and smaller microbes, and suddenly we could photograph disease-causing viruses and prions (dead, deformed proteins). Know thy enemy! Microbes that we haven't been able to grow in Petri dishes and thus didn't even know were part of our microbiomes are now being discovered using advanced DNA sequencing. The technologies of microbial exploration and control march on.

As scientific knowledge of microbiology increased, societies developed tools for combatting the germ insurgence that had always existed but that we were only beginning to understand. Communities constructed sanitation systems and instituted garbage collection. Decades later, we began to pasteurize everything potentially poisonous, from raw milk and cheese to apple cider. By the late 20th century, using hand sanitizer by the gallon wasn't at all unusual. Collectively, these major hygiene campaigns have done a wonderful job of ridding the developed world of disease-carrying germs. "Cleanliness is next to godliness" has resulted in spectacular increases in life expectancy, and infant mortality has plummeted over the past century, dropping from about 1 in 10 to 1 in 200.

However, we now realize that this eradication of microbes in our external and internal environments has had unexpected consequences. Despite the increased lifespans and reduced infant mortality that have partly resulted from such improvements, in recent decades the medical establishment has seen an increase in allergies and autoimmune diseases in the industrialized world. Asthma rates have risen from about 1% of all children to over 10%. Many blame microbe eradication, due to something called "The Hygiene Hypothesis,"[20] which suggests that early exposure to *more* germs builds better immunity.

There may be something to this hypothesis. As our lives have become increasingly sanitary, our resilience in the face of germs (and their influence on our microbiomes) seems to have degraded. While the rates of nearly all infectious diseases continue to decline, the opposite is occurring in the realm of non-infectious chronic diseases that we now know are at least associated with the state of the immune system and the microbiome, where many components of that immune system are formed. For example, in the past five years, we have witnessed unprecedented increases in childhood obesity, in addition to the continuing adult obesity epidemic. The rates of inflammatory bowel diseases, mental health disorders such as depression and anxiety, and even autism continue to increase rapidly. Chronic diseases, many that are primarily gastrointestinal, or which have a gastrointestinal component, are on the rise. Could it be that we have compromised our immune systems in an effort to save ourselves from germs? We haven't changed genetically in 50 years, but our disease susceptibilities have, because it turns out that when it comes to our seemingly successful war on microbes, we may be both the victors and the victims of collateral damage.

But it's not just about fungi, either. In many if not most cases, dysbiosis is the result of complex interactions between fungi and bacteria. There is rarely a single culprit. The trick, therefore, is not to eradicate a potential "bad guy" microbe, but to keep it in balance with its fellow microbial citizens so that it can play its part without becoming too abundant or developing more pathogenic qualities. Even potentially pathogenic fungi such as *Candida* can have a beneficial role to play, but let them overgrow and dysbiosis can be the result.

This is why it is so important to control fungal growth in any way you can. Fungi can be the wild card in dysbiosis and the most immediate factor that introduces instability. The better we understand fungi and learn to manipulate them, the more successful we will be in treating conditions, both mild (like a bout of diarrhea or chronic IBS symptoms) and serious (like Crohn's disease), that involve microbiome imbalance.

SIBO and SIFO

SIBO (small intestinal bacterial overgrowth) is one of the latest conditions people in the health world are talking about. Many popular health books and websites blame SIBO for just about every symptom of poor health. But SIBO and its fungal counterpart, SIFO (you can probably guess that stands for small intestinal fungal overgrowth), are serious problems. Once thought to be a rare condition, SIBO is now easier to diagnose, and it is turning out to be more common than once thought.[21] And SIFO, while even less understood, is now a proven culprit in many people's stubborn GI symptoms.[22]

Normally, most of your gut bacteria live in your colon, but with both SIBO and SIFO, microbes grow up into the small intestine until this upper part of your GI tract is populated with microbes that aren't meant to be there. Your small intestine is not the proper environment for these bacteria and fungi, and their presence can cause inflammation of the small intestine and a wide range of gastrointestinal symptoms like diarrhea, gas, bloating, nausea, burping, indigestion, and problems with nutrient absorption.

While several different bacteria are known to occur in cases of SIBO, *Candida* is to blame in most if not all cases of SIFO, and several recent studies have identified that among patients with unexplained GI symptoms, approximately 25% had SIFO when tested.[23]

What is causing these wandering microbes? Evidence points to two common causes: One cause is small intestinal dysmotility, a condition in which the small intestine is not moving food along the GI tract as quickly or efficiently as it should due to impaired muscle activity. Dysmotility is often blamed for functional disorders like IBS. The second cause is the widespread use of proton pump inhibitors (PPIs).[24] These are acid-blocking medications commonly prescribed for acid reflux. Both SIBO and SIFO may be unintended consequences of these two things, but they may have other causes we haven't yet discovered.

Do you have SIBO, SIFO, or both? Popular health websites may try to "diagnose" you by asking if you have certain symptoms. But beware: Even though one study demonstrated that patients with SIFO are most likely to suffer from nausea and patients with SIBO were more likely to experience abdominal pain and gas, the presence of any of these symptoms does not prove you have SIFO or SIBO.[25] There are many other causes of these symptoms, and the only truly reliable way to diagnose SIBO or SIFO is via a laboratory test.

If you have unexplained GI symptoms that don't respond to dietary shifts, you may want to ask your doctor about getting a test for SIFO or SIBO. However, since the current standard treatment for these conditions is to take antibiotics or antifungal medications, which come with their own risks of increased dysbiosis, dietary and lifestyle interventions (such as the Mycobiome Diet) are a preferable treatment, as long as they effectively reduce or eliminate your symptoms.

DO YOU HAVE DYSBIOSIS?

Is this imbalanced state happening in your gut? Are you dysbiotic? There are many conditions and situations that can put you at a greater risk for dysbiosis, so let's assess your risk. Check all the items that apply to you:

Dysbiosis Risk Checklist[26]

- ☐ Were you a C-section baby?
- ☐ Were you ever hospitalized as a child?
- ☐ Were you fed with a bottle rather than breastfed?
- ☐ Did you have colic as a baby?
- ☐ Did you take antibiotics multiple times as a child?
- ☐ Did you grow up in a home without any animals?
- ☐ Did you grow up in an exceptionally clean, hygienic environment?
- ☐ Did your family always use a dishwasher rather than washing dishes by hand?
- ☐ Have you taken antibiotics multiple times as an adult?
- ☐ Did you ever have a *C. difficile* infection?
- ☐ Do you or did you ever have asthma and/or allergies?
- ☐ Do you have a diagnosed autoimmune disease, such as Crohn's disease, ulcerative colitis, rheumatoid arthritis, lupus, psoriasis, or celiac disease?
- ☐ Are you or were you ever very overweight?
- ☐ Do you eat a high-sugar diet?
- ☐ Are you under a lot of stress for prolonged periods of time?
- ☐ Would you describe yourself as mostly sedentary during the day (like working at a desk or spending many hours at home sitting)?
- ☐ Are you over 50 years old?

If you checked even one of these boxes, but especially if you checked more than three, you are at greater risk for dysbiosis. It doesn't mean you have it right now. You may have suffered from dysbiosis in the past that has resolved. For example, someone who was born by C-section and on antibiotics as a child may have been deprived of an intrinsically diverse and robust microbiome but may have lived a healthy lifestyle for many years and has now overcome any microbiome imbalance. Another person may have had excellent microbiome beginnings but has since lived an unhealthy lifestyle and has eaten a high-sugar, low-nutrient diet for many years. This person may have a serious case of dysbiosis.

Dysbiosis is quite common. And while I can't diagnose you through a book, let alone by a checklist, you can get a pretty good idea of the favorable or unfavorable balance in your microbiome by having been diagnosed with certain health conditions, or more simply, by assessing your general symptoms. These are clues, not diagnoses, but they are a beginning and can help set you on a path to improving the health of your microbiome, and by extension, many aspects of *your* health: your digestion, your immune system, and even your mental health.

DYSBIOSIS AND HEALTH DYSFUNCTION

Many serious health issues have been associated with dysbiosis. In some of them, we know dysbiosis is probably a trigger or contributor, but in many of them we are not entirely sure whether the dysbiosis leads to the condition or the condition leads to the dysbiosis. More likely, there is a bi-directional influence—a sort of give-and-take kind of development over time, as the microbiome becomes more imbalanced and other functions begin to decline, each feeding into the other.

The following health conditions have been associated with dysbiosis, even though some of them have no apparent connection with the GI tract—further evidence of the microbiome's influence throughout the entire body. If you have been diagnosed with any of the following conditions, you likely have at least some level of dysbiosis.[27] Check any diagnoses you have currently:

Common Conditions Related to Dysbiosis Checklist

☐ Allergies (environmental[28] and food allergies[29])
☐ Asthma[30]
☐ Atopic dermatitis[31]
☐ Autism[32]
☐ Yeast infections (candidiasis) like thrush, athlete's foot, jock itch, or vaginal yeast infections[33]
☐ Celiac disease[34]
☐ Chronic fatigue syndrome[35]
☐ Prediabetes, metabolic syndrome, or type 2 diabetes[36]

- ☐ Gastric ulcer related to the bacteria *H. pylori*[37]
- ☐ Gastroesophageal reflux disease (GERD), which is a serious chronic form of acid reflux[38]
- ☐ Heart disease, atherosclerosis (hardening of the arteries)[39]
- ☐ Immunosuppression (as with cancer treatment or HIV)[40]
- ☐ Inflammatory bowel diseases (like Crohn's disease and ulcerative colitis)[41]
- ☐ Irritable bowel syndrome (IBS) and other functional bowel disorders (like functional constipation and gastroparesis)[42]
- ☐ Low energy, feeling tired all the time even with enough sleep[43]
- ☐ Malabsorption, or inability to absorb sufficient nutrition from food[44]
- ☐ Metabolic syndrome[45]
- ☐ Migraines[46]
- ☐ Multiple sclerosis[47]
- ☐ Obesity[48]
- ☐ Psychiatric disorders such as attention-deficit/hyperactivity disorder (ADHD), schizophrenia, clinical depression, anxiety disorders, bipolar disorder, or obsessive-compulsive disorder[49]
- ☐ Rheumatoid arthritis (or other diseases characterized by chronic inflammation)[50]
- ☐ SIBO or SIFO (small intestinal bacterial/fungal overgrowth)[51]
- ☐ Systemic Lupus Erythematosus[52]

But even if you don't have a diagnosis or an obviously serious health condition, you could still have dysbiosis that could turn into something worse if you don't address it. Having a few of the following symptoms (some people have many) means you are more likely than average to be in a state of current and active dysbiosis, and your microbiome could probably use some attention. Check any of the following symptoms you currently have:

Dysbiosis Symptom Checklist

- ☐ Anxious or panicky feelings, feeling nervous for no obvious reason[53]
- ☐ Bloating, gas, stomach pain after eating, constipation, diarrhea[54]
- ☐ Chronic headaches[55]
- ☐ Chronic itching (skin, ears, rectum), rashes, and other skin disruptions[56]
- ☐ Depression, anxiety, irritability, or mood swings[57]

- ☐ Heartburn or reflux[58]
- ☐ High blood sugar, or high A1c, suggesting a prediabetic state[59]
- ☐ Hormonal issues (especially PMS and perimenopausal symptoms)[60]
- ☐ Irresistible sugar or refined carb cravings[61]
- ☐ Joint pain and other musculoskeletal problems[62]
- ☐ Low energy, chronic fatigue[63]
- ☐ Post-adolescent acne[64]
- ☐ Feelings of sadness or depression for no apparent reason[65]
- ☐ Seasonal allergies[66]
- ☐ Sudden, unexplained weight gain, or inability to lose weight (weight loss resistance)[67]

The gut microbiome is linked to every one of these symptoms, and while they could all potentially be caused by something else and the presence of them does not prove dysbiosis, it is likely that dysbiosis is either a contributing factor or has resulted from the conditions causing the symptoms and is then in turn making your symptoms worse.

If you have determined that you probably do have some level of dysbiosis, there is a lot you can do, even without medical intervention, to rebalance and maintain your microbiome for improved health. There is also plenty you could *stop doing*. Let's consider what you may be doing that could be profoundly disruptive to your microbiome, particularly in terms of its contribution to conditions that allow for fungal overgrowth. It won't do you much good to try to fix your microbiome imbalance if you are currently doing things to cause it at the same time. You may have to do some of these things, such as take certain prescriptions, but knowing what can cause or worsen dysbiosis can help you make decisions about the things you do that are not medically necessary.

WHAT CAN CAUSE OR WORSEN DYSBIOSIS?

A lot of things people do every day can cause or worsen imbalance in the microbiome. If you recognize that you are doing any of these things, you may be able to stop doing them as a first step toward getting your microbiome back to a healthy balance—this can help the Mycobiome Diet to work even better for you. Or, if you must do them, know that you may need to be even more proactive in increasing the health of your microbiome:

Taking antibiotics: Let's say you get strep throat or bronchitis or pneumonia and you need an antibiotic. Antibiotic means antibacterial, and these medications wipe out bacteria—not just the pathogenic bacteria causing your illness, but many of the good guys as well. Meanwhile, your immune system is also busy trying to get that infection under control, which gives pathogenic fungi an opportunity to move in and take over undetected. This is why people often get digestive disturbance (such as diarrhea) after taking antibiotics—an overgrowth of the opportunistic yeast *Candida albicans* is often the culprit. Of course, sometimes antibiotics are necessary—even critically important or life-saving. Other times, they may be prescribed "just in case," but you may be able to heal from whatever mild infection you have without them. Ask your doctor to advise you whether antibiotics are necessary.

Taking antifungals: Antifungals can be just as disruptive as antibiotics because they remove fungi that could be contributing to healthy microbiome balance. The complete obliteration of fungi—even *Candida*—in various symbiotic processes can cause a chain reaction that results in dysbiosis.

Taking certain other medications: Many other over-the-counter and prescription drugs have been shown to cause or worsen dysbiosis. Talk to your doctor before stopping any prescribed medication, but you should know that the following kinds of medications could be contributing to microbiome imbalance. (Note: The cited studies did not necessarily involve the particular branded drugs named below. I am providing these examples here just so you will have an idea of what kinds of drugs fall into each category.)

- **Acid-reducing drugs,** especially proton pump inhibitors[68] like omeprazole (e.g., Prilosec) but also H2 (or histamine-2) blockers like ranitidine, cimetidine, nizatidine, and famotidine (e.g., Zantac, Tagamet, and Pepcid); and antacids (e.g., Tums and Rolaids).[69] You may be able to resolve reflux and acid indigestion with diet rather than medication.
- **Nonsteroidal anti-inflammatory drugs (NSAIDs)** like ibuprofen (e.g., Advil and Motrin), naproxen (e.g., Aleve and Naprosyn), aspirin (e.g., Bayer and Bufferin), and COX-2 inhibitors such as celecoxib and valdecoxib (e.g., Celebrex and Vioxx). The Mycobiome Diet is an anti-inflammatory diet that could help you to reduce your use of these pain relievers.
- **Hormone-manipulating drugs** like birth control pills and IUDs and hormone replacement therapies (such as estrogen replacement). You may

need these, but they could be contributing to dysbiosis. The Mycobiome Diet could help to counteract this effect.

- **Corticosteroids:** Often necessary, but these should not be taken long-term for many reasons, including microbiome disruption.
- **Diabetes drugs** such as metformin and insulin. If you take these, you most likely need to take them, but in the case of type 2 diabetes, a balanced diet that helps to regulate blood sugar could eventually reduce your need for these drugs. Never stop them without your doctor's okay!
- **Antipsychotics[70] and anticancer/chemotherapy drugs:** As with some of these other categories, these are likely to be necessary if you have a prescription for them, so don't stop taking them! But being on these medications can be a good reason to adhere strictly to the Mycobiome Diet (with your doctor's approval).

Exposure to certain environmental factors: It isn't just pharmaceuticals that can mess with your microbiome. There is also evidence that personal care products like mouthwash, shampoo, skin cream, and soap can disrupt microbiome balance. So can chemical exposures to things like pollution, heavy metals, plastic compounds, and chlorine. Anything toxic that goes into or onto your body is a potential microbiome disruptor.

Bad habits: Many of the things you do every day—or just the way you live your life—can contribute to either a healthy, diverse, robust microbiome, or an imbalanced microbiome run by pathogenic bacteria and fungi. Consider your current level of stress, how much sleep you get, how much junk food and refined sugar you eat, how much saturated and trans fats and fatty meat you eat, how much fiber you eat, and how much exercise you get. These can all directly impact the microbiome. (The Mycobiome Diet will help to improve conditions brought on by all these habits.)

What's in Your Microbiome?

Thanks to the recent advancement in next generation DNA analysis, new tools are out there that can be used to help characterize your gut microbiome and thus identify what steps you can take to help restore balance. These steps include tests that can tell you what microbes you have in your microbiome. The results could lead to a better understanding of what is causing your dysbiosis and, in the future, more targeted treatments and personalized medicine. This field is still new, but exciting.

Although different companies market in-home test kits that you can easily find on the Internet, I am (in the spirit of full transparency) the cofounder of a company called BIOHM Health that offers a Gut Report based on a fecal sample you send in. If you are interested in learning more about this service, see the information in the Appendix. But know that this test is not in any way required to do the Mycobiome Diet and will not change your results on the diet in any way. It is simply for those who want a little more information about the composition of their own microbiome.

A FEW THINGS TO DO RIGHT NOW

In most cases, you don't need a doctor to tell you that you have dysbiosis. If you have it, you probably know it is due to symptoms that impact your life. You certainly don't need a medical diagnosis to follow the program in this book—it is likely to improve your health no matter what aspect of your microbiome is out of balance. Why not start right now, even before you start the Mycobiome Diet? Here are a few simple things you can think about as you get ready to address your dysbiosis:

Don't overhype hygiene. Traditional wisdom may advise that it is healthy to be clean, but the truth is that the microbes in and on your body come from the outside, and the more you have, the more robust your health is likely to be. That means being dirty might not be so bad after all, and conversely, excessive cleanliness might be detrimental to your health, especially when you were a child. As a dad raising kids in Kuwait, I can tell you a story about my older son and his playmate as an example of the benefits of getting a little dirty. "Tom" was a neighborhood friend (both he and my son were 6 or 7 years old) who was forced to wear white gloves when playing outside. Apparently, his father was trying to show him exactly how dirty things were out there! As it turned out, Tom was the one who was always getting sick, while my son was the one getting filthy . . . and staying healthy. Exposure to lots of different microbes (good and bad) is essential for priming and training your immune system, so that later on, in adulthood and whenever it is challenged by pathogens, it's able to distinguish between harmless organisms that it should ignore and live with, and dangerous pathogens that it needs to respond to and eradicate.

Hang out with animals. Some interesting research suggests that children brought up in environments that are typically considered to be less clean have more microbiome diversity and, in many cases, better health with fewer allergies, less asthma, and more vigorous immune systems. Specifically, children on dairy farms have more contact with animals, are sometimes inside barns and stables, and tend to consume unprocessed, unpasteurized raw milk products. One study discovered that these children had a much lower risk of developing allergies, eczema, and asthma than children raised in more hygienic (or typical) environments.[71] Another study looked at the microbiomes of infants born into homes with pets, and showed that the presence of animals in the household also contributed to greater microbiome diversity, which could contribute to a reduction in future allergies.[72]

Another example comes from a 2015 study in which researchers quantified the reduction in risk of asthma for children growing up with dogs.[73] The investigators examined records of more than one million children born in Sweden between 2001 and 2010. Of the 275,000 or so school-age children in the study group, the children of dog-owning families had a 13% lower chance of developing asthma than their peers who grew up without a dog.[74]

Go outside. If you don't consider yourself an "outdoor person," it can be tempting to break out the antibacterial wipes at the first sign of dirt, but this is really doing yourself (and your overall health) a disservice. Spending time outdoors is meant to be a little messy, so enjoy it—garden and put your hands in the dirt, lie on the grass, climb a tree, or just run around outside with kids, knowing that by letting yourself get back to nature, you're also welcoming more beneficial microbes to take up residence.

Exercise more. With all its benefits, our modern lifestyle has a drawback that is difficult to overcome: A sedentary lifestyle. Kids sit for most of the day in school, then come home and watch TV or play video games or sit at their computers. Adults are no better off, spending many hours each day at computers while at work, then at home in the evenings they are watching TV or at the computer again. We all know that exercise is good and that a sedentary lifestyle can lead to poor health, weight gain, and associated disorders—as well as specifically impact the microbiome in some detrimental ways.[75] That's why there are so many gyms and fitness centers and exercise programs. The problem is using them!

This makes me think of the many happy hours I spent playing outside with my friends when I was a young boy. The only condition my mother gave me was to "come home before the sun sets." I know things are different now, and it's not as safe as it once was to play outside unsupervised. Back in those days, we didn't have all the video games, computers, and smart phones kids have now. Instead, we ran around, played football, chased each other, and just played.

Recent studies show that a lack of exercise can lead to dysbiosis, while exercise increases microbial diversity. One of these studies investigated the effect of exercise on the gut microbiomes of professional athletes compared to a control group matched for physical size, age, and gender.[76] Their data showed that athletes had a higher diversity of gut microorganisms (representing 22 distinct phyla, compared to the 6 or 7 dominant phyla most people have). Another critical finding by these authors is that athletes had lower inflammation than nonathletes in a control group. The athletes were also fitter, had better body composition, and had healthier markers of metabolism.

Exercising outdoors, with exposure to the variety of microbes in your environment that are different from the ones you can get indoors, can increase the benefits even more. Recent studies have shown that recreational activities such as hiking allow you to pick up bacteria that abound in the natural environment.[77] I try to go out and hike as much as possible and enjoy nature with my grandchildren, knowing it is benefiting more than my family relationships. It is benefiting my microbiome. For more about exercise and my recommendations, see Chapter 7.

You may already have some great ideas about how you can begin to mitigate your own dysbiosis by altering the lifestyle habits and exposures I've just told you about, and in Chapter 5, I'll give you even more information about what science says can legitimately help with dysbiosis in general and fungal overgrowth in particular. But first, let's look at one of the most notorious bad guy fungus known to human guts all over the world—the one that you may want to be particularly focused on getting back under control, and the one most likely to be instrumental in the health issues you would like to resolve: *Candida.*

Candida Unmasked

If your gut could display "Most Wanted" posters, they would probably be of this guy: *Candida albicans.* When people talk about "*Candida,*" they often mean the fungus *Candida albicans,* and when they say, "I have *Candida,*" what they usually mean is that they have (or think they have) candidiasis, which is an infection due to the overgrowth of certain *Candida* yeasts. *Candida albicans* is the most studied fungus in humans because it is easy to culture in a lab and is the fungus most responsible for causing serious infections in humans. Although about half of all adults have some *Candida* in their gastrointestinal tracts and probably almost all adults have some *Candida* somewhere in them or on them, it doesn't necessarily cause a problem . . . if it doesn't grow out of control. When it does, those *Candida* thugs can take over, creating potentially mild to serious health issues like vaginal candidiasis or systemic blood infections that can be fatal. *Candida albicans* doesn't mess around.

But *Candida albicans* is not the only member of the *Candida* genus to cause a stir inside the human body. In the United States, various *Candida* species (including *Candida albicans*) are responsible for the vast majority of fungal infections. (*Aspergillus* is the runner-up.) *Candida* species are the fourth most common cause of hospital-acquired infections in the United States,[78] and one study reported a 40% mortality rate in patients who contracted an infection with *Candida* while in the hospital[79] even when the patient was being treated for it.

There are more than 100 species of *Candida,* but only 20 of them are known infectors of humans. Five of the species are the most common—approximately 95% of *Candida* infections are caused by these five bad guys:

Candida albicans: This is the species most often responsible for fungal infections worldwide. It's not only responsible for annoying mild infections like thrush, but also for deep-seated infections that are hard to resolve and pose a serious threat, like candidemia (a blood-stream infection), pyelonephritis (a kidney infection), peritonitis (an infection in the abdominal cavity), and meningitis.[80] In fact, nearly 50% of all *Candida* infections worldwide are caused by this species.

Candida glabrata: This species has recently become more of a problem. It's responsible for 20% of the bloodstream infections in the United States, and like *Candida albicans* it can be invasive and serious. Older people are especially susceptible to this fungus and it is one cause of urinary tract infections.[81] The rise in the incidence of infections from *Candida glabrata* has been attributed to the widespread use of fluconazole (the trade name is Diflucan). This is an antifungal drug that was introduced in the 1990s to treat fungal infections in AIDS patients and others with compromised immunity—*Candida glabrata* is mostly resistant to this drug, so when fluconazole eliminated the competition, *Candida glabrata* was given room to thrive.[82]

Candida tropicalis: This fungus is also on the rise and has become a more frequent cause of candidiasis, especially in people with acute leukemia or those undergoing bone marrow transplants. It can also cause gastrointestinal and systemic infections and has been associated with severe myalgia (muscle pain) and myositis[83] (muscle inflammation and degeneration). A recent study by my group[84] showed that Crohn's disease patients have a disproportionately high amount of this fungus, which aggravates gastrointestinal symptoms due to its overgrowth and its collaboration with the bacteria *Escherichia coli* and *Serratia marcescens* to make the disease even worse.

Candida parapsilosis: This fungus is the second most common species seen in blood cultures in Europe. It colonizes the skin, and one study showed that 40% of health care workers, such as nurses and doctors, had this fungus on their skin. *C. parapsilosis* tends to form biofilms on catheters and other implanted medical devices,[85] and the microbes that produce these biofilms seem to be stubbornly resistant to antifungal medications.

Candida krusei: This species is less pervasive than the four species I've already described, but we are keeping an eye on this one because it tends to be particularly resistant to fluconazole (an inborn characteristic). That means when it strikes, it is hard to resolve. Most *Candida* species are responsive to this medication—*C. albicans,* for example, is very likely to be successfully controlled by fluconazole. Not so with *C. krusei,* which can cause bloodstream infections, diarrhea in newborns, and endophthalmitis[86] (a serious infection of the inner eye).

New Kid on the Block

Mycologists like myself continue to discover new *Candida* species all the time, and we are always on the lookout for those that could impact human health. In 2016, the Centers for Disease Control and Prevention (CDC) published an alert that a new multidrug-resistant species called *Candida auris* was causing invasive infections. Researchers are calling *C. auris* "the new kid on the block," since there is much we don't know about it yet and it may have the potential to become significant. It was originally isolated in 2008 from a Japanese patient's ear canal and has since caused serious invasive infections with a high mortality rate (approaching 60%).

Not only is it resistant to most antifungal drugs on the market, but it can use the skin as a breeding ground. It appears to have emerged independently in four separate populations on five continents. It has now been found in Japan, South Korea, India, Kuwait, South Africa, Pakistan, the United Kingdom, and most recently in Venezuela, Colombia, and the United States.[87] It has been detected in health care settings, and some testing our group completed showed that *C. auris* (as well as *C. parapsilosis* and *C. glabrata*) could live for seven days on both moist or dry surfaces. Interestingly, when we compared the frequencies of recovery (survival) of *Candida* species against bacterial pathogens from dry hospital surfaces, our data showed that there were no significant differences in the percent recovery of *Candida* species versus other pathogens. For moist surfaces, however, *Candida* species were significantly more likely to survive than other pathogens.[88]

Because this yeast can stay on the skin and spread to other patients, it has led, in some extreme cases in the United Kingdom, to the closing of entire hospital wards. We are currently developing skin colonization models, investigational drugs, and hospital disinfectants so that we can have better ways to control this particular species of *Candida*. In the meantime, the CDC has described this emerging *Candida* species, with its aggressive resistance to antifungal medications, as "concerning."[89] Indeed.

CANDIDA MYTHS AND TRUTHS

But wait . . . what about all the *other* problems you've heard about that are caused by *Candida?* If you spend some time browsing popular alternative health sites online, you will probably see *Candida* blamed for just about every vague health symptom there is: fatigue, constipation and diarrhea, bloating, gas, stomach aches, sinus infections, rashes, joint pain, brain fog, irritability, mood swings, food allergies, nutrient deficiencies, depression, anxiety, a weakened immune system, sugar cravings, acne, body odor, bad breath, insomnia, itchy eyes, itchy ears, a low libido, panic attacks, clumsiness, a poor memory, chemical sensitivity, light sensitivity, water retention, and even autoimmune diseases.

Really? Do *Candida* species of fungus *really* cause all those issues? It's enough to make a person doubt that *Candida* overgrowth, or candidiasis (infection caused by *Candida*) is a real thing at all. Is "candida" just a fake diagnosis proliferated by opportunistic "health" websites posting clickbait for more advertising profit? Is it one of those things alternative medicine practitioners like to blame everything on? If you ask your doctor about it, will you get that *look* that implies, "Have you been on the Internet too much lately?" Is candidiasis only a problem in extreme health situations like in Crohn's, HIV, or cancer patients, or only in infants and the elderly? Or is it likely to impact people who are not severely ill and are functioning in their lives but just don't feel quite as good as they would like to feel?

Before I answer, let me tell you a story.

Shortly after I first came to the United States as a young man, I attended my very first medical conference in the United States entitled "*Candida* and Candidiasis." It was in Baltimore, Maryland, and I remember being particularly interested in one of the speakers who was talking about the importance of *Candida*. This was in 1992, and back then, medical professionals didn't pay a lot of attention to yeasts and other fungi in humans, except when they caused obvious problems like invasive infections, thrush, or vaginitis.

This speaker was arguing that *Candida* may be more of a problem, and more prevalent, than the current thinking suggested. He was a doctor who particularly wanted to draw attention to the dramatic increase in *Candida*-caused infections in the HIV-infected patients who were just starting to be seen in the late 1980s.

He also talked about other common issues related to *Candida*, including digestive issues *Candida* can trigger or aggravate. He pointed out that in 1991, isolating a *Candida* or even an unspecified yeast from a patient was considered to be of no consequence by the medical community at large—that physicians rarely requested the identification of yeast isolates obtained from a patient and thought that "yeast" was likely a contaminant of the lab results and of no clinical significance.

He pointed out that when a patient comes to see a doctor with a fever, the doctor's first response is typically to prescribe an antibiotic—even though antibiotics make people *more* vulnerable to *Candida* infection, since the antibiotic wipes out both the bad bacteria and the good bacteria that help to control *Candida.* Even more alarming to him was that even when a fever did not subside while on the antibiotic, the doctor would typically change the antibiotic to another one, rather than consider that the problem might be fungal in nature. He said, "They just do not think fungus."

As a young scientist studying fungus, I was fascinated. This doctor was passionate in his delivery. He implored the medical mycology community to develop better educational programs to increase the awareness in the general medical community about the importance of considering *Candida* as the source of many health issues. He begged the pharmaceutical industry to establish research and development programs for the discovery of effective and safe new drugs to address this problem, pointing to the fact that the "gold standard" for treating invasive fungal infections was a drug called amphotericin B that was extremely toxic and was referred to by physicians as "amphoterrible" or "shake and bake," because the patients started shivering while the drug was being administered through their veins. He called upon the federal government to increase funding for research to better understand what makes *Candida* cause disease, because this could provide more and better insight into what we should be targeting in order to stop the spread of these pathogenic fungi and control dangers that can come from them.

When I looked around me, I could see that some members of the audience were intently listening, but it was also clear that many others were skeptical, dismissive, or even disbelieving. After the session, some doctors admitted they didn't take this field seriously. But the phrase he used kept coming back to me: "They just do not think fungus."

As I look back on this experience with a broader perspective, I believe that part of the problem was that this was the era when health books were being published that did not utilize good science to support their claims. This included more than one book about *Candida*, each of which conveyed the message that *Candida* was responsible for that general feeling of unwellness people have when they aren't as healthy as they could be. They also included a long list of vague symptoms (you can still find lists like this on the Internet), from short attention span to menstrual problems.

Nevertheless, for years, the "yeast syndrome" has been discussed in journals and books and television talk shows. An early proponent, Dr. William Crook, stated that "The yeast connection is a term to indicate the relationship of superficial yeast infections in your digestive tract or [elsewhere] to fatigue, headache, depression, PMS, irritability, and other symptoms that can make you feel sick all over." Further, he suggested that preventing *Candida* overgrowth in the gut can alleviate symptoms of manic depression, schizophrenia, ADHD, and autism.[90]

To my knowledge, none of these claims have been proven by randomized, placebo-controlled clinical trials. While there is research to support that dysbiosis in general may be related to all of these problems, this research does not specifically implicate *Candida*. This early popular literature was neither a helpful contribution to mycology nor a conduit for a self-reflective analysis of the study of mycology, because it cast suspicion on *Candida* and perhaps made doctors even less likely to "think of fungus," or at least take it seriously.

There is still much we don't know about the role of *Candida* in human health, and there are many health conditions we do know are caused by or are greatly aggravated by *Candida*. Considering its potential to do serious harm and its proven notoriety as an opportunistic pathogen, it certainly can't hurt to get it under control—and it almost certainly will help with at least some, if not many, symptoms of microbiome imbalance. Just because *Candida* is the subject of some pseudoscience does *not* mean that it is not a legitimate threat to health, and it also does not mean that *Candida* cannot be blamed for certain symptoms in people who are not severely ill or immunocompromised.

Reflecting back on this "first contact" I had with fungal research in the United States, I am grateful that our understanding of *Candida* has come so far. I had already been interested in *Candida* since the early 1970s, and this doctor was presenting credible medical data. It was clear to me that the field of fungal infections was in its infancy in the 1980s, and I saw this as an exciting opportunity to contribute to our understanding of the pathogenesis of fungal infections and to help patients who may be suffering silently due to the effect of fungi.

There is still much for us to learn and understand, but we do know a lot more now than we did then about what makes *Candida* cause or worsen disease. We have a number of effective and safe antifungals, although we need to continue our efforts to discover novel agents that are effective against emerging antifungal resistant strains and species like *C. auris.* Another welcome change is that the Infectious Diseases Society of America has put in place guidelines that urge doctors to take the presence of *Candida* seriously, and that laboratories should identify it so that it can be treated. We are starting to see the light at the end of the tunnel, as our recent publications are showing.[91] We have also made a significant advancement in our understanding of *Candida* and its relationship with the gastrointestinal tract, as well as how to manipulate it with diet and certain supplements (which I will discuss more specifically throughout the second half of this book).

WHAT MAKES *CANDIDA* SO BAD?

Candida is an interesting organism from a research standpoint. When *Candida* sets up shop in the gastrointestinal tract, it might not cause inflammation. It might remain neutral (commensal). On the other hand, it might cause inflammation, even without noticeable overgrowth. It has the potential to play multiple roles.[92]

But when *Candida* decides to play the "bad guy," it can cause a lot of trouble, especially in the ways it can interact with both bacteria and other fungi to create harmful biofilms and secrete metabolites and enzymes that can lead to damage of the gut lining. *Candida* is also notorious for inhibiting good bacteria, such as *Lactobacillus,* especially when *Candida* has overgrown or is too abundant. Both these actions—damaging the gut lining and inhibiting the action of beneficial microbes—can have a cascade of negative health effects.

It is well known that in a healthy gut, bacteria such as *Lactobacillus* play an effective role in keeping *Candida* under control. They do this by secreting substances that inhibit *Candida* from sticking to the lining of the GI tract, and that also keep it from forming hyphae (tentacle-like structures that make *Candida* more harmful).[93] However, when *Candida* overgrows, the tables are turned. After antibiotic therapy, for example, when all bacteria have been wiped out, including beneficial bacteria like *Lactobacillus, Candida* can prevent the regrowth of *Lactobacillus,* altering the recovery of the bacterial microbiota after antibiotic treatment is stopped.

This effect isn't limited to *Lactobacillus.* Recent studies indicate that *Candida,* even when present at a low level in the intestinal microbiome, has the potential to influence the way the microbiome reassembles itself after antibiotics.[94] You may feel better, but *Candida* may still be inhibiting the good bacteria you need for optimal health. In a very real sense, *Candida* "protects its turf" by controlling the proliferation of the good bacteria that would normally control the *Candida*.[95]

Candida is particularly dangerous for human health because of particular qualities it has, called "virulence factors" or "pathogenicity factors." The following are some of *Candida*'s notable virulence factors:

Stickiness. In order for a microbe to cause infection, it must be able to stick to (or adhere to) tissues. My team and others have demonstrated that *Candida* is very efficient in adhering to human cells, especially mucosal tissue, such as inside the mouth.[96]

Shapeshifting. Another interesting property of *Candida* species in general (and of *C. albicans* in particular), is that *Candida* species can change shape to become more invasive. *Candida* species have a yeast form and a branching, filament-like or tentacle-like form. The filamental form is best at penetrating tissue, but the yeast form can also cause infection—whichever form is more conducive for the environment is the form that *Candida* will become.

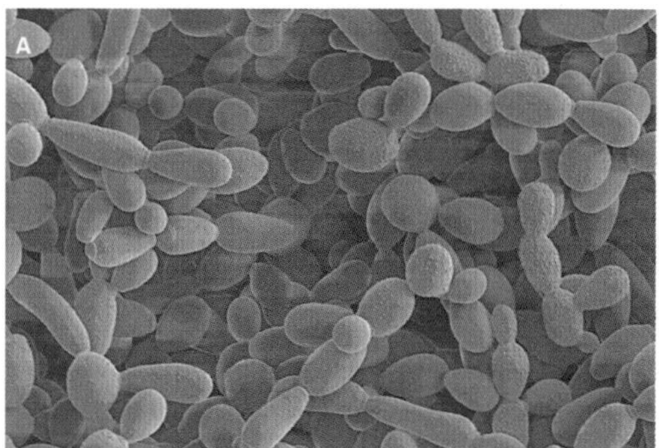

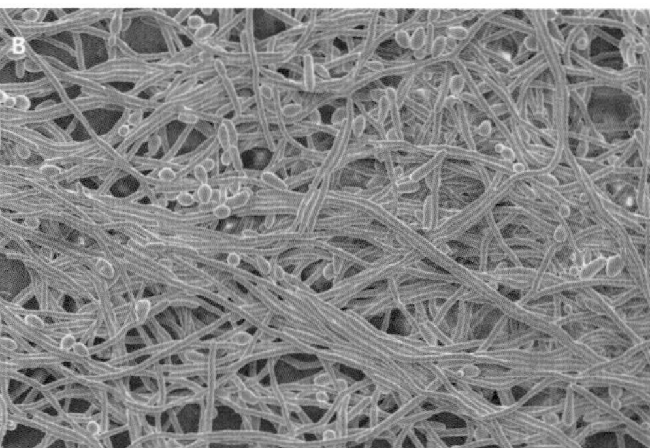

Scanning electron microscopy images showing how *Candida albicans* cells can exist either as a yeast—oval-shaped budding cells (A)—or form thread-like structures called hyphae, or filaments (B). The ability of *Candida* to form hyphae is a virulence factor that helps it to invade host tissues.

Enzyme production for tissue destruction. Another thing *Candida* can do is manufacture and secrete two types of enzymes. The first is phospholipases, which break down the lipids in the host cell membrane; and the second is proteinases, which break down the protein portion of the cell. Both of these enzymes can weaken host cells to make it easier for *Candida* to invade.

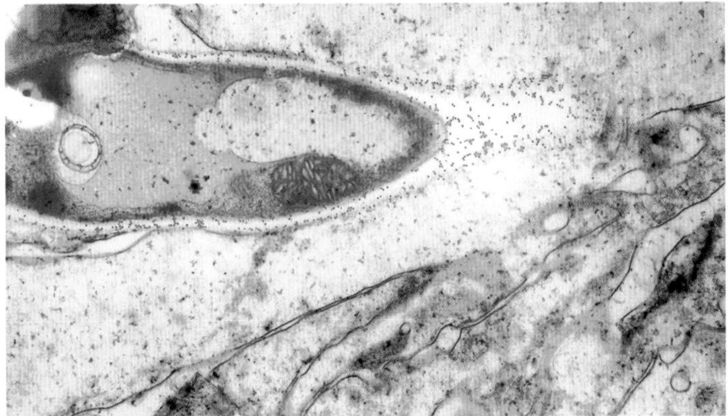

Phospholipase-B enzyme during *Candida albicans* invasion of gastrointestinal tract. Blue dots show phospholipase secretion forging the way for the fungi invasion of intestinal cells. Living in Ohio, I am reminded of a snow plow clearing the way for cars.

Biofilm formation. One of the most ingenious of *Candida*'s virulence factors is its ability to form biofilms, or protective plaques that shield it from the immune system. This provides *Candida* (and some of its virulent bacterial cronies) some distinct advantages, which I will describe more fully in Chapter 4.

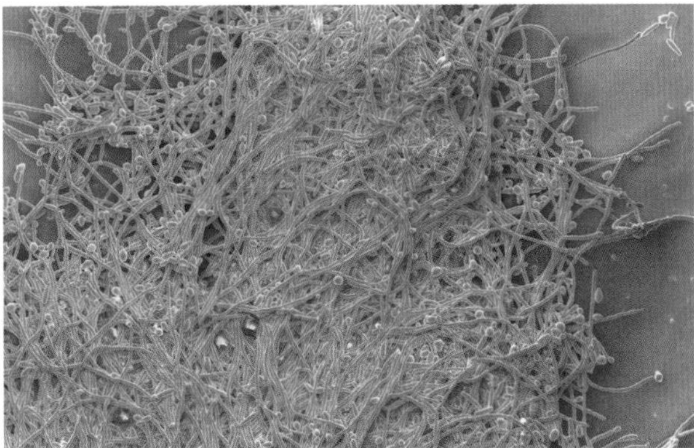

Candida albicans forming a thick biofilm on catheter material. Biofilms consist mainly of filaments that help this fungus invade and break down human tissue, such as the gastrointestinal lining.

RISK FACTORS FOR *CANDIDA* OVERGROWTH

Are you at risk for *Candida* overgrowth? There has been a lot of research linking increased *Candida* and related infections with various situations, therapies, and conditions. Some risk factors are out of your control, but some you can certainly control.

Candida Overgrowth Risk Factors	
Factors You (Mostly) Can Control	**Factors You (Mostly) Can't Control**
Diets high in simple carbs and sugar	Genetic predisposition
Vitamin deficiencies	Infancy
Diets low in fiber and resistant starch	Old age
Diets low in antioxidants	Antibiotic use
Pregnancy	Staying in a hospital—the longer the stay, the greater the risk
Contraceptive use	Using corticosteroids
Wearing synthetic or tight clothes	Using acid blocker medications
Unsanitary manicure/pedicure	Having a wound or burn
Intravenous drug use	Having a surgical procedure
Douching, especially overuse	Having an intravascular catheter, implanted medical device, or respirator

The following factors may put you at more risk:

You are already colonized by *Candida*.[97] You can't get a *Candida* infection if you don't already have *Candida* in or on your body. When *Candida* lives on your skin, it is more likely to infect you if you get an injury that breaks the skin barrier or if you have a catheter inserted. When *Candida* lives in your GI tract, it can migrate into other areas of your body if the integrity of your gut barrier is compromised. In the 1960s, a German scientist did a test on himself to prove that *Candida* can breach the gut barrier.[98] He drank a test tube full of *Candida* in liquid (like a milkshake). Very quickly, he became sick. He then took a sample of his own blood, and sure enough, it was full of *Candida,* proving that *Candida* can indeed move from the gut into the blood, where it can cause an infection.

Obviously, we can't (or shouldn't) do experiments like this today, but the results were certainly interesting! The fact alone that *Candida* can so easily move from benign locations to places in the body that can cause serious infection is a good reason to actively reduce or eliminate *Candida* from your body through lifestyle interventions as much as possible.

You take antibiotics. One study showed that the number of different antibiotics a patient has been exposed to over a lifetime is one of the most significant risk factors for *Candida* infection,[99] and another study showed that 94% of patients with *Candida* infections had been previously exposed to antibiotics, with 61% of them treated with more than four different types.[100] Risk rises with broader-spectrum antibiotics and longer exposure to antibiotics.[101]

You take certain drugs. Steroids, immunosuppressive drugs, and H2 blockers in particular can raise the risk of *Candida* infection by lowering the body's immune response.

You have an implanted medical device, catheter, or other apparatus that has access to the inside of your body, including being on a ventilator and being fed intravenously. When something breaches the barrier between your outside and your inside, you are at greater risk for a *Candida* infection, especially a dangerous bloodstream infection.[102]

You undergo surgery. Every time a surgeon works inside your body, you are at a greater risk of *Candida* infection.[103]

You are critically ill and experience extended hospital stays. One study showed that many critically ill (but not immunosuppressed) patients staying in ICUs for long periods become colonized with *Candida,* even if they didn't develop infections.[104] My team conducted a study to determine whether the mycobiome changes in patients after admission to the ICU. We took samples from people on the day of admission to the ICU, to determine what they came in with. Then we took samples again after seven-day hospital stays. Our results clearly showed that time in the ICU was indeed associated with changes in the patient's fungal community, including an overall increase in the abundance of *Candida albicans.*[105]

CANDIDA'S (PROVEN) ILL EFFECTS

Aside from the more obvious yeast-related health issues (like athlete's foot, thrush, vaginitis, and the like), *Candida* can cause or worsen many other health issues, such as these:

Antibiotic-associated diarrhea: This can occur when antibiotics have killed off the bulk of beneficial bacteria in the colon. *Candida* probably causes diarrhea by stimulating the secretion of water, sodium, and potassium into the small intestine. People who develop *Candida*-associated diarrhea are more likely to be elderly, hospitalized, or immunosuppressed,[106] but it can certainly happen to anyone.

IBD and maybe IBS: Quite a lot of research has linked *Candida* to inflammatory bowel diseases (IBDs) such as Crohn's disease (CD) and ulcerative colitis (UC). One study reported that the fecal mycobiome in patients with IBD was substantially different from that of healthy control subjects.[107] Another study demonstrated that a significant fungal colonization of the colon is more frequent in patients with a long history of UC than in patients with a short history of this disease, and that antifungal treatment reduces the inflammation of the colon during the course of UC in humans.[108] My group characterized the gut bacterial microbiota and the mycobiome in multiple families with CD and their healthy relatives. We showed that *Candida tropicalis* and the bacteria *Serratia marcescens* and *Escherichia coli* were associated with CD microbiome imbalance. We also demonstrated that these three species work together.[109] Of course, the presence of *Candida* isn't proof that *Candida* is a cause. And although there isn't yet definitive proof that *Candida* is a cause of symptoms associated with irritable bowel syndrome,[110] evidence is mounting. One study showed the waste products of yeast and yeast antigens could possibly be a trigger for irritable bowel syndrome symptoms.[111]

***Candida* arthritis:** This severe condition most typically affects the hips and knees and in a few cases, shoulders, ankles, elbows, wrists, toes, and vertebrae. Most victims had a previous bloodstream or other invasive *Candida* infection, and the *Candida* subsequently settled into the joints, causing infection and pain. *Candida* arthritis can erode and destroy bone, narrow joint space, increase fracture risk, and cause pain.[112]

Allergies: There is some evidence to support the theory that colonization with *Candida* can trigger allergic reactions. In 1992, a study[113] was able to establish an allergic response to *Aspergillus fumigatus*, another opportunistic fungal pathogen, in the lungs of mice with increased *Candida*.[114]

Inflammation in the GI tract: There has also been some interesting research linking *Candida* to inflammation and delayed lesion healing in the gastrointestinal tract and associations with Crohn's disease, ulcerative colitis, gastric ulcers, duodenal ulcers, perforated ulcers, and peritonitis.[115]

Many serious infections: A research project revealed all the following *Candida*-related infections in critically ill but non-immunosuppressed patients: blood infections, skin infections, vaginal infections, cystitis, abdominal infections, bronchitis, heart infections, bone infections, brain infections, kidney infections, and infections of the vascular system.[116]

Nail infections: Among people with fungal nail infections, which occur more frequently in the aging population, *Candida albicans* can be a cause, although it is an uncommon one.[117] It is responsible for nearly 2% of nail infections, particularly in the finger nails.

THE *CANDIDA* SOLUTION

Since beneficial bacteria in the microbiome help keep *Candida* under control, it makes sense that optimizing your microbiome is the best possible therapy for your mycobiome and for keeping *Candida* operating as a contributing member of your microbiome society. That means doing everything you can to balance your gut via the factors that you can control. Now that you understand *Candida*'s potential for harm, you will be better prepared to defeat it. But *Candida* has some potent allies. Let's meet them because, as they say, it's best to know thy enemy.

Partners in Crime: When Fungi and Bacteria Conspire Against You

In 1974, my advisor handed me a paper that changed the course of my career. It was a paper about rabbits, showing that when they were given antibiotics (to kill bacteria), they were more likely to develop *Candida* infections (caused by fungus). This triggered something in my brain—I realized that what affects bacteria also affects fungus in a chain reaction of dysfunction that eventually affects the health of the host (in that case, the rabbit). As I learned more, I recognized how often and in how many different ways fungi and bacteria work together—for their mutual benefit and yours, for their mutual benefit but not yours, and even in competition with each other and you. Fungi and bacteria have agendas. They form communities. They change within those communities, according to changes in their environments. Their interactions are complex and fascinating, but more important, their interactions can *directly affect you*. You simply can't look at bacteria without considering fungi, and you can't look at fungi without considering bacteria, and you can't look at either one (or both) without considering what their interactions mean for the person who hosts them.

THE QUEST FOR POWER: BACTERIAL-FUNGAL INTERACTION (BFI)

Bacterial-fungal interaction (BFI) is a term for the many complex ways that fungi and bacteria tend to form physically and metabolically interdependent groups that behave completely differently than any single microbe would behave on its own. Think of it like a big group of people thrown together under a single roof—like in a college dormitory or a small business or a commune or even at a family reunion. Each person comes into the environment as an individual with a certain way of interacting with the world as an individual, but once they get together and form a community—even a temporary one—their behaviors tend to change. When they go home for a family Thanksgiving or interact in the breakroom at work or move into a house together, those individuals will inevitably shift their dynamic and behave a little differently, in the context of the group. Some of these interactions will be positive. People working together may inhibit their natural antisocial reactions to facilitate group harmony and a more productive work environment. Some interactions may be negative. Family members may push each other's buttons and get in arguments during the Thanksgiving holiday. Relationships can grow or suffer. Group dynamics are complex and sometimes unpredictable.

Microbes are much the same. They form "families" or communities and then they interact and develop new behaviors. These interactions can be mutually beneficial, or they can be competitive. Sometimes the interactions are disorderly (like that family Thanksgiving) and sometimes they are quite well organized and symbiotic (like a successful small business), with all the microbes contributing to the greater good to accomplish tasks they couldn't do alone. (This is called syntrophism.)

We have learned how to manipulate BFIs for our own benefit in certain areas, such as in agriculture, environmental protection, food processing, biotechnology, and of course, medicine[118] and human health. To use a nutrition example, let's say you eat a bowl of brown rice. Inside your gut, the fungus *Candida* breaks down the starch in the rice, which liberates simpler sugars. These are then fermented by the bacteria *Prevotella* and *Ruminococcus*, resulting in fermentation by-products that feed the bacteria *Methanobrevibacter*. The by-products of *Methanobrevibacter*'s digestion result in even simpler sugars, which *Candida* can then turn around and consume, to complete the circle (this is also an example of how *Candida* can actually have a beneficial function). *Candida* couldn't get the sugar it needed without helping bacteria break it down enough, and meanwhile, you also benefit in various ways from those by-products that are released in your system—the by-products of microbial digestion, or fermentation, of the food you eat can be enzymes that, either directly or through a cooperative process with other microbes, help you to better assimilate the nutrients in your food while also ensuring the balance and survival of the microbial community. It's a win-win-win interaction among bacteria, fungi, and you.

But throw in a disruptive factor, and the benefits can disintegrate. Medication can be a disruptive factor. For example, a recent study showed that antifungal treatment for *Candida* caused worsening of inflammatory diseases such as colitis and allergic airway diseases (such as asthma and allergic rhinitis, in which allergies negatively impact breathing).[119] Removing *Candida* from the system is like pulling out a block from the middle of a very tall and complex block tower. It might have been a block of the wrong color, or a block with a crack in it, and that one little block may not seem to be doing much, but because it is part of a complex whole, taking it away can cause the whole tower to collapse. Similarly, when antibiotics remove both pathogenic and beneficial bacteria, the good bacteria that control the abundance of bad microbes, both fungal and bacterial, aren't around to check overgrowth. In this case, the small numbers of *Candida* species participating civilly can turn into a mob—and one dangerous element of *Candida* mob mischief is the contribution to the construction of biofilms.

BIOFILMS EXPOSED

The scientist in me would define the word *biofilm* as: "An organized, complex, spatially heterogeneous microbial community enclosed in a matrix of exopolymeric material composed of polysaccharides, proteins, and DNA, that attaches to an inanimate object or an organic surface; and that enables the influx of nutrients, the disposal of waste, and the formation of micro-niches." But to be a little less technical about it, I would also describe biofilms as structures that are like houses. A biofilm has a matrix of material that is not living. This is like the frame of a house. But inside the biofilm, there are residents, like the people living within a house. Biofilms are strong and secure, like a house with a locked front door and good insulation. They "open the door" for food delivery and to take out the trash, but they don't let in elements that might harm the residents, such as antibiotics, antifungals, or even your own immune system. In fact, not even desiccation, oxidation, or radiation can penetrate the exterior easily, which is why it is so difficult to treat infections that are biofilm-associated.

Unfortunately, in many cases, the residents in these biofilm "houses" are more like criminal elements than friendly neighbors; the trash they release and the residents they protect are most interested in causing trouble. Fungal pathogens can even shed "decoy" cells to distract the immune system, release anti-inflammatory signals to trick the immune system, and create camouflage molecules on the surface of biofilm that make it "invisible" to the immune system[120]—pretty sneaky.

But biofilms are hardly mysterious. You have already seen plenty of them because they are everywhere—you only need look at the slime you scrub from around your sink drains, or the slick slimy surface of stones in a garden pond or on the sides of boats in the water. You can feel them on your teeth in the morning before you brush, and when you brush your teeth, you are removing the biofilm we call plaque. You can also have biofilms anywhere you have a mucosal surface. You have mucosal surfaces along the entire length of your gastrointestinal tract from mouth to anal canal, inside your nose and sinuses, on all your internal organs, inside your reproductive organs, and in your lungs. The mucus layer on many mucosal surfaces sometimes protects the surfaces from biofilms forming on them, but in some cases, microbes use the mucin in mucous to attach and begin building biofilms. When the microbiome is healthy and vigorous, the mucosal layer tends to form a better barrier against pathogenic bacteria.

Biofilms aren't always bad. Good bacteria and fungi can cooperate to form biofilms that can actually promote wellness. When that happens, you won't notice because your body is working correctly, and you feel fine. An example would be biofilms in the GI tract, which can contain beneficial communities of microbes (like *Bifidobacteria* and *Lactobacillus*) that protect against pathogens and that support digestive health by breaking down food through fermentation. These beneficial biofilms take up space, thereby preventing the formation of biofilms housing more pathogenic microbes—the bad guys can't move in when healthy, beneficial biofilms are already taking up all the real estate.

The bad biofilms are the ones that cause problems, of course, especially in people with compromised immunity, wounds, surgical sites, or significant inflammation, or who are taking antibiotics—but pathogenic biofilm formation can happen to anybody. These biofilms can be insidious in many ways, and when they are bad, the majority involve *Candida* species, especially our now-familiar nemesis, *Candida albicans*.[121] *Candida* species are particularly

The Making of a Biofilm

Biofilms form in four distinct developmental stages:

The early phase: This phase takes from 1 to 11 hours to complete. The biofilm begins when a microbe adheres or sticks to a surface (whether a device or a tissue) and begins to multiply or grow to form what we call a microcolony (going from few cells to many cells). By 11 hours, a microbial community forms, with cells clumping together on the surface where the first microbe attached.

The intermediate phase: This phase occurs between 12 to 14 hours after initial formation. During this phase, the newly formed community begins to secrete sticky materials made of sugars and proteins, building their "house." This secretion forms the matrix—a sort of gelatinous blob in which the microbial cells are embedded, not unlike a Jell-O salad with fruit cocktail suspended in the gelatin.

The maturation phase: During this third phase, the amount of extracellular, gelatinous material increases until all the microbes in the community are fully embedded (the Jell-O salad is finished).[122] The cells within this mature biofilm have a three-dimensional structure and the biofilm provides the microbes within it a source of nutrients. It also acts as a sewer system to excrete waste, and it protects the microbes against the elements and potential harm, such as from antibiotic or antifungal drugs and the immune system. The biofilm is a complete and protected environment, constructed by the microbes that live within it and are now a part of it.

The dispersal phase: During this final phase of this "family," the "kids" are all grown up and ready to move out. Cells start to break away from the mature biofilm in search of new surfaces to stick to, so they can form biofilms of their own. If the biofilm is a good one, this is a positive development because it means even more surfaces will be covered with beneficial microbes. If it is a biofilm made by pathogenic microbes, this migration is bad news for you because it means even more pathogenic biofilms in your system.

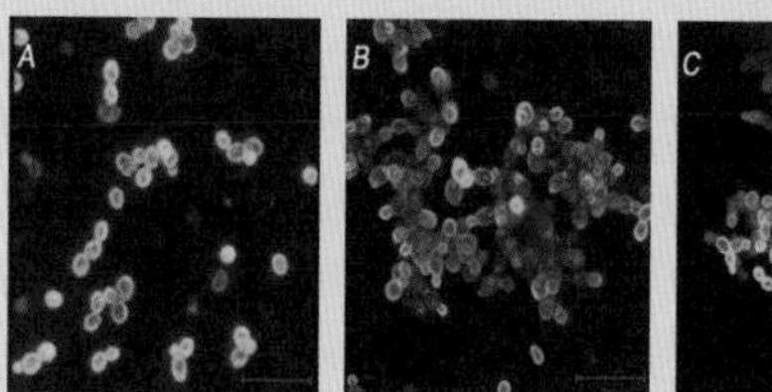

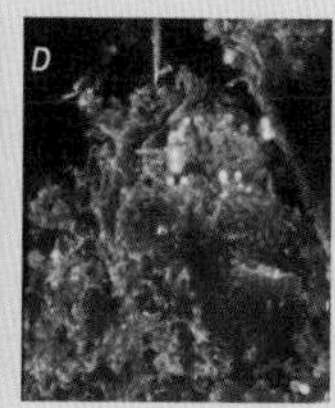

D

Confocal scanning laser raicroscopy images showing the phases of biofilm development over 48 hours. Early phase consisting of two steps: adhesion (90 minutes, A), and microcolony formation (6 hours, B). This is followed by intermediate phase (12 hours, C), and culminates in mature phase (48 hours, D).

good at forming biofilms, compared to bacteria. Studies have shown that *Candida* biofilms are thicker than bacterial biofilms and even more impervious.

Biofilms provide pathogenic microbes with a sheltered environment to proliferate and become more virulent—for example, *Candida* can change its shape into its more virulent filamental form when safe and secure inside a biofilm. And like in any family or close-knit community that exists over a long period of time, the individual microbes in a biofilm grow and reproduce in a predictable pattern, starting out small and vulnerable and then maturing, improving the "house," reproducing, and finally sending their offspring out to set up house somewhere else. The more robust the biofilm, the more likely it will be to spread—for better or for worse.

BIOFILMS IN THE GASTROINTESTINAL TRACT

Biofilms can form in many different places, but one of the most dangerous for you and me is the gastrointestinal tract. When biofilms form in the human gut, refered to as "digestive plaque," they can result in serious infections that antibiotics can't always resolve, and these pathogenic organisms can travel from the gut into the bloodstream. But even when they remain in the gut, they can result in serious conditions.

One example is Crohn's disease. My team has discovered, while studying the bacterial and fungal communities that reside in the guts of Crohn's disease patients,[123] that two pathogenic bacteria—*Serratia marcescens* and *Escherichia coli*—work together with *Candida tropicalis* to form robust biofilms that keep them protected from antibiotics and the immune system. While in this biofilm, *Candida* can change its shape to its filamental form, allowing it to more easily break down the protective mucin layer of the gastrointestinal lining (where the biofilm is adhered), damaging it and causing inflammation that can worsen the symptoms of Crohn's disease. It can also breach the intestinal lining in order to invade other parts of the body.

Another example is colon cancer. Several studies have demonstrated a link between biofilms and colon cancer.[124] One study looked at the interaction between two bacteria—*Escherichia coli* and *Bacteroides fragilis* (two of the pathogenic bacteria that the Mycobiome Diet reduces). Together, these bacteria formed biofilms on the inner surface of the gastrointestinal tract in colon cancer patients, suggesting that microbiome health is linked to colon cancer

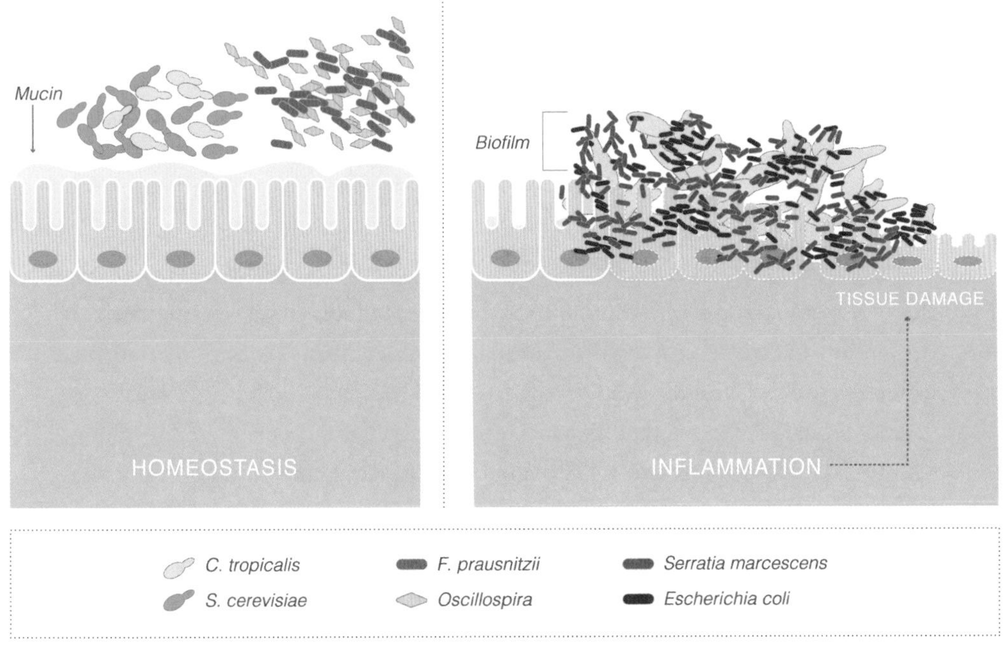

Biofilms formed on the GI tract in the presence of healthy microbiota compared to imbalanced fungal and bacterial communities.

development.[125] Other studies have shown that these biofilms lead to the disruption of a healthy mucosal barrier,[126] and that this biofilm formation was linked to colon cancer in humans.[127]

But even in people without a serious diagnosed disease, gastrointestinal biofilms that cause inflammation and infection could be forming. Having such formations conspiring beneath the cover of biofilms is clearly not in the best interest of human health. The combined resources of these bad guys can seriously compromise your wellness by:

- Weakening your internal defenses
- Making you resistant to antibiotic and antifungal therapies
- Compromising your intestinal barrier (which can lead to gut permeability or "leaky gut syndrome")
- Producing enzymes that can break down the mucin protecting the gut lining, causing lesions in the digestive tract

- Increasing systemic inflammation, rate of oxidative damage, and cell death, all of which lead to weight gain, depressed immunity, and poor health . . . or even cancer

Is there anything we can do to stop them? This is perhaps the most important question of all.

WEAPONS IN THE FIGHT AGAINST BIOFILMS

Because of the danger of biofilms, there has been a lot of research into their prevention and treatment. My team and I have been fighting biofilms on many different fronts. I have received grants from the National Institutes of Health to find better ways to combat biofilms, and my team and I have tested all the antifungals that are commercially available. We found certain ones that are better at inhibiting biofilms (such as caspofungin, anidulafungin, and micafungin). I also founded a company called Great Lakes Pharmaceuticals that developed a solution (called B-Lock) for the problem of biofilm formation on catheters in medical settings, which is now being considered for approval by the European Union (typically EU approval paves the way for approval in the United States).

But much of that work is still in process. What can you do about biofilms right now, especially the ones that may be in your gut—the ones that cause so many problems? Science has been less effective at targeting these, due to the fact that researchers previously did not recognize the importance of doing so. However, now that mainstream science is recognizing this important health obstacle, there is some interesting and provocative research showing that certain foods and supplements could literally break down biofilms so pathogenic microbes can be eliminated by drug therapy and the immune system. I have included many of these foods in the Mycobiome Diet, and my team has identified select probiotic strains that are particularly good at antagonizing pathogens and breaking down gut biofilms, including the most difficult mixed-species types. I recently published a scientific paper on this,[128] in which my team evaluated the ability of a novel probiotic (BIOHM Probiotic) to prevent and treat polymicrobial biofilms formed by *C. tropicalis* with *E. coli* and *S. marcescens*, three pathogens that tend to be elevated in Crohn's disease patients.[129] Our data showed that the probiotic was effective at preventing and inhibiting biofilms formed by these pathogens. The probiotic also inhibited *Candida albicans* germination. Based on these results, we proposed that the designed probiotic may be useful in the management of biofilm-associated gastrointestinal diseases including Crohn's and colorectal cancer.

There has also been some research into the encouragement of healthy biofilms, which inhibit pathogenic biofilms—something the Mycobiome Diet also encourages. This means we can fight biofilms in two ways: by breaking down the bad ones and building up the good ones—and you have the power to control those actions simply by altering what you eat and how you live.

I have put everything we know about what can legitimately reduce the power and potency of pathogenic biofilms into the Mycobiome Diet. As you will see in the next chapter, there are particular foods and food components as well as lifestyle behaviors that have been shown to impact biofilms in a way that can benefit your health. Let's look at what those are, and then we will jump right into the program and get you on track to make over your microbiome, optimize your mycobiome, dissolve harmful biofilms, and start feeling better as soon as possible.

Scientific Answers to Finagling Your Fungi

Your microbiome is a product of what you eat, how you live, where you live, and what you are exposed to, today, yesterday, and all the way back to before you were born. It is like a continuously shifting map of your life, with some elements (metaphorical major highways and historical landmarks) remaining consistent, and others (newly constructed roads, bridges, bike paths, and housing developments) constantly changing to reflect what you are doing right now. That means you can shift many important aspects of your microbiome in major ways that in turn can significantly improve your own health.

But you don't want to waste time on crazy unproven lifestyle changes that are difficult and aren't going to make a difference. In this chapter, I'm all about showing you the *proof*—there is fascinating evidence about the influence of macronutrients, micronutrients, phytochemicals, specific foods, specific dietary styles, and lifestyle behaviors on the health and diversity of your microbiome, on fungal abundance, and on biofilm formation. What you do to your microbiome today determines what your microbiome can do for you tomorrow, so knowledge, in this case, is literally power over your own health. After reading this chapter, you'll know even more about how to foster a healthy and balanced microbiome, so the Mycobiome Diet will make much more sense to you. You'll know exactly why I've highlighted certain foods and discouraged others—and why I can predict you will feel the difference in just a few days, or even in 24 hours.

Two Basic Truths

Your gut balance is what it is because of what you eat (and ate): The foods you eat shape your microbiome.[130] Vegetarians and healthy omnivores and people who eat a typical Western diet that's high in animal fats and sugars all have very different microbiomes because the microbes within them have adapted to the incoming food types. Vegetarians have more intestinal microbes suited for starch digestion, and heavy meat eaters have more microbes suited to bile digestion. When you eat foods that are considered *prebiotic* (such as vegetables and whole grains), you are providing the best food source for microbes that benefit your health. When you eat a lot of meat and animal fat, you are providing the best food for bile-tolerant microbes that have some benefits but also tend to be much more inflammatory. When you eat a lot of sugar and refined carbs, you are providing the best food for *Candida,* which can (as you have learned) cause many health problems for you. Microbes that are good at digesting vegetables and grains won't survive very well in someone who hardly eats any carbs. Likewise, bile-digesting microbes won't survive very well in someone who mostly eats plant foods. Everything you eat feeds somebody in your microbiome—the question is, are you feeding the good guys or the bad guys? You have an opportunity with every meal to encourage the growth of beneficial microbes, or to encourage the growth of harmful microbes. Your choice.

The microbiome you started with is persistent but is also changeable: The particular microbes that have adapted to you and your diet and lifestyle tend to have either health benefits for you (like the production of short-chain fatty acids (SCFAs), digestive enzymes, or nutrient assimilation) or can make you more prone to certain health problems (such as inflammatory conditions or infections). If you change your diet, such as choosing to eat more vegetables and fiber, or more junk food and sugar, your microbiome will shift in response.[131] If you only change it for a short time and then go back to your original diet, your microbiome will revert, too. If you are a vegetarian and switch to a carnivorous diet, or if you are a heavy meat eater and switch to a vegetarian diet, your microbiome will change within 24 hours[132]—but as soon as you go back to your original diet, your microbiome will revert back to the way it was before (we saw this happening in our clinical trial, in those who went back to their original diets after following the Mycobiome Diet for four weeks). The longer you sustain a dietary change, the more lasting your microbiome shifts will be. The dietary habits you have practiced for most of your life have had the most influence on your current microbiome configuration, and there are some aspects of your microbiome that were established in the first few years of life and will likely never change.[133] However, there are also some predictable and reproducible shifts in specific beneficial or pathogenic microbes that are pretty reliable with certain kinds of dietary changes.[134] Bodies adapt, and so do microbiomes, but not unless you force the adaptation through consistent long-term dietary and lifestyle changes.

HOW YOUR GUT BALANCE REACTS TO MACRONUTRIENTS

At a very basic level, nutrition influences your microbiome health. The three basic macronutrients—protein, fat, carbs—and where you choose to get them from matter.[135] If you've ever been told not to eat one of the three macronutrients, read on to see why they are all equally important—their sources as well as their amounts—for microbiome health.

Protein Power

You need protein to build the structures of your body, but not all proteins are the same as far as your microbiome is concerned. Many studies have demonstrated that protein from animal sources is more likely to encourage more pathogenic bacteria, with the exception of whey (a by-product of cheese making), which has a beneficial effect, and casein (also from milk). Research shows that casein tends to reduce intestinal inflammation by reducing inflammatory bacteria and increasing the production of anti-inflammatory SCFAs.[136]

Plant-based proteins in particular appear to encourage beneficial bacteria. One study showed that those on a diet based primarily on animal products lost more microbial diversity and many beneficial bacterial species, and increased their risk of inflammatory bowel diseases like Crohn's disease and ulcerative colitis. Many other studies support the benefits of plant protein on the microbiome, suggesting that, in general, you will most benefit your microbiome by getting more protein from plants and dairy products, and less protein from animal meat.

Fat Chances

You need fat for energy, cell growth, nutrient absorption, and to keep your hormonal system running smoothly. However, you don't need to overdo it. High-fat diets generally have a deleterious effect on microbiome health, and this effect is most pronounced in diets high in saturated fat. However, monounsaturated fats (like those prominent in fatty fish such as salmon and certain plant foods like olives and walnuts) seem to have a neutral effect on microbiome health. For example, one study compared microbiome-induced inflammation in mice fed lard to mice fed fish oil. The lard-fed mice had microbiome changes that increased inflammation, while the fish-oil mice did not.[137] This implies that vegetable and seafood fat are better for your microbiome, as well as your inflammation level, than saturated animal fat.

By contrast, low-fat diets have generally been shown to improve microbiome health. This is interesting because current diet trends such as a ketogenic diet and a paleo diet emphasize fats, including saturated fats, and claim that these diets are beneficial to health. They may have some benefits for some people, but those benefits do not seem to apply to the microbiome, at least in terms of reliable scientific evidence. Basically, you need fat, but the best kinds come from seafood and plants . . . and even then, you don't need too much.

The Carb Conundrum

The category of carbohydrates is the most complex and the most well researched, in terms of its influence on the microbiome. You may have heard (especially if you follow low-carb-type nutrition information in the media) that "humans don't need carbs," and that "humans can't digest grains." Maybe humans don't need carbs (although it would be awfully difficult to live without getting any), but the most beneficial microbes inside the human gut rely on fiber and resistant starch (a type of starch you can't digest but your microbiome can) for their fuel source. And those come from foods rich in carbohydrates.

In fact, people who eat a high-fat diet tend to increase the numbers of bacteria in the small intestine that facilitate fat absorption, leading to inflammation and weight gain, but people who eat a lower-fat, higher-carb diet rich in fiber and vegetables (the "good carbs") have much higher levels of beneficial bacteria such as *Bifidobacteria* and *Lactobacillus.* Carbs are the fuel sources for these beneficial microbes, so if you aren't eating very many carbs from plants, you may be reducing the diversity of your microbiome and encouraging the growth of more microbes that can put you at risk for health issues such as obesity and inflammatory bowel disease.

But wait . . . before you run off to start carb-loading, the picture is a little more complicated. There are many different kinds of carbs, and when you eat too many of them all at once, especially simple starches and sugars, you are feeding *Candida,* which can spike in abundance within 24 hours of a high-carb meal. That means a carb free-for-all isn't good for you, either. How do you navigate the confusing landscape of carbs?

Let's start with some carb basics. There are two types of carbohydrates:

those that are digestible (starch and sugar) and those that are indigestible (fiber and resistant starch). Your body reacts very differently to each of these.

What's Worse Than Sugar?

Research shows that artificial sweeteners have a detrimental effect on the microbiome. This may be counterintuitive since they are meant to replace sugar and don't contain sugar, but they change the microbiome in ways that can induce glucose intolerance and put you at greater risk for metabolic syndrome and type 2 diabetes.[138] Mice fed artificial sweetener developed intestinal dysbiosis with increases in pathogenic *Bacteroides* species and reduction of beneficial *Lactobacillus reuteri.* Artificial sweeteners may be even more likely to induce glucose intolerance than pure sugar.

We obtained further evidence that artificial sweeteners could negatively affect the gut microbiome in a study we conducted to determine the effect of Splenda on the microbiome using a mouse model. Our results showed that this sweetener promoted gut microbiome imbalance. Specifically, consumption of Splenda promoted expansion of the bacterial phylum Proteobacteria (an increase in this phylum is a red flag for inflammation), as well as an overgrowth of *E. coli.*[139]

Digestible carbs like the starchy parts of grains and the sugars in fruit and dairy products get digested in the small intestine (although their digestion begins in the mouth, with chewing). Your gut microbes can and do digest these sugars, and some of your beneficial gut bacteria also do well on fuel from digestible carbs.[140] But you digest most of this type of carbohydrate before it reaches the large intestine, where most of your gut microbes live. Some of these carbs come from nutrient-dense foods like whole grains, vegetables, and fruit, while others come from nutrient-poor foods like refined white flour, white rice, and white sugar. They are all digestible carbs, although with varying nutrient levels.

Although you and your microbes may be able to digest sugar, don't forget that *Candida,* and especially *Candida albicans,* is sugar's biggest fan. In fact, *Candida* has the ability to sense sugar, and is hot on sugar's trail like a bloodhound after a scent—specifically in the forms of glucose, fructose, and mannose.[141] If you eat too much sugar—more than you can easily digest—*Candida* is sure to find it, consume it, and multiply. Think about that the next time you eye that vending machine!

Of course, if you eat some sugar now and then, you will probably be okay. Normally, your good gut bacteria will keep the *Candida* numbers down, and a healthy environment in your large intestine is not conducive to *Candida albicans* overgrowth. But let's say you just had a course of antibiotics, which has vastly reduced your good bacteria. Feed *Candida albicans* a bunch of sugar in this scenario, and it can quickly grow out of control. Or imagine that you eat way too much sugar day after day after day. At some point, you're just rooting for *Candida* to take out the good guys, especially if your sugary, white-floury treats keep you too full to eat much fiber or resistant starch (contained in foods such as vegetables, legumes, and whole grains). Then, not only are you feeding *Candida,* but you are starving the microbes that manage *Candida.* That's a perfect storm.

Milk Please, No Cookies

Interestingly, while sugar can have a detrimental effect on the microbiome due to increasing *Candida,* lactose (milk sugar) seems to be particularly beneficial. Lactose decreases the abundance of the pathogenic bacterium *Clostridium* and increases anti-inflammatory SCFAs. Both of these changes are helpful to those with irritable bowel syndrome. This is somewhat surprising, since many people associate dairy products with digestive problems and irritable bowel syndrome-type symptoms.[142] Low-fat and nonfat dairy products may be the best for the microbiome because they are rich in milk sugars and casein, the beneficial milk protein, but not in the dairy fats that can have a more negative, inflammatory effect on the microbiome (similar to the fat from meat).

Indigestible carbs, by contrast, pass through the small intestine undigested and move into the large intestine, where most of your microbes live. Indigestible carbs come from high-fiber foods like vegetables, whole grains, legumes, and fruit; resistant starch–rich foods like potatoes, sweet potatoes, plantains, winter squashes, oats, corn,[143] barley;[144] and whole grains like brown rice, whole wheat, and spelt. (Many of these foods contain both fiber and resistant starch.)

You can't digest them, but your microbiome can, fermenting them and creating by-products that benefit you, such as digestive enzymes and substances that support your immune function, reduce inflammation, support hormonal balance, and much more. This is a great example of symbiosis: You eat things you can't digest to feed your microbiome, which will then produce substances that make you healthier.

Diets high in indigestible carbs tend to result in a greater microbiome diversity, a lower abundance of pathogenic bacteria like certain species of *Clostridium* and *Enterococcus,* and a greater abundance of beneficial bacteria like *Bifidobacterium* and *Lactobacillus.* By contrast, research has shown that people who don't consume very much dietary fiber tend to produce fewer anti-inflammatory SCFAs.

This is why fiber-rich whole grains and vegetables with resistant starches are genuinely *good carbs* for your microbiome. Contrast this to simple sugars and starches that can be a source of energy for you but, in excess, can be detrimental to the health and balance of your microbiome, not just because of their lack of nutrients, but because of how much *Candida* thrives on them.[145]

Pre-, Pro-, and Postbiotics

Prebiotics feed beneficial bacteria and fungi. Probiotics are beneficial bacteria and fungi. These terms are well established and frequently used. Postbiotics, however, are something new. When probiotics ferment prebiotics, they produce fermentation products such as anti-inflammatory short-chain fatty acids (SCFAs) and butyrate, which provides energy to cells. Postbiotics are these very compounds—the fermentation by-products that probiotics produce. Scientists are just beginning to produce them in supplement form for therapeutic use so that people can get the benefits of these fermentation products even if their microbiome is not producing them naturally. This is a relatively new technology that may become more widespread if it proves to be useful in treating gastrointestinal conditions. Keep an eye out for it.

OTHER DIETARY INFLUENCES

Two other notable food categories that have been studied in terms of their microbiome effect are fermented foods that actually contain beneficial microbes, and polyphenols, which are compounds found in plants that benefit human health in many ways. The latter is perhaps the most exciting for our purposes, as many have been shown to dissolve biofilms.

Fermented foods: Foods such as yogurt, kombucha, kefir, miso, tempeh, sauerkraut, kimchi, and other pickled vegetables, help to replenish the microbiome with beneficial species (probiotics). Although some of these will be transient, passing through without colonizing or colonizing only for short periods, they can have a temporary benefit by inhibiting the colonization, growth, or virulence of pathogenic bacteria. With a steady influx of prebiotics and probiotics, some ingested probiotics may colonize the large intestine longer term but will probably not establish permanent residence. However, that may not be necessary,[146] as transient probiotics have demonstrated health benefits—while they are visiting, they may crowd out the bad guys and stimulate resident populations.

Polyphenols: Many foods containing phytochemicals fall under the category of polyphenols. Polyphenols have antioxidant, anti-inflammatory, and anticarcinogenic properties, but have also demonstrated anti-biofilm activity,[147] with the ability to actually dissolve or break through biofilms. This means they are good for you *and* your microbiome.

A surprising number of these compounds have this biofilm-busting capability, so to keep pathogenic bacteria and fungi under better control and thwart their biofilm-constructing plans, I suggest using these food compounds frequently in your diet. Following is a list of phytochemicals (mostly polyphenols) and the foods that contain them that are proven biofilm breakers. Note that many of these compounds occur in the same foods—especially extra-potent green tea,[148] garlic, turmeric, and berries,[149] and certain herbs and spices. These are some of the compounds (and foods) specifically featured in the Mycobiome Diet:

- **Ajoene:** This compound is contained in garlic and has particularly strong antibacterial power. It has been shown to inhibit the growth of *E. coli*.[150]
- **Allicin:** All the onion family vegetables contain allicin. It is especially available in crushed garlic, but onions, shallots, leeks, and chives also contain some. It acts similarly to ajoene.[151]
- **Allyl isothiocyanate:** This is in cruciferous vegetables, especially bok choy, broccoli, Brussels sprouts, cabbage, cauliflower, horseradish, kale, kohlrabi, mustard greens, radishes, rutabaga, turnips, and watercress.
- **Camellia sinensis:** Find this in all true tea, including green tea, black tea, oolong tea, and white tea.
- **Carvacrol:** Thyme oil, oregano oil, and wild bergamot all contain this compound. These are essential oils, so only types approved as edible should be consumed, and only in small amounts, more like a supplement than a food. Carvacrol is also in tequila (but alcohol has other negative effects on the microbiome, so I suggest you don't overdo it!).

- **Catechins and epicatechins:** Green tea, apples, blackberries, dark chocolate, cocoa, red wine, black grapes, raspberries, blackberries, cherries, guava, pears, fava beans, sweet potatoes, and purple potatoes all contain these compounds.
- **Cinnamaldehyde:** Get this from cinnamon and cassia.
- **Curcumin:** This trendy and powerful anti-inflammatory phytochemical has also demonstrated antibacterial, antiviral, and antifungal activity, particularly against *Candida* species.[152] Note that I encourage including it in your diet *at least* three times a week via its best source, turmeric. It's easy to find in dried form, but some stores also stock the fresh root.
- **Ellagic acid:** Raspberries have the most, but other foods with ellagic acid include strawberries, grapes, blackberries, cranberries,[153] pomegranates, guava, pecans, and walnuts.
- **Epigallocatechin:** Green tea, white tea, oolong tea, strawberries, raspberries, blackberries, plums, peaches, kiwi, and avocado are all good sources.
- **Eugenol:** This one is in cloves, cinnamon, basil, and nutmeg.
- **Gallic acid:** Many foods contain gallic acid, including blueberries, walnuts, apples, flaxseed, tea, sumac, and watercress.
- **Gallocatechin:** Chocolate, cocoa, coffee, cranberries,[154] pears, apples, legumes like lentils and chickpeas, many nuts, red and green grapes, grape juice, wine, and tea all contain gallocatechin.
- **Linoleic acid:** This biofilm inhibitor is abundant in plant-based oils, especially safflower oil, grapeseed oil, hemp oil, wheatgerm oil, walnut oil, soybean oil, and sesame oil. It's also in sunflower seeds, hemp seeds, and almonds.
- **Pterostilbene:** This compound is similar to resveratrol and occurs in many of the same food sources: blueberries, almonds, mulberries, peanuts, red wine, red grapes, grape leaves, and cocoa.
- **Punicalagin:** Pomegranates and pomegranate juice contain this.
- **Quercetin:** Leafy greens, broccoli, red onions, and peppers contain quercetin.
- **Resveratrol:** Many foods contain this popular phytochemical known for its many antioxidant benefits. It's also a biofilm-breaker. Get it from red wine, red grape juice, fresh grapes, peanuts, peanut butter, pistachios, cocoa powder, dark chocolate, strawberries, blueberries, red currants, cranberries, lingonberries, and mulberries.

- **Sulforaphane:** Many foods contain sulforaphane, which promotes the production of Nrf2, a protein that helps to slow aging. It is also anti-inflammatory, anticarcinogenic, boosts the brain-enhancing brain-derived neurotrophic factor (BNDF), and is cardioprotective, among other benefits in addition to its action against biofilms. The best sources are the cruciferous vegetables, especially broccoli sprouts (these have the highest amount), but also broccoli, cauliflower, kale, Brussels sprouts, cabbage, bok choy, collard greens, mustard greens, watercress, arugula, and turnips.
- **Tannic acid:** Grapes and persimmons contain this substance.
- **Thymol:** This compound comes from the thyme plant.
- **Umbelliferone:** Find this one in celery, cumin, fennel, and parsley.
- **Ursolic acid:** This chemical occurs in apple and cranberry skins—it is the naturally occurring waxy substance that makes apples shine when you polish them. There is also some in basil, blueberries, cherries, pomegranates, and plums (it is most concentrated in prunes). In addition to its ability to dissolve biofilms, it is being studied for its tumor-inhibiting action in breast cancer.[155]
- **Vanillin:** Vanilla beans contain this, but so do oats, whole-grain flour, cocoa, olive oil, vinegar, olives, and surprisingly, alcohol-free beer.[156]

A FEW MORE MICROBIOME SUPERSTARS

Beyond polyphenols and the other biofilm inhibitors mentioned previously, as well as the fiber- and resistant-starch foods, plant and dairy protein foods, and plant fats, there are some other specific foods that have demonstrated positive effects on the microbiome. These are some of the other foods I've included in the Mycobiome Diet. Let's look at a few more microbiome-friendly foods:

Soy: Soy foods like tofu, tempeh, and soy milk are controversial, as many people believe they interfere with hormone production and could cause thyroid problems. While I have not seen convincing evidence proving that soy foods are dangerous for human health, there is good evidence that soy foods are good foods for your microbiome. Soy foods interact with your microbiome to increase levels of beneficial *Bifidobacterium* species and *Lactobacillus* species as well as reduce pathogenic bacteria populations.[157] Overall, these influences could lower disease risk and promote health, which is why I include soy foods as an optional protein source in the Mycobiome Diet.

Apple cider vinegar: Another biofilm-dissolving food, it's the acetic acid (not the acidity *per se*) in apple cider vinegar that has been proven to eradicate biofilms without damaging tissue.[158]

Pistachios: Nuts are a good source of fiber and micronutrients, but pistachios in particular have demonstrated significant microbiome benefits. In a study comparing the influence on the microbiome of pistachios and almonds, pistachios showed a much stronger effect, increasing more of the beneficial butyrate-producing bacteria.[159] While almonds are good, pistachios are one of the best nut choices.

Walnuts: Like pistachios, walnuts have demonstrated benefits to the microbiome. They are rich in omega-3 fatty acids and antioxidants. One study using rats compared diets with the same amount of fat, fiber, and protein, but with one diet using walnuts to meet those numbers, and the other using corn oil, casein, and cellulose fiber.[160] The group eating the walnuts had significantly greater microbiome diversity (more species), including an increase in beneficial species and a reduction in inflammatory species. Another study looked at humans and what happens when they eat walnuts, or don't eat walnuts.[161] As with the rats, walnut consumption significantly improved microbiome health by increasing probiotic species and species that produce butyric acid, while decreasing more inflammatory species. This happened based on a daily intake of 43 grams of walnuts (a little bit less than half a cup) over eight weeks (this is one reason I recommend walnuts on the Mycobiome Diet, although this amount is somewhat high for those focusing on weight loss, due to the amount of polyunsaturated fats and calories they contain).

Mushrooms: According to multiple studies, mushrooms not only contain prebiotic fiber but contain many bioactive substances and polysaccharides that are all prebiotic. Some mushroom metabolites stimulate immune cells, reverse dysbiosis caused by a high-fat diet, improve the gut barrier, and increase microbiome diversity.[162]

Coconut oil: Multiple studies have shown the anti-inflammatory benefits of medium-chain triglycerides (MCTs) from coconut oil, which can reduce intestinal inflammation, especially in people with Crohn's disease.[163] Several studies have demonstrated a positive effect from coconut oil on the gut microbiota of people with obesity.[164] I recommend regular consumption of coconut oil unless your doctor has advised you to limit your saturated fat intake.

SPECIFIC DIETS

Sure, specific food compounds have specific effects, but what about whole dietary strategies? Science has something to say about these as well, although precisely isolating what certain diets actually are always makes this information a little less exact. Even so, an increasing amount of research is now looking at the influence of particular dietary patterns on human health. The evidence sometimes seems contradictory, in part because every diet has its good and bad qualities. It all depends on your perspective and what you are trying to accomplish. With that in mind, let's take a look at some of the most popular diets, specifically through the lens of the microbiome:

Paleo diet: The idea is a good one: Eat only whole, natural, seasonal foods you had to gather or hunt on your own, and live as naturally as possible inspired by paleolithic life, and you will be healthier. Research examining the microbiomes of isolated indigenous populations do show a dramatically higher microbial diversity than the people in Western developed societies have lost.[165] While the way the so-called paleo diet is often practiced in the United States today is far from actual ancient diets, ideally it should be a natural, seasonal, whole-food diet, which comes with many microbiome benefits due to the high plant food content. However, the problem with this diet in its modern form is that it excludes whole grains and legumes, and their valuable prebiotic content.[166] It also typically excludes all dairy products, which also have microbiome benefits. It may also, in some forms, contain a lot of red meat, which is known to increase inflammatory bacterial species in the microbiome. As with vegetarian diets, it's all in how you practice it.

Mediterranean diet: This diet is low in red meat, high in seafood and whole grains as well as vegetables and fruits, and includes many sources of polyphenols and prebiotics, all qualities that benefit the health of the microbiome.[167] Microbiome-friendly elements include seafood, olive oil, green vegetables, intact whole grains in moderate amounts, and optional alcohol use no more than three times per week. Less favorable elements include too many carbohydrates and grains. One recent study showed an increased prevalence and abundance of *Candida* in participants who ate a Mediterranean diet.[168] Some practicing this diet may also use it to justify daily alcohol intake, which may or may not help some people with certain health aspects, but which has been proven to decrease microbial diversity.

Vegetarian, vegan, WFPB diets: Vegetarian diets don't contain any animal meat. Vegan diets exclude all products that come from animals, including dairy products, eggs, and sometimes even honey. Whole food plant based (WFPB) diets contain whole plant foods only, with no processed foods. In general, these strategies are all microbe-beneficial due to the high intake of plant protein, plant fat, fiber, and resistant starch. Of course, some "junk food vegetarians" may end up eating a lot of processed food, fried food, and sugar, which has a detrimental effect and can increase *Candida*. Ultimately, the gut-friendliness of these diets is typically high but could depend on how you practice them.

Low-calorie diet: The benefits of restricting energy intake along with increasing dietary fiber has been shown to increase microbial diversity 25% or more, especially in those with a low baseline diversity.[169] The problem with very low-calorie diets is that they can result in nutrient deficiencies.

Popular Diets That Are Not Microbiome-Friendly

While certain severe health issues can justify extreme diets, some popular diets have a markedly negative effect on the microbiome, mostly because they severely reduce prebiotics, polyphenols, and diet diversity. If microbiome health is your goal, these diets may not serve you:

Elimination diets: Although elimination diets can be good to practice over short periods of time to isolate intolerances and sensitivities to certain foods, over the long-term their restrictive nature can result in severe nutrient deficiencies and malnutrition, which can negatively impact the microbiome.[170]

Low-FODMAP diet: This diet is popular with people who have irritable bowel syndrome (IBS). It eliminates many different sources of fermentable (indigestible) carbohydrates like fiber and resistant starch, in an effort to reduce gastrointestinal symptoms. However, this also reduces microbiome food, and various studies have demonstrated that in IBS patients, a low-FODMAP (fermentable, oligosaccharides, disaccharides, monosaccharides, and polyols) diet significantly reduces beneficial *Bifidobacterium* species as well as microbiome diversity, while a high-FODMAP diet results in much greater bacterial diversity, especially of species that produce butyrate, a short-chain fatty acid (SCFA) that is essential for a healthy intact colon and gut lining. SCFAs increase energy production in the colon, shore up the gut lining, and may even guard against colon cancer.[171]

Low-carb and ketogenic diets: Diets high in fat and low in complex carbs that completely exclude major categories of beneficial prebiotics like whole grains, legumes, and starchy vegetables are the antithesis of a microbiome-friendly diet. There has been one study looking at diets with low microbiota-accessible carbohydrates (MACs), and it showed poor production of anti-inflammatory SCFAs and more dysbiosis. These diets in effect starve the microbiome and predispose people to chronic disease by inhibiting the immune system, since many immune system components are produced by a healthy microbiome.[172]

LIFESTYLE INFLUENCES

Food has the most obvious and direct influence on the microbiome, but lifestyle also has the potential to alter microbiome balance. The following are some of the habits scientists have investigated in terms of their influence on the microbiome. I have also considered them in formulating the lifestyle portion of the Mycobiome Diet (Chapter 7 contains more detailed lifestyle guidance):

Stress: Research has demonstrated that stress impacts the gut directly through the gut-brain axis, altering the microbiome. This alteration includes reducing the abundance of beneficial *Lactobacillus*.[173] Since 75% of Americans say they suffer from symptoms of stress,[174] this is a significant observation. Stress can also promote inflammation through microbiome alteration.[175] One study refers to this connection as "Mind-Microbe Balance."[176]

Sedentary lifestyle: Exercise has positive effects on the microbiome, increasing the abundance of microbes that help to produce SCFAs, which reduce inflammation, both in the gut and systemically. These positive changes disappear in people who stop exercising.[177]

Smoking: Smoking influences the microbiome, specifically by increasing potentially harmful *Bacteroides* and *Prevotella*.[178]

Sleep disruption: Sleep disturbances, especially chronic ones like you would have if you traveled to other time zones frequently or worked the night shift, can contribute to intestinal dysbiosis as well as increased incidence of obesity, metabolic syndrome, and inflammatory bowel disease, with a likely underlying cause of microbiome shifts.[179] Interestingly, one study showed that sleep disturbances did not alter the microbiome in mice fed a standard healthy diet but did significantly alter the microbiome in mice fed a high-fat, high-sugar diet, suggesting that a poor diet can worsen the effects of poor sleep and a good diet can lessen them.[180]

Because of the significant influence of these lifestyle factors, it is important that, in addition to adopting a diet that encourages a beneficial microbiome balance, you also adopt a healthier lifestyle that includes stress reduction, sufficient high-quality sleep, and moderate exercise.

As you move forward with the Mycobiome Diet, remember that your purpose is to optimize microbiome health in general, and mycobiome health specifically. But humans are complex and there are many influences on health. Every person reacts to foods, to some extent, in an individual way. This has to do with genetics, environment, and of course, your unique microbiome signature. Some foods that benefit the microbiome may have a detrimental effect on some people in other ways (such as whole-grain wheat on someone with celiac disease or a sudden increase in fiber intake on someone with a functional bowel disorder like IBS). Just because a research study says something is good doesn't mean it will be good for you right now. You must know your own needs and predispositions to food reactions, and you should always check with your primary care physician when you try something new.

However, it is my belief that in general and for most people, because the microbiome is so broadly influential to health, prioritizing microbiome health is a sound overall wellness strategy with a cascade of positive effects. Let's start making those positive, health-boosting changes in *your* microbiome.

PART TWO

MYCOBIOME MASTERY

6

The Mycobiome Diet Plan

Now that you know what your microbiome needs and what foods best nourish it (and you), it's time to put that knowledge into practice. With the help of some experts in nutrition and using my knowledge of the microbiome and its many influences, I have carefully formulated the Mycobiome Diet to optimize the health and diversity of your microbiome by feeding beneficial microbes, discouraging pathogenic microbes, dissolving biofilms, and generally giving your microbial populations the resources they need to work out their differences and strengthen their communities, in their own favor, and in yours. There are no phases, no stages, and no steps, other than an easy week to start and then a longer plan to help you learn how to eat for your microbiome on your own. This is a style of eating you can practice for life. It's not restrictive. It is customizable based on how you like to eat, and it is nutritionally complete—in fact, it is not just complete, but nutritionally optimal . . . not to mention delicious!

This diet is filled with the foods your beneficial microbes love, as well as food proven to bust through biofilms and your most annoying symptoms, from gastrointestinal distress to excess weight to fatigue and foggy thinking. Everything relevant that I know about microbiome health in general and mycobiome health in particular is integrated into the guidelines and other aspects of this dietary strategy.

We'll start with a bird's-eye view and some general rules about the do's and don'ts of eating for a more robust and balanced mycobiome and microbiome.

THE MYCOBIOME DIET RULES

The Mycobiome Diet is:

- Nutritionally balanced
- Whole-food based
- Low-glycemic
- Rich in fiber and resistant starches
- Low in sugar
- Full of good mono- and polyunsaturated plant fats
- Low in saturated fat and animal fat
- Full of satisfying lean plant protein and animal protein primarily from seafood, with a bit of poultry thrown in for those who like it
- Suitable for omnivores, vegetarians, and those who must be gluten-free or who prefer to avoid grains
- Flexible, diverse, and customizable

The basics are as follows:

Eat mostly whole food. Do not eat any processed food, "fast food," or packaged foods with more than three ingredients. If the ingredients label lists chemicals and additives, don't eat that food. If the bag, box, or can says something like "brown rice" as a single ingredient, or "organic garbanzo beans, water, sea salt," those are acceptable foods. Although the following foods are not exactly whole foods, they are okay on this diet:

- Mixed foods in which all or most of the ingredients are whole foods—like a packaged soup mix of dried beans, brown rice, and spices.
- Grain products that are 100% whole grain, such as 100% whole wheat tortillas, bread, bagels, or pita, even if they come in a package. These may contain more than three ingredients, but the most important element is that all grain ingredients are whole.
- Fermented foods like sauerkraut, kimchi, and low-fat or nonfat yogurt. The probiotic benefits of these foods makes them worthwhile, but look for lacto-fermented brands rather than those containing vinegar, as they have a better probiotic content.
- Nut-based and coconut-based milk, yogurt, and cheese. These may have multiple ingredients, but they are okay if they are unsweetened. They

make good alternatives to full-fat milk products, or to prevent overuse of dairy products.

- Condiments like soy sauce, chili paste, sriracha, and the like. Do not use condiments with added sugar. These condiments can add flavor and interest to microbiome-beneficial foods you might not otherwise enjoy.

Most of your foods should come from the produce section, the bulk bins, the seafood counter, and the dairy case. Note that in the recipe section, whenever we include a food that typically comes in packaged form and that may be difficult to find in a mostly unprocessed state (such as almond milk or marinara sauce), we provide simple instructions for how to make these things yourself. If you do this, you can probably avoid almost all processed foods if you choose. However, if you can find pure, simple versions of these foods in the store, of course you can use them, as this is more convenient.

Have a protein at every meal and every snack. Every time you eat, include a protein from the Proteins list (food lists start on page 95). Even if you are having just a small snack, always include protein instead of opting for a carb-rich or sweet snack. Protein choices include tuna, a hard-boiled egg, or hummus and whole-grain crackers instead of cookies or potato chips. Protein is important not just for maintaining and building muscle and other structures in the body, but for helping you to feel full so you aren't tempted to overeat simple carbohydrates or sugary foods that increase *Candida.* Remember that high-carb meals immediately increase *Candida* abundance, but diets rich in amino acids from proteins are associated with lower levels of *Candida.*

Have an oil- or fat-rich food with every meal and snack. The oils and fats on the Mycobiome Diet (see Oils/Fats list, page 98) are primarily from plant foods, eggs, and seafood, with monounsaturated and polyunsaturated fatty acids dominating over saturated fats. Your oil/fat at each meal and snack can be added (such as olive oil drizzled over vegetables) or it can be from a fat-rich food (such as nuts, avocado, tofu, or salmon). Like protein, fat makes food more satiating, meaning you are less likely to overeat simple carbohydrate foods that can spike *Candida.* Remember that *Candida* is inhibited by a diet high in healthy fats.

Have a resistant starch food with every meal. You can also include these with snacks, but this is optional. This category (see Resistant Starch Foods, page 98) is manna from heaven for your microbes. These prebiotic foods are rich in indigestible carbohydrates that pass through your small intestine and into your large intestine, providing a feast for your beneficial microbes. Many of these foods are also rich in fiber. Just don't overdo it. More is not better. One serving per meal is all you need to keep your microbes happy and keep *Candida* under control. Don't skip that serving, though. Your microbes depend on it.

Note that while there are gluten-containing grains in this category, you do not need to eat them, or any grains. There are plenty of other plant-based sources of fiber and resistant starch. However, if whole grains don't bother you, then eat them. They are fine sources of prebiotics and excellent sources of fiber.

HOW MUCH AND HOW OFTEN

The Mycobiome Diet includes four categories of foods:

- Foods to include in your diet *every day.*
- Foods to include in your diet *at least three times a week* (but daily is also okay).
- Foods to limit. You can eat them once in a while, but do not eat them every day.
- Foods to exclude. Do not eat these foods! They are conducive to the growth of pathogenic microbes and the suppression of beneficial microbes. These foods can lead to dysbiosis.

Let's take a look at the foods in each of these categories.

FOODS TO EAT EVERY DAY

Be sure to include each of the following food categories, as well as you possibly can, in the amount indicated. Make these foods a habit and part of your core diet. (Serving sizes for the specific foods within a category are indicated in the food lists, starting on page 95.) Note that the first five categories correspond to a food list, and your choices should come from these food lists:

Proteins: Eat at least three servings but no more than five servings of any protein on the Proteins food list, including at least one serving of protein with every meal and snack.

Oils/fats: Eat 2 to 4 tablespoons of any oil or fat from the Oils/Fats food list, including at least 1 tablespoon of oil or fat or one serving of a fat-rich food with every meal and snack. Note: If you are vegan, you may add more oil, as needed, but limit yourself to the oils and fats on the Oils/Fats food list—flaxseed oil is one great option, as it can stand in for fish oil.

Resistant starch foods: Eat at least three servings per day for omnivores, and six servings per day for those who do not eat animal products, from the Resistant Starch food list, including one to two servings with every meal. Including resistant starch as a snack is optional. Note: For vegetarians and vegans, to ensure sufficient protein at least two of your resistant starch servings should consist of legumes.

Cruciferous vegetables: At least 1 cup per day (no maximum) from the food list. Have these at any time of day. You will get the most beneficial impact from cruciferous vegetables like broccoli, kale, cabbage, cauliflower, and Brussels sprouts if you eat them cooked or fermented rather than raw.

Mycobiome-friendly (MF) vegetables: At least 2 cups per day (no maximum) from the food list. Have these at any time of day. Note: Both cruciferous and mycobiome-friendly (MF) vegetables have no limits in the amount you can eat, so if you get hungry between meals or need larger portions, you can always eat more of any food from these categories, rather than adding more protein, fat, or carbohydrate foods.

Apple cider vinegar: Have at least 1 tablespoon per day. You can have more, if you like. Bust those biofilms! Note: Raw apple cider vinegar is the best option, and if you choose to drink it mixed in water (as some people do), use a straw. The acidic vinegar could wear away your dental enamel over time, so try not to let it touch your teeth.

FOODS TO EAT AT LEAST THREE TIMES A WEEK

You can have any of the following foods daily, but you should eat them at least three times per week. I find it's easiest to do this every other day, such as on a Monday, Wednesday, and Friday, or on a Tuesday, Thursday, and Saturday, just to help stay organized.

Fish/seafood: Have a 4- to 6-ounce serving of any fish or seafood from the animal protein sub-list of the Proteins list, at least three times per week. I highly recommend including fish and seafood in your diet because of the cardioprotective properties of eicosapentaenoic acid (EPA) and docosahexaenoic acid (DHA). Research also shows that the fat from fish and other seafood is not associated with an increase in inflammation-causing microbes, as is saturated fat from other animal foods.

Vegetarian/Vegan Alert

If you do not eat seafood, it is very important for you to have a good plant-based source of alpha-linolenic acid (ALA), which the body converts to EPA and DHA, at least three times per week, or preferably every day. The following can replace one serving of fish or seafood:

- 1 tablespoon flaxseed oil (this is the richest source of ALA—mix it into any food or drink if the taste is too strong for you)
- 2 tablespoons ground flaxseeds
- 4 to 6 ounces tofu or other approved soy products (see the food list)
- ¼ cup walnuts

Note that any of these vegetarian options can count as a fat serving in any meal or snack, or it can be extra, on top of the fat requirement, if you feel you need more healthy fats in your diet (some people do better with more fat, some with less).

Pistachios and/or walnuts: Have at least 2 tablespoons or up to ¼ cup three times per week. Note that this will count as a fat serving. If you do not eat animal products, you can have up to ¼ cup daily.

Berries: Have at least 1 cup three times per week, or up to 1 cup per day from the Berries list.

Fermented foods: Have at least three servings per week from the Fermented Foods list.

Green tea: Have at least 3 cups over the course of the week, but a daily cup is ideal. Note that if you cannot drink green tea because you are too sensitive to the small amount of caffeine it contains, you may substitute a daily cup of berries, which contain many of the same compounds (although in lower amounts).

Ground turmeric: Have 1 teaspoon minimum at least three times per week. Daily is ideal. It's easy to mix turmeric into any cooked food or use it to make Golden Milk (page 255). Also note that a compound called piperine in black pepper increases the absorption of the curcumin in turmeric that is responsible for the potent anti-inflammatory action, so always add a pinch of black pepper to any food or drink containing turmeric. (The recipe for Golden Milk contains black pepper for this reason.)

Garlic: Have 1 to 2 cloves fresh, at least three times per week, but a daily dose is ideal. Fresh raw garlic is the form with the best microbiome-enhancing, biofilm-breaking properties. I like to include it in salad dressings for the most potent effect. It's still good for you if you cook it, but raw is best for breaking through those biofilms. Garlic powder, garlic salt, and granulated garlic do not count toward this requirement.

Garlic versus *Candida albicans*

I've been investigating ways to inhibit *Candida* since early in my career. Garlic has been one particular focus of my research. Years ago, I studied how a garlic extract might impact the growth of *Candida albicans*,[181] and sure enough, garlic affected this yeast in multiple ways, including by compromising the structure and integrity of the yeast cells and inhibiting their growth. Garlic treatment can damage *Candida* cells so that they appear deformed, with their outer protective layer breaking up, leading to leakage of important cell contents and eventual cell death. This is why I encourage eating fresh garlic every day on the Mycobiome Diet.

Ginger: Add at least 1 teaspoon dried ground ginger to cooked dishes or 1 tablespoon fresh grated ginger in food three times a week. You can also make fresh ginger tea—simply add slices of raw ginger to boiling water and steep for 10 minutes.

FOODS TO LIMIT

You can have these foods (although they are entirely optional), but do not have them more than specified here. They are fine, even potentially beneficial, in small amounts, but can become damaging to microbiome health in excess.

Alcohol: Don't have any more than three servings per week of any alcohol, and preferably never more than one serving in a day. Choose only unsweetened varieties, such as wine (dry red wine preferred, serving size 4 ounces), beer (serving size 12 ounces), or spirits (serving size 2 ounces) without any sweet mixers. Again, it is fine to exclude alcohol completely. Too much has been proven to harm the microbiome.[182]

Added sweeteners: You'll see in the next section that certain added sweeteners should be excluded completely because of their *Candida*-encouraging properties. However, there are two natural sweeteners that have been shown to benefit the microbiome when consumed in small amounts: real maple syrup and raw honey. These are the *only* accepted added sweeteners, and they are only for those who feel they absolutely must have a sweetening option for certain foods, such as tea or oatmeal. It's important, however, not to overdo these foods. Use up to but no more than 1 tablespoon per day. One teaspoon is better. None is best.

You Can Retrain Your Sweet Tooth

Think you can't live without sugar? Always remember that *Candida* loves any simple sugars! Sweeteners are never required, and in fact, I recommend training your palate to be more sensitive to sweetness, which will happen much more rapidly if you exclude all added sweeteners and get your sweet tastes only from fruit and spices like cinnamon. When I was a child growing up in the Mediterranean region, I used to have so much sugar in my tea that my parents joked that I had a cup of sugar with a hint of tea. However, now I do not use any sweetener in my tea and wouldn't want to because I enjoy the nice flavor of the tea itself. It may not seem easy at first to wean yourself off sugar, but it won't take long for your palate to adjust, and you will taste the flavors of food more intensely and enjoy your food even more. After a few days to a few weeks, you probably won't crave it anymore. People in our study generally noted that sugar cravings abated after two weeks on the Mycobiome Diet.

Coffee and/or black tea: You don't have to give up your morning coffee, although I recommend limiting yourself to 1 or 2 cups of coffee or black tea per day, for the sake of your digestion. There are some microbiome benefits to both coffee and black tea. As long as you get your minimum 3 cups of green tea per week, you can add these in, too. I encourage organic coffee because crops can be heavily sprayed with pesticides, herbicides, insecticides, fungicides, and chemical fertilizers. Also, organic coffee contains more chlorogenic acid and trigonelline than standard coffee (and also slightly more caffeine).[183] Both compounds have been linked to reduced incidence of diabetes and cancer. Chlorogenic acid is a polyphenol, and trigonelline is an alkaloid that has antimicrobial effects, and its status as a phytoestrogen may reduce the risk of reproductive cancers in women.[184] However, don't add any sweeteners other than the allowed amount of raw honey or real maple syrup as specified previously, or better yet, don't sweeten them at all.

FOODS TO EXCLUDE COMPLETELY

The foods in this category have no place in the regular diet of anyone seeking a more robust and beneficially populated microbiome. Avoid these as well as you can. We all make mistakes and the occasional inclusion of these foods isn't going to harm you, but the more diligent you are with the Mycobiome Diet, the faster your microbiome will respond.

No added sugar (except for real maple syrup and raw honey, as specified previously). These foods are not only nutrient-sparse but can contribute to blood sugar instability in some people, and also to excessive calorie intake. *Candida* loves these sugars, so keep it at bay by keeping them out of your diet. I know mistakes happen but do your best to go sugar-free and you will feel better in all kinds of ways. The sweeteners to exclude are:

- Agave syrup/agave nectar
- Artificial sweeteners, which are slayers of beneficial bacteria and have a proven association with excessive weight gain (ironically) and also with dysbiosis
- Beet sugar
- Brown rice syrup
- Brown sugar
- Cane sugar (all forms)
- Coconut sugar
- Corn syrup (including high fructose corn syrup)
- Date sugar
- Glucose (and any food additive ending in *-ose*)
- Imitation maple syrup
- Maple sugar
- Molasses
- Raw sugar
- Sugar syrup

No refined grain products. This very broad category may make up a large part of your current diet. But if you want to eat for microbiome health (and your own health), it's time to get rid of these. They include:

- Any bread or bread product (bread, bagels, English muffins, rolls, breadsticks, pizza crust, pita bread, etc.) or pasta that is not made with 100% whole grains
- Any baked goods with added refined sweetener (doughnuts, cookies, cake, muffins, etc.)
- White rice
- Gluten-free bakery products (bread, bagels, pizza crust, etc.) made with any refined grains, such as white rice flour
- Instant/quick oats (100% whole-grain oats, including old-fashioned and steel-cut oats, or Irish oats are fine)

When in doubt, avoid it. Read the label, especially for bread products. Many say "whole-grain" or "multigrain" but contain refined flour. This is very important, as *Candida* loves refined grains as much as pure sugar. If the label says "100% whole grain" and there are no refined grains in the ingredients list, these products are okay. Sprouted grain products are usually a safe bet.

No oils or fats, or fat-rich foods, other than those on the Oils/Fats list. That means no:

- Vegetable oils not listed on the Oils/Fats list, including corn, soybean, sunflower, and all-purpose vegetable oil.
- Butter
- Full-fat dairy products like cream, half-and-half, whole milk, cream cheese, whipped cream, or full-fat dairy cheese. Or ice cream, of course.
- Lard

No processed, cured meat, such as bacon, sausage, ham, or deli meats. Use fresh meat only—and preferably, seafood.

No processed or packaged food with more than three ingredients, unless all the ingredients themselves are natural whole foods. For example, packaged plain brown rice is fine, but a package of flavored rice with sauce is not.

Here is a handy cheat sheet so you can see all the rules in one place. Use the check-off list to keep track of your requirements as you fulfill them. These are good reminders to put on your refrigerator or pantry door.

MYCOBIOME DIET RULES SUMMARY

Eat mostly whole food. No processed foods or packaged foods with more than three ingredients.

Have protein from the list with every meal and snack. (No processed or cured meat.)

Have an oil/fat or fatty food from the list with every meal and snack.

Have a resistant starch food from the list with every meal. This is optional for snacks.

Foods to Eat Every Day

- **Coconut or extra-virgin olive oil,** at least 1 tablespoon.
- **Resistant starch foods,** 1 to 2 cups.
- **Cruciferous vegetables,** at least 1 cup with no maximum.
- **Mycobiome-friendly vegetables**, at least 2 cups.
- **Apple cider vinegar,** at least 1 tablespoon.
- **Optional: eggs (2), poultry (like chicken and turkey—6 ounces), low-fat or nonfat dairy products (1 cup), tofu and tempeh (4 to 6 ounces), edamame (1 cup),** two servings maximum.

Foods to Eat Three to Seven Times Per Week (amounts are per day)

- **Fish/seafood,** up to 6 ounces.
- **Ground turmeric,** at least 1 teaspoon.
- **Ginger,** at least 1 teaspoon dried and ground or 1 tablespoon fresh grated.
- **Garlic,** 1 to 2 cloves.
- **Pistachios and/or walnuts,** ¼ cup.
- **Green tea,** at least 1 cup.
- **Fermented foods,** ½ cup.

Foods to Limit

- **Alcohol,** no more than 3 times a week. Or exclude completely.
- **Real maple syrup or raw honey,** no more than 1 tablespoon per day. Less is better.
- **Coffee and/or black tea.** Prioritize organic varieties.

Foods to Exclude Completely

- **No added sugar** sweeteners (except for real maple syrup and raw honey).
- **No refined grains.**
- **No processed, cured meat.**
- **No processed or packaged food** with more than three ingredients.
- **No oils or fats,** other than those allowed, including butter.
- **No full-fat dairy products.**

THE MYCOBIOME DIET DAILY AND WEEKLY FOOD TRACKERS

I have created two trackers to help you keep track of all your daily and weekly requirements. The first is a daily tracker. Use it to keep track of your daily requirements and to tally the daily totals. You can make copies of the tracker provided here, or you can make your own version. The second is a weekly tracker. Use it to ensure you get everything required into your week. You can make copies of the tracker provided here, or you can make your own version.

DAILY MYCOBIOME DIET TRACKER

DATE:__________________

	Breakfast	Lunch	Snack	Dinner
Did you include these per-meal requirements?	Protein Fat/oil Resistant starch	Protein Fat/oil Resistant starch	Protein Fat/oil	Protein Fat/oil Resistant starch
Did you include these per-day requirements?	Cruciferous vegetable MF vegetable Apple cider vinegar	Cruciferous vegetable MF vegetable Apple cider vinegar	Cruciferous vegetable MF vegetable Apple cider vinegar	Cruciferous vegetable MF vegetable Apple cider vinegar
Did you include any of these 3×/week requirements?	Fish/seafood (or veg options: flaxseed, soy food, or walnuts) Fermented food Pistachios/walnuts Berries Green tea Turmeric Garlic	Fish/seafood (or veg options: flaxseed, soy food, or walnuts) Fermented food Pistachios/walnuts Berries Green tea Turmeric Garlic	Fish/seafood (or veg options: flaxseed, soy food, or walnuts) Fermented food Pistachios/walnuts Berries Green tea Turmeric Garlic	Fish/seafood (or veg options: flaxseed, soy food, or walnuts) Fermented food Pistachios/walnuts Berries Green tea Turmeric Garlic
Did you include any of these limited foods?	Alcohol Real maple syrup Raw honey	Alcohol Real maple syrup Raw honey	Alcohol Real maple syrup Raw honey	Alcohol Real maple syrup Raw honey

Some people like to use these trackers exactly as is, and some people like to personalize them for their own use. You can think of these trackers as trainers that help you get used to the diet. Eventually, eating the Mycobiome Diet foods will become habit and you won't have to keep track anymore (unless you want to!).

cont'd	**Breakfast**	**Lunch**	**Snack**	**Dinner**
If you ate an excluded food today, list what it was and why you think you ate it:	Refined grain product Oil/fat not on the list Processed/cured meat Full-fat dairy Added sweetener (except for maple syrup or honey) Packaged/processed/junk food Why do you think this happened? ______ ______ ______	Refined grain product Oil/fat not on the list Processed/cured meat Full-fat dairy Added sweetener (except for maple syrup or honey) Packaged/processed/junk food Why do you think this happened? ______ ______ ______	Refined grain product Oil/fat not on the list Processed/cured meat Full-fat dairy Added sweetener (except for maple syrup or honey) Packaged/processed/junk food Why do you think this happened? ______ ______ ______	Refined grain product Oil/fat not on the list Processed/cured meat Full-fat dairy Added sweetener (except for maple syrup or honey) Packaged/processed/junk food Why do you think this happened? ______ ______ ______

DAILY TALLY OF REQUIRED ELEMENTS

4 servings protein
4 servings fat/oil
3 to 6 servings resistant starch

1 cup minimum cruciferous vegetables
2 cups minimum MF vegetables
1 tablespoon minimum apple cider vinegar

WEEKLY MYCOBIOME DIET TRACKER

Please fill this out at the end of the week, using your daily tracker pages for reference.

WEEKLY TALLY

DID YOU MEET ALL DAILY REQUIREMENTS THIS WEEK (check all that apply)?

- ☐ Protein at every meal
- ☐ Oil/fat at every meal
- ☐ Resistant starch at every meal
- ☐ Daily cruciferous vegetable requirement
- ☐ Daily MF vegetable requirement
- ☐ Daily apple cider vinegar requirement

DID YOU INCLUDE ALL REQUIRED WEEKLY FOODS?

- ☐ 3 servings fish or seafood (or veg options: flaxseed, soy food, or walnuts)
- ☐ 3 servings minimum fermented food
- ☐ 3 servings pistachios and/or walnuts
- ☐ 3 servings berries
- ☐ 3 cups minimum green tea (or three additional servings berries)
- ☐ 3 teaspoons minimum ground turmeric
- ☐ 3 cloves minimum garlic

LIMITED FOODS:

ALCOHOL. What type and how much for the week?________________________

REAL MAPLE SYRUP OR RAW HONEY. What type and how much for the week?

____

HOW DID YOU DO THIS WEEK? Note whether you stayed on plan or not. Describe any symptoms that may crop up, such as any digestive upset, fatigue, or headaches that can come with dietary transitions, as well as weight changes if you choose to keep track of those: ______________________________________

____

____

____

____

____

____

____

WEIGHT? ________

YOUR COMPLETE MYCOBIOME DIET FOOD LIST

Now for the fun part—all the great foods you get to eat! Bookmark this list so you can easily find it whenever you want to check if a food is a part of the Mycobiome Diet or not. As you meet your daily and weekly requirements, always make your choices from the foods listed here.

What about Foods Not on This List?

Any foods not found on the Foods to Exclude Completely list (page 89), and any food not mentioned here on the Your Complete Mycobiome Diet Food List (such as fruits other than berries and other meats like beef, pork, and lamb) are allowed in moderation. However, all required foods must be prioritized and included in your diet as specified. Only then, and only if you are genuinely still hungry, should you consider other food choices. For example:

- As long as you eat fish at least three times per week and fulfill your protein requirement at each meal with the foods on the list only, you could add other animal proteins as extra protein beyond what this diet requires. Lower-fat sources are most conducive to microbiome and mycobiome health, so add in other meats sparingly and choose lean cuts of beef and pork (and never processed meat or cured meat).
- As long as you eat all the required vegetable servings per day, you could also add in an apple or some mango for snack or dessert, put a banana in your smoothie, or add in any other fruit or vegetables not on the lists. However, overeating fruit can encourage the growth of *Candida,* so add it in small amounts only, if you like it. The best reason to add a little fruit is to fuel a vigorous workout.

Restrictions always apply. For example, full-fat dairy products, cured meat, and refined grain products are not allowed, even after you have met your requirements.

Proteins

Remember to include one protein serving at every meal and every snack.

Animal protein. Serving size 4 to 6 ounces or two eggs. Add other fresh meats only when your protein requirement is fulfilled.

- Chicken
- Eggs
- Fish, all kinds (such as cod, halibut, mahi-mahi, salmon, tilapia, tuna, etc.)
- Shellfish, all kinds (such as crab, lobster, oysters, scallops, shrimp, etc.)
- Turkey

Dairy products, nonfat or low-fat (1%) only.

- Cheese (such as nonfat feta or part-skim fresh mozzarella—serving size 2 ounces)
- Cottage cheese (serving size 6 ounces)
- Milk (serving size 1 cup)
- Yogurt, unsweetened (plain; serving size 6 ounces)

Soy protein. Do not use packaged, processed soy products such as store-bought "veggie burgers" or "veggie hot dogs," although you can certainly make your own veggie burgers using tofu or tempeh.

- Edamame (doubles as a resistant starch; 4 ounces)
- Soy milk (unsweetened only; 1 cup)
- Soy milk yogurt (unsweetened only; 6 ounces)
- Tempeh (doubles as a fermented food; 4 ounces)
- Tofu (preferred non-GMO, organic—doubles as a fat serving; 4 ounces)

Worried About Soy?

Soy has had a lot of bad press. Many soy products are highly processed, and soy is a heavily sprayed crop. Many foods also contain soy protein isolates, which are highly processed. Soy is also a phytoestrogen that some people fear has negative hormonal consequences (although research suggests they have health benefits, and I have seen no peer-reviewed articles suggesting that consuming soy is associated with any proof of health problems). However, organic soy products like edamame, tofu, soy milk, and organic fermented soy products like tempeh and miso, are not highly processed. They are high in protein, and contain healthy fats (including omega-3 fatty acids). Soy is proven to be good for your heart, it contains fiber, and it also contains isoflavones—those phytoestrogens—that may actually be helpful for postmenopausal heart disease prevention, easing hot flashes, preventing certain cancers, and possibly even reducing bone loss.[185] Soy is also excellent microbiome food.[186] Unless your doctor has told you that you cannot have soy for health reasons, then natural, minimally processed organic whole soy products are nothing to worry about. If you are a vegetarian or a vegan, they can be an important source of nutrition.

Legumes. Serving size: 1 cup fresh, ½ cup peanuts or cooked legumes. All types of legumes are allowed, including any legumes not on this list, but these are the most common.

Note: Any of these can double as a resistant starch, except for peanuts, which can double as a fat serving.

- Adzuki beans
- Black beans
- Black soybeans
- Black-eyed peas
- Chickpeas
- Edamame
- Great Northern beans
- Green beans
- Kidney beans
- Lentils
- Lima beans
- Mung beans
- Navy beans
- Peanuts
- Peas (green, split, etc.)
- Pink beans
- Pinto beans
- Red beans
- White beans

Nuts and seeds. Serving size: 2 tablespoons to ¼ cup. Unsweetened nut and seed butter is allowed (serving size: 1 to 2 tablespoons). Note the range in serving sizes—have at least the minimum, but no more than the maximum. Your choice may depend on your hunger and your calorie needs.

Note: Any of these can double as a fat serving. Also note that botanically, some of the listed nuts are actually seeds or drupes, but we are going by the common designations.

Nuts:

- Almonds
- Brazil nuts
- Cashews
- Hazelnuts
- Macadamia nuts
- Pecans
- Pine nuts
- Pistachios
- Walnuts

Seeds:

- Chia seeds
- Flaxseeds
- Hemp seeds
- Pumpkin seeds
- Sesame seeds
- Sunflower seeds

Oils/Fats

Remember to include one serving at every meal and every snack.

Oils that are good to consume raw (serving size: 1 to 2 tablespoons):

- Avocado oil
- Extra-virgin olive oil
- Flaxseed oil
- Hemp oil
- Nut oils, raw, cold-pressed (like walnut, almond, hazelnut, or macadamia oil)
- Sesame oil (plain or toasted)

Oils that are good to use for cooking (serving size: 1 to 2 tablespoons):

- Avocado oil
- Coconut oil (and coconut milk and coconut butter)
- "Extra light" olive oil
- Ghee (clarified butter)
- Grapeseed oil
- Macadamia nut oil
- Peanut oil
- Safflower oil
- Sesame oil

Coconut products:

- Coconut milk, canned (serving size: ½ cup)
- Coconut oil (serving size: 1 to 2 tablespoons)
- Coconut "butter" (serving size: 1 to 2 tablespoons)

Fat-rich foods that can double as both a fat and a protein:

- Eggs, whole (serving size: 2 eggs)
- Fatty fish (serving size: 4 to 6 ounces)
- Nuts, seeds, and peanuts (serving size: 2 tablespoons to ¼ cup—see Nuts list)
- Nut and seed butters and peanut butter, all types (serving size: 1 to 2 tablespoons)
- Tempeh and tofu (serving size: 4 ounces)

Resistant Starch Foods

Remember to include three portions per day for omnivores, or six portions per day for people who do not eat animal products, with a minimum of two servings comprised of legumes for vegetarians and vegans—soy products count as legumes.

Note: All legumes can also count as a protein serving. Also note: The box on page 100 contains more information about how to maximize the resistant starch content in legumes and starchy vegetables.

- Bananas, on the unripe side—as they ripen, their resistant starch gradually turns to sugar, so try to get the greenish ones (serving size: 1 small or ½ large)
- Barley, whole grain (serving size: ½ cup cooked)
- Corn, whole grain—not corn by-products like corn oil or corn syrup (serving size: ½ cup whole-grain cornmeal, 4 ounces cooked polenta, or 1 cup cooked fresh corn)
- Legumes, all types, fresh, such as edamame, lima beans, or green beans (serving size: 1 cup); or legumes, dried, soaked, and cooked or canned (serving size: ½ cup). Note that one serving of legumes can do double duty as a resistant starch and a protein.
- Oats, 100% whole grain "old-fashioned" or steel-cut (serving size: ½ cup measured before cooking)
- Potatoes, all kinds, including sweet potatoes and yams (serving size: about ½ cup, or 6 ounces, cooked and mashed)
- Rice, 100% whole grain only (serving size: ½ cup cooked)
- Other grains that have varying levels of resistant starch as well as fiber and many other health properties.[187] Only choose products made with these grains if they are 100% whole grain without any "white flour" or refined flour (serving size: 2 ounces of a bread product, or of a pasta weighed before cooking):
    - Multi-grain products, if 100% whole grain only
    - Sprouted grain products, if 100% whole grain only
    - Amaranth
    - Barley
    - Millet
    - Quinoa
    - Rye
    - Spelt
    - Wheat
    - Winter squashes, all types (serving size: ½ cup cooked)

How to Maximize Your Resistant Starches

When certain foods such as potatoes, rice, and pasta are cooked and then cooled, they undergo a process called starch retrogradation, which means the starches form a different structure when heated, and yet another structure when subsequently cooled. This heated-then-cooled-starch structure makes the starch even more resistant to digestion, so that it passes through the small intestine and feeds the microbes in the large intestine, becoming an even more available prebiotic. When practical, take advantage of this phenomenon by making batches of potatoes, sweet potatoes, oatmeal, brown rice, and whole-grain pasta, then storing them in the refrigerator and eating them throughout the week. (Reheating these foods does not reduce the resistant starch content and may even increase it more.)

Cruciferous Vegetables

Remember to have at least 1 cup per day, no maximum. If you cook these, measure before cooking—the 1 cup requirement is for the vegetables in their raw state.

All types, including:

- Arugula
- Bok choy
- Broccoli
- Broccoli rabe
- Broccoli sprouts
- Brussels sprouts
- Cabbage
- Cauliflower
- Chinese broccoli
- Chinese cabbage
- Collard greens
- Daikon
- Kale
- Kohlrabi
- Maca
- Mizuna
- Mustard greens
- Napa cabbage
- Radishes
- Rutabaga
- Tatsoi
- Turnip greens
- Turnips
- Watercress

Other Mycobiome-Friendly (MF) Vegetables

Remember to have at least 2 cups of these per day, measured in their raw state, so measure before cooking—no maximum.

- Artichokes
- Asparagus
- Beet greens
- Celery

- Chicory
- Chives
- Cucumber
- Dandelion greens
- Eggplant
- Endive
- Garlic
- Grape leaves
- Leeks
- Lettuces, all types
- Mushrooms, all types
- Onions
- Parsley
- Parsnip
- Peppers, all types (sweet and hot)
- Purslane
- Radicchio
- Scallions/green onions
- Shallots
- Sorrel
- Spinach
- Swiss chard
- Tomatoes

Berries

Remember to have at least 1 cup three times per week, or up to 1 cup daily—you may also substitute an additional cup of berries three times per week if you cannot drink green tea.

- Acai berries
- Black raspberries
- Blackberries
- Blueberries
- Boysenberries
- Cranberries
- Elderberries
- Goji berries (if they are dried, use ¼ cup)
- Gooseberries
- Huckleberries
- Lingonberries
- Mulberries
- Raspberries
- Strawberries

Fermented Foods

Remember to have between one and three servings per week—serving size is ½ cup unless otherwise indicated below.

- Beet kvass
- Kefir
- Kimchi (serving size: ¼ cup)
- Kombucha
- Miso soup
- Pickled vegetables (lacto-fermented)
- Pickles (lacto-fermented, such as Bubbies brand—not conventional vinegar pickles)
- Sauerkraut (serving size ¼ cup)
- Tempeh (serving size 4 ounces—this doubles as a protein)

- Yogurt (unsweetened only, nonfat dairy-based, or plant-based such as almond or coconut; serving size: 6 ounces—this doubles as a protein)

Herbs and Spices

Although this is not a required group, herbs and spices make food more interesting and flavorful. Many also contain potent antioxidants and other phytochemicals like polyphenols that have great microbiome benefits. Add any of these to the foods you prepare and enjoy!

- Black pepper
- Cayenne pepper
- Herbs, dried and fresh, all
- Sea salt
- Seasoning mixes without additives or sugar (containing only natural herbs and/or spices)
- Spices, dried and fresh, all

Beverages

Serving size: 1 cup.

- Coffee, organic
- Herbal tea, all types
- Kefir, lassi, or other yogurt drinks, unsweetened only
- Kombucha (naturally fermented, no sugar added after fermentation)
- Milk, low-fat or nonfat only
- Nut, coconut, or grain milk, unsweetened only
- Sparkling water, unsweetened
- Tea, all types (black, green, white, oolong, etc.)
- Water with fresh fruit added (lemon, lime, berries, etc.), unsweetened
- Water, preferably purified or spring water
- Wine, beer, and other alcoholic drinks, unsweetened only, no more than one serving three times per week

THE MYCOBIOME DIET SAMPLE MEAL PLAN

There are many ways to do the Mycobiome Diet, because the only requirements are to eat the foods on the food list in the amounts and frequency specified. However, some people like a little more direction, or want to lean in gradually as they adjust to a new way of eating. For these reasons, I have provided a plan for you.

This plan has two steps. First, begin with the seven-day meal plan. This plan requires only basic cooking—nothing too complicated—and uses only simple recipes that can be easily explained within the plan's grid format. This is the plan we used in our Mycobiome Diet trial. It will help you get used to how the Mycobiome Diet works, because it includes all the necessary elements, like protein, oil/fat, and resistant starch at each meal, as well as the daily elements and the foods you need at least three times per week. It's all included and mapped out for you.

This plan will also help you ease in to the diet. If you aren't currently eating a lot of vegetables, fiber, or resistant starch, you may notice gas and bloating at the beginning of this diet. If you tend to eat more fat and meat (such as on a low-carb diet), your microbiome is likely populated by bile-tolerant microbes that help you to digest this kind of diet. These microbes also tend to be inflammatory. The anti-inflammatory microbes associated with normal weight and good health are the types that digest fiber and resistant starch, so you need to cultivate those by feeding them. That is what you will be doing on this diet. Just know that at first, when you don't have many of these mircobes, you might feel a little uncomfortable. Rest assured that this will pass. Ease into the fiber-rich foods and be sure to chew all plant foods thoroughly. For more information about other ways to help you ease into the Mycobiome Diet, especially if you are having some symptons of digestive distress, see the Carley's Corner boxes in Chapter 9.

You will start to feel much better as you integrate these gut-friendly foods into your diet and encourage healthy microbiome balance by keeping pathogenic fungi like *Candida* under control, nourishing the bacteria that help with this control, and dissolving biofilms that are harboring pathogenic bacteria. You may begin losing extra weight you've been carrying, and you may notice that some of your chronic symptoms (such as digestive issues) begin to resolve. Although this seven-day plan includes all your requirements, track these on the food tracker charts (see pages 92–93) so you can get in the habit of including all of these necessary and microbiome-friendly elements.

You can do this plan once, twice, three times, or more, but at some point, once you have all the elements down, you can "graduate" to step two, the 20-day plan.

The step two plan takes you through three meals and one snack per day based on the recipes starting on page 149. This plan is a bit looser. It allows for more customization. Because not every recipe contains all of your per-meal requirements, I cue you about what nutritional components you need to add to each meal (such as a protein, an oil/fat, or a resistant starch), so you can get in all your requirements. But I leave it up to you which specific ingredients you want to add. For example, if you need to add a protein to a meal, you might decide on some salmon, some baked tofu, or two eggs. If you need to add a resistant starch, you might go for some potatoes, lentils, or quinoa. If you need to add an oil/fat, you may prefer to use extra-virgin olive oil, coconut oil, or some walnuts. The more you start choosing from these categories on your own, the more comfortable you will get with this style of eating. This is training for eating for the rest of your life in a way that nourishes and nurtures a healthy and robust microbiome.

The 20-day plan also includes reminders for green tea (be sure to get three cups in per week) and the other daily requirements, but you will probably want to continue to track your requirements in the food tracker until those microbiome-friendly foods become second nature.

You can continue to do the 20-day plan more than once, or you can mix-and-match it with the 7-day plan, or you can begin incorporating your own favorites into the rotation. By this point, you should be feeling great! You will be in the habit of eating what best fuels your beneficial microbes and controls your pathogenic microbes. Although you can loosen the reins a bit once you feel good, your weight has stabilized, and your symptoms have abated, stick with the basic concepts of the Mycobiome Diet for life:

- A protein, oil/fat, and resistant starch at every meal.
- A variety of vegetables every day.
- Frequent consumption of seafood, berries, fermented foods, green tea, apple cider vinegar, pistachios and walnuts, garlic, and turmeric.
- Avoid processed foods, refined sweeteners, refined grains, cured meat, and high-fat meat (except for fatty fish).
- Moderate, at most, alcohol consumption.

Make these guidelines a part of your everyday life and your microbiome will thrive. So will you. And remember: Everything you do for your microbiome includes better mycobiome control. Keep those fungi working for you, not against you!

Finally, if you already feel comfortable with the food lists and you don't like following specific plans, that's fine, too. You can also ignore the plans completely and do it your own way from the beginning. These plans are here for guidance and inspiration, but what really matters is that you stick to the approved foods, omit the excluded foods, and follow the other guidelines I've already described. Keep those food lists handy!

THE SEVEN-DAY MYCOBIOME DIET MEAL PLANNER

This is the plan our test subjects used as we tested the effects of the Mycobiome Diet. It is not different than the 20-day plan in terms of effect, but the foods are simpler to prepare, and it includes a variety of foods with all of the necessary Mycobiome Diet requirements. This keeps track of everything for you. You can do it once, or as many times as you like, as you get comfortable with your new style of eating.

Note that there are plant-based options for all animal products, and gluten-free or grain-free options for all grain products. These varations are meant to accommodate various eating styles, preferences, or requirements.

As a reminder, you may always use any seasoning on the food list, including sea salt, pepper, and all natural unsweetened herbs and spices.

This meal plan generally serves one, but you can easily double anything to serve two, or to save a second portion for another meal.

DAY 1	
BREAKFAST	Omelet made with 2 eggs (or 4 ounces of scrambled tofu) mixed with about ½ cup each spinach, mushrooms, and onions (or to taste), sprinkled with 1 tablespoon nonfat feta cheese (optional) or 1 tablespoon nutritional yeast 1 slice 100% whole-grain toast topped with 1 tablespoon olive oil (or 4 ounces potatoes, shredded and sautéed in oil) 1 cup green tea (or 1 cup berries)
LUNCH	Big salad with vegetables (choose from all vegetable lists), protein (salmon, shrimp, chicken, beans, tofu, etc.—if using an animal protein, add ½ to 1 cup of any approved grain, legume, or starchy vegetable) dressed with 1 tablespoon extra virgin olive oil and unlimited apple cider vinegar
SNACK	½ cup hummus with raw carrots and broccoli florets 1 cup kombucha

DINNER	Black bean soup: To make two servings, warm up one can drained, rinsed black beans, 2 cloves fresh garlic minced, 1 chopped white onion, 1 can diced tomatoes (or 2 fresh chopped tomatoes), 1 teaspoon cumin, ½ teaspoon turmeric, and ¼ cup chopped fresh cilantro or parsley. Add salt and pepper to taste. Puree if desired, or puree half for a creamy-chunky soup. Top with avocado cubes or a dollop of low-fat yogurt and a sprinkle of cumin. Roasted blue or purple potatoes drizzled with 1 teaspoon extra-virgin olive oil or warm coconut oil 2 cups broccoli mixed with 1 minced garlic clove and 1 teaspoon minced ginger sautéed in 2 teaspoons toasted sesame oil
EVENING	Lemon, berry, or any other herbal tea
DAY 2	
BREAKFAST	1 cup berries and 1 sliced banana (on the unripe side), mixed with ½ cup plain nonfat yogurt (such as Greek yogurt—dairy or plant-based) or cottage cheese and ¼ cup pistachios 1 cup black coffee or any tea
LUNCH	Big salad with vegetables (choose from all vegetable lists), protein (salmon, shrimp, chicken, beans, tofu, etc.—if using an animal protein, add ½ to 1 cup of any approved grain, legume, or starchy vegetable) dressed with 1 tablespoon extra virgin olive oil and unlimited apple cider vinegar
SNACK	Leftover black bean soup with a tablespoon of nonfat Greek yogurt (dairy or plant-based)
DINNER	4 to 6 ounces roasted turkey breast (or baked tempeh drizzled with soy sauce) 1 cup mashed sweet potatoes (or from 1 sweet potato) 1 to 2 cups cabbage sautéed in coconut oil or warmed sauerkraut
EVENING	1 mug of Golden Milk (use the recipe on page 255 or look for premixed powder in the health food store) or turmeric tea
DAY 3	
BREAKFAST	Smoothie with 2 cups berries, ½ cup silken tofu, juice of ½ lemon, plus ½ cup ice and enough additional water to make it pourable (start with ¼ cup) 1 ounce 100% whole-grain crackers or 4 ounces leftover mashed sweet potatoes 1 cup green tea (or 1 additional cup berries)
LUNCH	Big salad with vegetables (choose from all vegetable lists), protein (salmon, shrimp, chicken, beans, tofu, etc.—if using an animal protein, add ½ to 1 cup of any approved grain, legume, or starchy vegetable) dressed with 1 tablespoon extra virgin olive oil and unlimited apple cider vinegar
SNACK	¼ cup walnuts and ½ cup red grapes
DINNER	Plantain "nachos": 1 cup thinly sliced green plantain fried in 1 tablespoon coconut oil or ghee until golden brown and crispy, topped with ½ cup pinto beans, ¼ avocado cubed (or ¼ cup freshly made guacamole), ¼ cup tomato salsa (add 1 clove fresh garlic, minced), 1 cup finely shredded cabbage, and 1 chopped green onion
EVENING	Lemon, berry, or any other herbal tea

DAY 4	
BREAKFAST	Chia seed or flaxseed pudding made by soaking overnight: ½ cup soy or nut milk, ½ cup pumpkin or butternut squash puree, and ¼ cup chia seeds or ground flaxseeds; top with ½ cup berries and dashes of cinnamon and turmeric 1 slice 100% whole-grain toast topped with 1 tablespoon olive oil or 4 ounces potatoes shredded and cooked in olive oil 1 cup black coffee or any tea
LUNCH	Big salad with vegetables (choose from all vegetable lists), protein (salmon, shrimp, chicken, beans, tofu, etc.—if using an animal protein, add ½ to 1 cup of any approved grain, legume, or starchy vegetable) dressed with 1 tablespoon extra virgin olive oil and unlimited apple cider vinegar
SNACK	1 large tomato sliced with basil leaves and 2 ounces of thinly sliced fresh mozzarella (if you don't eat cheese, substitute ¼ cup walnuts)
DINNER	6 ounces steamed fish (or tofu marinated in soy sauce and sesame oil) with fresh lemon juice Steamed asparagus, unlimited Bok choy (unlimited) sautéed in 1 tablespoon coconut oil or sesame oil ½ cup cooked brown basmati or jasmine rice, or 4 ounces of any kind of roasted potatoes
EVENING	1 mug of Golden Milk (use the recipe on page 255 or look for premixed powder in the health food store) or turmeric tea
DAY 5	
BREAKFAST	Smoothie made with 1 cup kefir or yogurt (dairy or plant-based), 1 banana (on the unripe side), 1 cup baby kale leaves, 2 tablespoons almond or any nut butter, and 1 teaspoon ground or fresh minced ginger, ½ cup of ice, plus enough water to make it pourable (start with ¼ cup) 1 cup green tea (or 1 cup berries)
LUNCH	Big salad with vegetables (choose from all vegetable lists), protein (salmon, shrimp, chicken, beans, tofu, etc.—if using an animal protein, add ½ to 1 cup of any approved grain, legume, or starchy vegetable) dressed with 1 tablespoon extra virgin olive oil and unlimited apple cider vinegar
SNACK	½ cup hummus with raw carrots and broccoli florets 1 cup kombucha
DINNER	6 ounces steamed shrimp (or steamed edamame) Coleslaw made from 1 cup chopped cabbage, ½ cup shaved Brussels sprouts, 1 grated carrot, 1 minced green onion, 1 minced garlic clove, and ½ cup nonfat plain yogurt (dairy or plant-based) ½ cup whole-grain thin rice noodles
EVENING	Lemon, berry, or any other herbal tea

DAY 6	
BREAKFAST	2 scrambled eggs or 4 ounces scrambled tofu cooked in any oil approved for cooking, with fresh asparagus mixed in or on the side ½ cup oats, cooked according to package directions, or 1 banana (on the unripe side) 1 cup black coffee or any tea
LUNCH	Big salad with vegetables (choose from all vegetable lists), protein (salmon, shrimp, chicken, beans, tofu, etc.—if using an animal protein, add ½ to 1 cup of any approved grain, legume, or starchy vegetable) dressed with 1 tablespoon extra virgin olive oil and unlimited apple cider vinegar
SNACK	Celery with nut butter, ¼ cup pistachios (or just use pistachio butter on the celery)
DINNER	Minestrone soup: To make two servings, sauté 1 chopped onion, 1 clove minced garlic, 1 stalk celery (chopped), and 1 carrot (thinly sliced) in 1 tablespoon olive oil. Add 1 can diced tomatoes, 1 can drained rinsed white beans, ½ cup cubed zucchini, a handful of fresh chopped basil, and 2 cups vegetable broth. Simmer until all the vegetables are soft. Top with a few cubes of toasted sprouted grain bread and sprinkle with a tablespoon of nonfat Parmesan or nondairy "Parmesan" (optional).
EVENING	1 mug of Golden Milk (use the recipe on page 255 or look for premixed powder in the health food store) or turmeric tea

DAY 7	
BREAKFAST	Smoothie with ½ cup mango, ½ cup pineapple, 1 banana (on the unripe side), 1 cup romaine lettuce leaves, ¼ cup wheat germ or raw whole-grain oats, 2 tablespoons flaxseeds or chia seeds, 1 tablespoon fresh lemon juice, ½ cup ice, plus enough water to make it pourable (start with ¼ cup) 1 cup green tea (or 1 cup berries)
LUNCH	Big salad with vegetables (choose from all vegetable lists), protein (salmon, shrimp, chicken, beans, tofu, etc.—if using an animal protein, add ½ to 1 cup of any approved grain, legume, or starchy vegetable) dressed with 1 tablespoon extra virgin olive oil and unlimited apple cider vinegar
SNACK	1 cup leftover minestrone soup
DINNER	4 to 6 ounces roast chicken (or baked tempeh drizzled with soy sauce and a bit of sesame oil) 1 cup mashed potatoes made with ½ to 1 tablespoon coconut oil or olive oil and mixed with ¼ cup chopped steamed spinach Small salad with watercress and sliced radishes, with ½ to 1 tablespoon olive oil, 1 tablespoon apple cider vinegar, and 1 clove minced garlic as a dressing
EVENING	Lemon, berry, or any other herbal tea

THE 20-DAY MYCOBIOME DIET PLANNER

You can find recipes for all these meals (other than the every-other-day big salad for lunch) starting on page 149. To help you get used to choosing these items for yourself, I have let you know what ingredients you need to add as a protein, oil/fat, or resistant starch in addition to the recipe, but you can pick anything you want from the food lists. For example, in the first recipe, the Cacao Oatmeal Bowls, you need to add a protein to complete your meal. You could add two scrambled eggs, a slice of baked tofu, leftover seafood or poultry from a previous meal, or you could stir some peanut butter into your oatmeal. You have more choices than you did during the 7-day plan, which will give you more independence and freedom as you get more skilled at balancing your meals to make them optimally microbiome-friendly.

A few additional things to note:

- For every breakfast, you can add one of your cups of green tea (or a cup of berries, if you can't have green tea), and/or a cup of black coffee or black tea. If you want to add some unsweetened low-fat milk or unsweetened almond or other plant milk to your coffee or tea, that's fine, too. Just be sure to get in your minimum 3 cups of green tea per week. See my note about coffee and black tea on page 88. I have placed reminders with each breakfast.
- For the days when you have a big salad for lunch, remember that you can use this meal to get in all your required daily vegetables, if you choose.
- You can have an optional glass of wine up to three times per week, with dinner.
- Every evening, you can choose to have an optional cup of herbal tea (ginger, peppermint, chamomile, etc.) or a cup of Golden Milk (recipe on page 255) or turmeric tea to get in your turmeric requirement. These are not included in the 20-day meal planner because they are optional.
- For plant-based eaters, every recipe that contains animal products includes a plant-based option.
- For gluten-free or grain-free eaters, every recipe that contains gluten or grain includes a gluten-free or grain-free option.
- Unlike the 7-day plan, this meal planner does not dole out your daily and 3×/week foods, so it's up to you to keep track of getting your:

- Daily cruciferous vegetable serving and mycobiome-friendly (MF) vegetable serving (the every-other-day lunch salad is a good place to get these in)
- Daily apple cider vinegar serving
- 3×/week fish/seafood servings
- 3×/week berry servings
- 3×/week fermented food servings
- 3×/week pistachios/walnut servings
- 3×/week green tea servings (or 1 cup berry serving)
- 3×/week turmeric servings
- 3×/week garlic servings

DAY 1	
BREAKFAST	Cacao Oatmeal Bowls (page 154) Add a protein Green tea, coffee, black tea, or cup of berries
LUNCH	Avocado and Green Tomato Salad (page 180) Add a protein Add a resistant starch
SNACK	Beet Hummus (page 262)
DINNER	Pistachio-Crusted Salmon with Asparagus (page 220) Add a resistant starch
DAY 2	
BREAKFAST	Egg Breakfast Cups (page 160) Add a resistant starch Green tea, coffee, black tea, or cup of berries
LUNCH	Big salad with vegetables, protein (salmon, shrimp, chicken, beans, tofu, etc.—if using an animal protein, add ½ to 1 cup of any approved grain, legume, or starchy vegetable) dressed with 1 tablespoon extra virgin olive oil and unlimited apple cider vinegar
SNACK	Blueberry Smoothie (page 253) Add a protein if using almond or coconut milk Add an oil/fat if *not* using coconut milk
DINNER	Cauliflower Steak Salad (page 209) Add a protein Add a resistant starch

DAY 3	
BREAKFAST	Cinnamon Apple Cranberry Quinoa Bowl (page 159) Add a protein Green tea, coffee, black tea, or cup of berries
LUNCH	Chicken Quinoa Soup (page 185)
SNACK	Roasted Curried Cauliflower (page 266) Add a protein
DINNER	Creamy Whole Wheat Pasta with Spinach (page 217) Add a protein
DAY 4	
BREAKFAST	Fresh Fig Yogurt Cups (page 165) Add a resistant starch Green tea, coffee, black tea, or cup of berries
LUNCH	Big salad with vegetables, protein (salmon, shrimp, chicken, beans, tofu, etc.—if using an animal protein, add ½ to 1 cup of any approved grain, legume, or starchy vegetable) dressed with 1 tablespoon extra virgin olive oil and unlimited apple cider vinegar
SNACK	Cantaloupe Ginger Granita (page 254) Add a protein Add an oil/fat
DINNER	Broccolini, Potato, and Mushroom Sauté (page 204) Add a protein
DAY 5	
BREAKFAST	Strawberry Breakfast Bake (page 173) Green tea, coffee, black tea, or cup of berries
LUNCH	Heritage Carrot Salad (page 191) Add a protein Add a resistant sftarch
SNACK	Sesame Almonds (page 265)
DINNER	Chicken and Potatoes with Rosemary (page 212)
DAY 6	
BREAKFAST	Golden Milk Yogurt Parfaits (page 166) Add a resistant starch Green tea, coffee, black tea, or cup of berries
LUNCH	Big salad with vegetables, protein (salmon, shrimp, chicken, beans, tofu, etc.—if using an animal protein, add ½ to 1 cup of any approved grain, legume, or starchy vegetable) dressed with 1 tablespoon extra virgin olive oil and unlimited apple cider vinegar
SNACK	Green Goddess Smoothie (page 257)
DINNER	Poke Bowl with Creamy Cilantro Dressing (page 223)

DAY 7	
BREAKFAST	Sweet Potato Hash and Fried Eggs (page 174)
LUNCH	Luscious Legume Salad (page 195) Add an oil/fat
SNACK	Seasoned Roasted Carrots (page 269) Add a protein
DINNER	Chicken and Vegetable Teriyaki (page 215)

DAY 8	
BREAKFAST	Roasted Strawberry Yogurt Cup with Pistachios (page 170) Add a resistant starch Green tea, coffee, black tea, or cup of berries
LUNCH	Big salad with vegetables, protein (salmon, shrimp, chicken, beans, tofu, etc.—if using an animal protein, add ½ to 1 cup of any approved grain, legume, or starchy vegetable) dressed with 1 tablespoon extra virgin olive oil and unlimited apple cider vinegar
SNACK	Tropical Mango Smoothie (page 258) Add a protein if using almond or coconut yogurt
DINNER	Grilled Veggie Dinner (page 219) Add a protein Add a resistant starch

DAY 9	
BREAKFAST	Sweet Potato "Toast" (page 177) Green tea, coffee, black tea, or cup of berries
LUNCH	Summer Salad (page 198) Add a resistant starch
SNACK	Spinach Mashed Potatoes (page 271) Add a protein
DINNER	Scallops with Pea Puree (page 226)

DAY 10	
BREAKFAST	Pomegranate Breakfast Panna Cotta (page 169) Add a resistant starch Green tea, coffee, black tea, or cup of berries
LUNCH	Big salad with vegetables, protein (salmon, shrimp, chicken, beans, tofu, etc.—if using an animal protein, add ½ to 1 cup of any approved grain, legume, or starchy vegetable) dressed with 1 tablespoon extra virgin olive oil and unlimited apple cider vinegar
SNACK	Very Berry Smoothie (page 261) Add a protein if you are using almond or coconut milk
DINNER	Cauli-Brussels Chicken Tikka Masala (page 207) Add a resistant starch

DAY 11	
BREAKFAST	Cacao Oatmeal Bowls (page 154) Green tea, coffee, black tea, or cup of berries
LUNCH	Broccoli Black Bean Quesadillas (page 183)
SNACK	Beet Hummus (page 262)
DINNER	Sweet Potato Falafel Bowl (page 234)
DAY 12	
BREAKFAST	Egg Breakfast Cups (page 160) Green tea, coffee, black tea, or cup of berries
LUNCH	Big salad with vegetables, protein (salmon, shrimp, chicken, beans, tofu, etc.—if using an animal protein, add ½ to 1 cup of any approved grain, legume, or starchy vegetable) dressed with 1 tablespoon extra virgin olive oil and unlimited apple cider vinegar
SNACK	Blueberry Smoothie (page 253)
DINNER	Spicy Salmon Salad (page 229) Add a resistant starch
DAY 13	
BREAKFAST	Cinnamon Apple Cranberry Quinoa Bowl (page 159)
LUNCH	Chickpea Vegetable Wrap (page 188)
SNACK	Roasted Curried Cauliflower (page 266)
DINNER	Whole Wheat Pasta with Zucchini and Broccolini (page 244)
DAY 14	
BREAKFAST	Fresh Fig Yogurt Cups (page 165) Green tea, coffee, black tea, or cup of berries
LUNCH	Big salad with vegetables, protein (salmon, shrimp, chicken, beans, tofu, etc.—if using an animal protein, add ½ to 1 cup of any approved grain, legume, or starchy vegetable) dressed with 1 tablespoon extra virgin olive oil and unlimited apple cider vinegar
SNACK	Cantaloupe Ginger Granita (page 254)
DINNER	Sweet & Sour Shrimp Bowl (page 230)
DAY 15	
BREAKFAST	Strawberry Breakfast Bake (page 173) Green tea, coffee, black tea, or cup of berries
LUNCH	Hummus Plate (page 192)
SNACK	Sesame Almonds (page 265)
DINNER	Sweet Potato Turkey Boats (page 232)

DAY 16	
BREAKFAST	Golden Milk Yogurt Parfaits (page 166) Green tea, coffee, black tea, or cup of berries
LUNCH	Big salad with vegetables, protein (salmon, shrimp, chicken, beans, tofu, etc.—if using an animal protein, add ½ to 1 cup of any approved grain, legume, or starchy vegetable) dressed with 1 tablespoon extra virgin olive oil and unlimited apple cider vinegar
SNACK	Green Goddess Smoothie (page 257)
DINNER	Zucchini and Corn Pizza (page 248)
DAY 17	
BREAKFAST	Sweet Potato Hash and Fried Eggs (page 174) Green tea, coffee, black tea, or cup of berries
LUNCH	Pea and Radish Salad (page 196) Add a resistant starch Add a protein, or increase the amount of green peas to 1 cup
SNACK	Seasoned Roasted Carrots (page 269)
DINNER	Thai Butternut Squash Soup (page 240) Add a protein
DAY 18	
BREAKFAST	Roasted Strawberry Yogurt Cup with Pistachios (page 170) Green tea, coffee, black tea, or cup of berries
LUNCH	Big salad with vegetables, protein (salmon, shrimp, chicken, beans, tofu, etc.—if using an animal protein, add ½ to 1 cup of any approved grain, legume, or starchy vegetable) dressed with 1 tablespoon extra virgin olive oil and unlimited apple cider vinegar
SNACK	Tropical Mango Smoothie (page 258)
DINNER	Vegetable Chili with Brown Rice (page 243)
DAY 19	
BREAKFAST	Sweet Potato "Toast" (page 177) Green tea, coffee, black tea, or cup of berries
LUNCH	Veggie Buddha Bowl (page 201)
SNACK	Spinach Mashed Potatoes (page 271)
DINNER	Turkey Meatballs with Tzatziki (page 237) Add a resistant starch

DAY 20	
BREAKFAST	Pomegranate Breakfast Panna Cotta (page 169) Green tea, coffee, black tea, or cup of berries
LUNCH	Big salad with vegetables, protein (salmon, shrimp, chicken, beans, tofu, etc.—if using an animal protein, add ½ to 1 cup of any approved grain, legume, or starchy vegetable) dressed with 1 tablespoon extra virgin olive oil and unlimited apple cider vinegar
SNACK	Very Berry Smoothie (page 261)
DINNER	Zucchini "Pasta" with Cherry Tomatoes (page 247) Add a resistant starch

MYCOBIOME DIET FAQS

As you become accustomed to this new way of eating, you will probably have questions. These are the most common questions I receive regarding the Mycobiome Diet. These answers should clarify the most common issues you may be wondering about.

Do I have to follow this exact meal plan?

No. This is just a sample to show you what is possible. As long as you follow all the guidelines, you can organize your meals and snacks in any way you choose.

What if I forget to eat a daily food, or am unable to eat a daily food for some reason?

Life happens! Just get back on track at the next meal. Don't let a mistake derail your progress. What you do most of the time is what will shape your microbiome and your mycobiome.

What if I eat an excluded food?

Again, life happens! Just get back on track for the next meal and try not to make any excluded food a habit. Many of these excluded foods can be hard to resist, so it's a good idea to break your dependence on these microbiome-compromising, *Candida*-encouraging foods.

What do I do if I have to go to a restaurant or I'm a guest at someone's home?

It can be difficult to live your "normal" life on some diet plans, but the Mycobiome Diet is designed to help you live fully without feeling deprived. Most restaurants will have compliant foods. Just ask if grain products are whole grain or not, and avoid all high-fat foods and refined grains and sugar. These days, many people request these kinds of accommodations. A few of the many options include big salads with a lot of veggies and lean meat (especially seafood—try a salmon or shrimp salad). Dress them with olive oil and vinegar, or bring your own favorite compliant dressing. Look for whole-grain pasta with vegetables and lean protein, sandwiches on whole-grain bread, tacos or burritos with lots of veggies and low-fat or no cheese, stir-fries, hearty soups, grilled lean meats, and seafood with sides of whole grains and vegetables. Most restaurants have healthy options that will fit your new lifestyle. For breakfast, you can always get oatmeal with fruit, or omelets with vegetables. When visiting a friend, all you have to do is politely decline any elements that don't fit with your preference, or just briefly mention that you are avoiding refined grains, sugar, and high-fat foods right now. And remember that if you do go off track every now and then, just get back on track again. If you've been following the Mycobiome Diet for a while, your body may object to foods with sugar or a lot of fat, but that's just a friendly reminder to stay on track. (Some of our test subjects in our clinical trial who went off the Mycobiome Diet study over Thanksgiving noticed ill effects that went away again after they went back on the diet.)

I've heard full-fat dairy is good for me. Why can't I have it?

Full-fat dairy products (especially from raw milk) have some health benefits, but when it comes to your microbiome and mycobiome health, they have an effect that is more negative than positive. All high-fat animal products encourage the growth of bacteria that are more inflammatory. However, since the protein and carbohydrates in dairy products have a positive microbiome effect in moderation, I advise eating only nonfat or low-fat dairy products with no more than 1% milk fat.

How do I include a fat source at every meal?

This should be easy to do. Just add olive oil or another approved oil listed to a vegetable, have some nut butter with a fruit or vegetable, or eat a food that naturally contains fat, like eggs or fatty fish. Do not use any fat source that is not on the oils/fats food list. I have specifically chosen only anti-inflammatory fat sources.

How do I put protein in every meal?

Protein comes in many forms (see the protein food list) so it should be easy to add some to every meal and snack, whether that means including some fish or other seafood, eggs, nonfat or low-fat dairy (like yogurt), poultry, or any vegetarian source of protein such as edamame, tofu, tempeh, unsweetened soy milk, plain soy yogurt, nuts or seeds, or nut or seed butters. Note that nuts and seeds are listed as approved proteins, and nut milks and nut-milk-based yogurts such as almond milk are fine to eat if they are unsweetened. However, nut-milk-based products are not good sources of protein. Soy milk and soy yogurt are, but almond milk and almond yogurt are not because the nut protein is too diluted.

Can one single food be both my protein and my fat, or protein and resistant starch?

Yes. Nuts, seeds, nut and seed butters, fatty fish, eggs, and tofu can all count as both a protein and a fat. Legumes count as both a protein and a resistant starch. These double-duty foods are marked in the food lists.

Why do I have to spread out my resistant starch servings over the day? Can't I have them all at once, like at dinner?

It is important, in order *not* to encourage the growth of harmful fungi (particularly *Candida*), to eat all starchy or higher-carbohydrate foods in small amounts throughout the day. This feeds the microbiome with prebiotics without overfeeding *Candida.*

How do I know what to put in my lunch salad?

I like to recommend having a big salad for lunch approximately every other day (or even every day), because this is an excellent opportunity to throw every required item in that you may miss at other meals. Start with 2 cups of leafy greens/lettuce and you have already met your mycobiome-friendly (MF) vegetable requirement for the day. Add other required vegetables, protein, olive oil, and apple cider vinegar, and you have checked off most of your boxes. Of course, you can also add anything else you like, if it is not on the excluded list. Fulfilling requirements at lunch allows more freedom at other meals. It's also an excellent opportunity to feed your microbiome in the middle of your busy day.

Can I have coffee?

Yes. There are some studies that have shown microbiome benefits from coffee. However, if you are able, choose organic coffee and be sure you also get your green tea for the day. Coffee is not a replacement for green tea. I talk more about this on page 88.

What other beverages can I have on this diet?

The only allowed beverages are water, coffee (unsweetened), tea (unsweetened, any type including herbal), nonfat or low-fat milk or nondairy milk (unsweetened), unsweetened kefir, yogurt drinks, lassi, and optional small amounts of alcohol as specified in the guidelines at the beginning of this chapter.

Can I be vegetarian or vegan and still follow this diet?

Yes. There are always plant-based options for every animal product.

Can I be gluten-free or grain-free and still follow this diet?

Yes, there are always gluten-free and grain-free options for every gluten-containing or grain-based product.

What do I do when I'm done with the Mycobiome Diet?

The purpose of the Mycobiome Diet is not to "go on" and then "go off" with some final destination in mind. This is training for a new way of eating that you can carry forward with you for the rest of your life. Your microbiome constantly shifts in response to what you eat, so if you keep eating to feed your beneficial microbes, you will continue to get healthier and stay that way for years to come.

Living a Fungi-Friendly Lifestyle

Eating for all parts of your microbiome is the best way to achieve better health, but there is some compelling research to show that other aspects of your life, from the environment you live in to sleep to stress to exercise, can significantly impact all the microbes in your gut. The pressures and stresses of our complex modern lives, not to mention the chemical pollutants we encounter and the degradation of our natural environments, may be the reason why so many people are now afflicted with chronic conditions like obesity,[188] inflammation and related gastrointestinal disorders like inflammatory bowel disease (IBD),[189] type 2 diabetes,[190] cancer,[191] and heart disease.[192] While genetics is certainly part of this equation, and diet is another big one of course, research continues to demonstrate the important role environmental and lifestyle factors[193] play on chronic diseases. Because so many of these diseases are also linked to dysbiosis in the microbiome, it makes sense to look at the big picture—environment, health issues, and the microbiome—to determine what you can do to make your environment and lifestyle habits work for you instead of against you.

This chapter takes a closer look at how you live your life. You can undermine the hard work you are doing to refurbish your gut health if you live a lifestyle that has a negative influence on microbial balance. Are your habits encouraging *Candida* overgrowth? Are you making life difficult for fungi-suppressing beneficial bacteria? Do that unused gym membership, that occasional cigarette, those sleepless nights encourage harmful biofilms and the proliferation of pathogenic microbes within? Let's find out by dipping into the world of lifestyle medicine to discover how fungi and bacteria may or may not be involved.[194]

EXERCISE BETTER

Every weekday morning I get up at 5 a.m. I start my day by feeding our dog Pixie, and then I go down to the basement to do my daily exercise. Pixie is a 10-year-old Pomeranian who refuses to walk after just a short while and demands to be carried. My dog walking days are therefore over. He obviously does not get very much exercise. I love this little dog very much, so I analyzed his microbiome and compared it with my daughter's dog, who never stops moving. I was not surprised to see that poor Pixie had elevated Proteobacteria, which is associated with inflammation. He also had high Firmicutes, which is not desirable either. By contrast, Shadow, my daughter's dog, had a well-balanced microbiome.

Despite Pixie's sedentary ways, I still make an effort to get moving without him. My exercise routine involves stretching, different elements of the yoga sun salutation (this takes about 15 minutes), then aerobic exercise on my elliptical trainer. I used to listen to the news while I did this, but that got too depressing (which is bad for the microbiome, as you will soon see), so now I watch old reruns of *I Love Lucy*. This provides me with a good workout and I start my day smiling and ready to go. (Good moods boost good microbes, because of the gut-brain connection.)

To get a little more exercise during the day, some years ago I started to take the stairs whenever I had to go up to my lab. Also, I have two labs—one for basic science at the School of Medicine at Case Western Reserve University, and a clinical lab at University Hospitals Cleveland Medical Center. These are in two different buildings, so I usually do about an hour and a half in the clinical lab, then walk over to my team at the science lab. This lab is on the fifth floor, and I take the stairs!

Earlier this year, I bought a standing desk, and although I'm not sure how many of the health claims these companies advertise are supported by research, I do know that it makes me feel good to spend my day moving all the time—sitting down, getting back up, standing, walking, and stair-climbing.

Why do I do all of this? The research is pretty clear that exercise has profound microbiome benefits as well as other benefits that are likely directly or peripherally related to microbiome health. Studies show that regular physical activity can treat multiple conditions that are inflammatory in nature.[195] People with type 2 diabetes, coronary artery disease, peripheral arterial disease, and obesity all show improvements in their immunological profiles when they start exercising regularly. In one study, when people with type 2 diabetes began doing both aerobic and resistance training (like weight lifting), they showed a decrease in the production of pro-inflammatory cytokines and an increase in anti-inflammatory cytokines.[196] Furthermore, moderate exercise has been shown to mitigate the effects of stress-induced intestinal barrier dysfunction—it is associated with the preservation of mucosal thickness, less intestinal permeability, and lower rates of bacterial translocation (as happens in "leaky gut syndrome").[197] Even a daily walk has some pretty potent microbiome-boosting power.

Interestingly, however, more is not better. Whereas moderate exercise has many positive effects, strenuous exercise can have negative effects on intestinal function. During extreme exercise, blood gets diverted away from the gastrointestinal system and goes where it is most urgently needed—to the heart, lungs, and muscles.[198] When this goes on for too long, homeostasis in the gut gets disrupted and intestinal cells called enterocytes can actually experience damage. Extreme endurance sports have an even more extreme effect and can lead to intestinal ischemia, which means the intestines are starved of blood, resulting in abdominal cramping and severe diarrhea.

I generally recommend what the American Heart Association as well as the US government's Physical Activity Guidelines for Americans recommend when it comes to exercise: a minimum of 150 minutes of moderate exercise every week. That translates to 30 minutes a day for 5 days, but you could exercise for shorter periods every day or for longer periods on fewer days. Just aim for those 150 minutes and you will be benefiting your microbiome and reducing your inflammation.[199] (By the way, the guidelines also state that children and adolescents ages 6 through 17 should be getting a full hour of moderate to vigorous physical activity *every day!* Get off the couch, kids!)

If you aren't in the habit yet, I understand—it can be hard to get motivated. When I am tempted to stay in bed, I try to talk myself into exercising by remembering how good it makes me feel. I tell myself I can sleep longer over the weekend. I would say this works 90% of the time. If you don't exercise 10 to 20% of the time, that's fine. Just try to compensate for it by moving more that day. The nice thing about a weekly exercise recommendation rather than a daily one is that you can skip a day or two and still get all your minutes in by the end of the week. Having an exercise buddy can also make you more accountable. Whatever it is that helps you get it done—exercising in the morning like I do, in the afternoon, after work, or even at night—that is the plan for you.

The Mycobiome Diet Exercise Recommendation

Engage in a minimum of 150 minutes of moderate exercise per week, including aerobic exercise, strength training, and some stretching.

SLEEP MORE (OR LESS)

According to the National Sleep Foundation, adults need 7 to 9 hours of sleep per night, although some people may be fine with 6 hours and a few may need 10 hours. They do not recommend that any adult sleep for less than 6 hours per night, or for more than 11 hours. They also advise that children and adolescents need slightly more sleep than adults, and that adults 65 years and older may need slightly less.[200]

I know many people who do not sleep well, and I know that aging is often associated with reduction in sleep length and quality. I'm not a young man anymore but, personally, I generally sleep pretty well. Sometimes I wake up in the middle of the night and start worrying about my grandchildren, or about work, or getting my grants funded and supporting the people who work in my lab. I always seem to be well-funded, but I worry about the future. The mind is a funny thing.

Sleep is another lifestyle element that is well known to directly impact the microbiome, and many studies have shown a link between sleep disruption and deprivation with microbial dysbiosis. In the study I referred to above, we asked participants about their sleep patterns—specifically, we asked them how many hours they slept each night. Nearly one third of the participants did not get enough sleep (seven to nine hours per night).

Many studies have demonstrated how sleep affects the body. So what happens when you don't get enough sleep, or you wake up frequently, or you sleep at irregular hours? Microbiome dysfunction happens. One study looked at how fragmented sleep affected mice. For four weeks, they disrupted the sleep of the mice, then allowed them to recover for two weeks. Sleep fragmentation changed their feeding behaviors, and the mice became more likely to become obese and develop insulin resistance—both conditions we know are related to the gut microbiome. These mice had increased levels of more pathogenic microbes and decreased levels of more favorable microbes, which led to inflammation in their visceral body fat (the more dangerous kind of inflammation, because this fat is stored deep inside around your vital organs). There is no doubt that sleep deprivation can increase your fat stores, your inflammation levels, your intestinal permeability, and your sensitivity to insulin,[201] putting you at greater risk for developing diabetes.

To get better sleep—and a healthier microbiome—here are some tried-and-true tips:

- Don't eat a large meal within three hours of going to bed, and avoid snacks at night. If you must have something, make it something light and easy to digest, like any resistant starch food.
- Don't look at any screens, including your television, your computer, and your phone, for at least one hour before going to sleep.
- If you are worried about something, talk to someone about it before you go to bed so that you can clear it out of your mind.
- Try not to get into arguments or start tackling big complex problems in the evenings after dinner.
- Create a bedtime routine. Whatever makes you feel calm and helps you wind down will work. Many people take a bath or a shower, listen to relaxing music, dim the lights, have quiet conversations with loved ones, or read a book. Spend an hour doing these things before turning in; they will help settle your body and mind.
- Listen to your body. If you feel tired, don't keep watching that show or answering e-mail. Take advantage of that tired feeling and go to bed.
- Keep a positive attitude about sleep. It helps!
- If you have serious problems sleeping and it is impacting your life, talk to your doctor about it.

Another remedy for sleep issues may be yoga. One study showed that in older adults with insomnia that impaired their daily functioning and quality of life, the practice of yoga resulted in significant improvements in a wide range of subjectively reported measures, including sleep quality, sleep efficiency, sleep duration, fatigue, depression, anxiety, stress, tension, anger, vitality, and an overall general feeling of well-being, as well as daily functioning in physical, emotional, and social roles.[202] That's a lot of benefit for a few sun salutations! If you don't already practice yoga, the best way to learn is to take a class for beginners, although you could also follow along with a yoga DVD or even a book.

The Mycobiome Diet Sleep Recommendation

Sleep for seven to nine hours each night. To discover your specific needs, listen to your body to determine what amount of sleep makes you feel the best. You should get enough so that you feel refreshed when you wake up and you don't get too tired during the middle of the day, but you shouldn't sleep so much that you have a hard time getting moving.

DON'T SMOKE

Does anybody need to be told, in this day and age, that smoking is bad for their health? I doubt it. Those who smoke admit they know that it is bad for them, but it is an addiction that is difficult to break. We also know smoking is most certainly bad for your microbiome.

As far as the research is concerned, there is very little doubt that smoking has a dramatic negative impact on microbial balance. Several studies have examined the microbiome configurations of smokers versus nonsmokers. One report surveyed all the literature on this subject between 2000 and 2016, and the studies revealed that in smokers, many pathogenic bacterial species were increased, while beneficial species were decreased. Smoking also decreased microbiome diversity.[203] Various theories suggested possible explanations for this effect, such as oxidative stress, increased intestinal permeability, reduced intestinal mucin (thinning the gastrointestinal lining), and pH shifts.

This survey noted that there were some parallels between the altered microbiomes of smokers and of people with both inflammatory bowel disease and obesity. In all cases, these microbiome shifts are likely to put people at greater risk for intestinal as well as systemic diseases, especially inflammatory bowel disease.

My group conducted a study comparing the mycobiome of the oral cavity in smokers and nonsmokers with the aim of determining the effect of smoking on microbial dysbiosis. Our data showed that smokers had a significantly higher abundance of *Candida albicans* as well as *Candida dubliniensis.*

There are so many reasons to quit this dangerous habit. If you can't do it for yourself, do it for your microbes!

The Mycobiome Diet Smoking Recommendation

Don't do it. If you need help quitting, talk to your doctor. There are many effective therapies.

GET YOUR NUTRIENTS

The interaction between micronutrients and the microbiome is interesting because our microbes depend on certain nutrients from us (that come from our diets),[204] but the microbiome also synthesizes certain nutrients that we depend on from them and impacts our mineral absorption. This is a relatively new area of research called metabolomics, which is the study of small molecules secreted by microbes as well as by humans. We still have much to learn, but we do know that the microbiome is negatively impacted by malnutrition, and that it is positively impacted by diets that include a wide range of vitamins, especially the B vitamins, vitamin K, and vitamins A, D, and E, as well as zinc. Deficiencies in these vitamins have a negative impact on immunity (especially cell responses) and have also been linked to the development of intestinal infections.[205]

In general, it's important to get complete nutrition by eating a wide range of whole foods. The Mycobiome Diet should provide you with everything you need, but a high-quality multivitamin could fill in any gaps. There may be other supplements that could benefit you, and I talk about that in Chapter 8.

The Mycobiome Diet Nutrient Recommendation

Get a wide range of nutrients from a diverse diet by eating many different items on the Mycobiome Diet food lists. The more variety of healthful whole foods you eat—especially vegetables and fruits—the more diverse and robust your microbiome will be.

DON'T TAKE UNNECESSARY MEDICATIONS

In the first part of the book, you learned about the negative impact of many prescription and over the counter drugs on the microbiome. Of course, such drugs are often required to address health problems. However, if they are not necessary, do your best to avoid them. I understand that sometimes the headache or the acid indigestion is so uncomfortable that an over-the-counter remedy is necessary. And of course, *never stop taking any prescribed medication without the approval of your doctor.* But if your medications are at your own option, the following list are the ones most harmful for your microbial balance (for the complete list with more information, see pages 33–35):

- Antibiotics and antifungals (often necessary, but ask your doctor)
- Acid-reducing medicines such as proton pump inhibitors, H2 blockers, and antacids (switching to the Mycobiome Diet may resolve your reflux problems without the need for continued medication, *but talk to your doctor before stopping any prescribed medication*)
- Nonsteroidal anti-inflammatory drugs like ibuprofen, naproxen, and aspirin, as well as COX-2 inhibitors
- Hormone-manipulating drugs like birth control and hormone replacement therapy
- Corticosteroids

The Mycobiome Diet Drug Recommendation

If you don't need a medication and your doctor agrees, don't take it.

STRESS MANAGEMENT

This is a big one—perhaps the most important lifestyle recommendation of all. Stress is a problem in our modern world and it comes at us from all corners. Not only are we busy, often putting in long hours doing difficult work, but inventions of convenience have isolated us from the kind of constant face-to-face human contact that used to be a stress-relieving part of daily life. We have families to tend to, children to care for, houses to clean, and bills to pay.

During one period in my life, when my wife and I were both working outside the home, we decided to split child care and housework evenly, dividing up our respective work hours and home hours. I know many people do this, and I felt fortunate—those times I spent with my children were among the happiest in my life. But they were also the most difficult! Parenting is a far more challenging job than any other profession, in my opinion. I can only begin to imagine how stressful it must be for those single parents who have to do it all themselves.

Stress has a profoundly negative impact on the human microbiome in general, and the mycobiome in particular, and it all has to do with the gut-brain axis (GBA). Recently, several researchers have expanded this to describe it as the microbiome-gut-brain axis, or the mycobiome-gut-brain axis.

The gut-brain axis or GBA is[206] a term used to describe the communication between the brain (the central nervous system, or CNS) and the gut (the enteric nervous system, or ENS). Biochemical and hormonal in nature, this communication involves signaling between the endocrine system (the hypothalamic-pituitary-adrenal axis, or HPA axis) and the autonomic nervous system (ANS). These are a lot of systems and acronyms and there won't be a test, but the main thing to know is that the brain talks to the gut, and the gut talks back to the brain through nervous system elements that are present in both areas. This communication is bidirectional[207]—it is a gut–brain conversation.

The result is that gut health and brain health are linked, in health and in dysfunction. The condition of your gut influences how you feel, how you present yourself, how motivated you are, and your cognitive function. The condition of your brain also influences your microbial composition and your level of dysbiosis. The HPA axis gets involved in any kind of stress response, pumping out cortisol, one of the primary stress hormones, to help the body deal with danger. Because of the GBA, there is always a gastrointestinal link to the stress response (this is why you may get "butterflies in your stomach," or a "nervous stomach," or stress-induced diarrhea).

There is a dysbiosis element in many neurological issues, including depression, schizophrenia, and autism spectrum disorder. And there is a neurological element in many gastrointestinal issues, including irritable bowel syndrome (often linked with anxiety and depression), inflammatory bowel disease, and ulcerative colitis,[208] just to name a few. Also, a decrease in microbial diversity can muffle the crosstalk and lessen the effectiveness of the relationships between the gastrointestinal and immune status, and the result can be greater susceptibility to chronic disease.[209] Our brains and guts are built to communicate. They are, in some ways, two parts of the same system.

Recent studies are also looking at the particular influence of fungi on the GBA. One study showed that mycobiome-related dysbiosis in particular caused visceral hypersensitivity, which is a science term for internal pain, usually associated with irritable bowel syndrome. The subsequent administration of *Saccharomyces boulardii* (a probiotic strain) improved the condition.[210] Just as with certain bacteria, fungi can also synthesize and release neurotransmitters. For example, *S. cerevisiae* and *Penicillium chrysogenum* can produce norepinephrine, which can activate the brain to decrease anxiety and increase brain activity and aggressive behavior. *Candida albicans* can produce histamine, which influences appetite, sleep-wake rhythm, and cognitive activity. Switching the direction, the neurotransmitter gamma-aminobutyric acid (GABA) can increase the virulence and form of *Candida albicans,* and serotonin, another neurotransmitter, can make *Candida albicans* less virulent.[211]

Another example is the way mycobiome composition seems to be related to central nervous system diseases.[212] For example, patients with anorexia nervosa tend to have several characteristic fungal species in their guts: *Aspergillus ruber, Penicillium solitum, Cladosporium bruhnei,* and *Tetratrichomonas* species. These are generally not in the guts of healthy people, so this is an unusual finding. Also, like patients with obesity, those with anorexia also seem to have less microbial diversity. Recent reports have demonstrated increased levels of *Candida* in people with autism and Rett syndrome (a neurological genetic disorder associated with abnormal gastrointestinal function and constipation).[213]

Many studies have demonstrated the microbiome effect on the stress response—improving gut health has been shown to calm anxiety-like behaviors in animals, and microbiome disruptions have been shown to cause anxiety-like behavior. This back-and-forth is highly complex, but the bottom line for our purposes here is that stress can increase dysbiosis, and dysbiosis can increase stress.

If you are following the Mycobiome Diet, you may notice that you feel calmer and even happier. This is due to the influence of improved microbiome health on your brain, via the GBA. But you can work this axis the other way as well—targeting your own stress can help to improve your microbiome balance even more.

I try very hard to minimize my own stress. I do this in many ways that are proven to be effective:

Yoga. In addition to my daily routine of sun salutations (and time on the elliptical machine), I do yoga every Sunday morning, which I find to be relaxing for both my body and my spirit. Specifically, I practice Satyananda yoga, which combines traditional physical yoga poses (asanas), breathing practices (pranayama), and meditation. This allows me to focus on the class and the practice, and I find I am not thinking about anything else. This is a nice break for my mind. Sometimes during the class, I get distracted thinking about work or family, but I try to pull my focus back to my practice. By the end of the class, I really feel great and I have a sense of inner peace and happiness.

Research shows that yoga reduces stress, and although there is not much information about yoga's direct impact on the microbiome, its reduction of stress will have an influence via the GBA. Studies have demonstrated that yoga, as well as meditation and tai chi, lead to a decrease in the expression of pro-inflammatory transcription factors, compared to a control group not practicing these techniques.[214] Another study showed that when both men and women 60 years and older practiced yoga twice a week for 12 weeks, they showed significant improvement in insomnia and sleep quality. They also reported reduced fatigue, improvements in depression and anxiety, and a generally elevated sense of well-being.[215]

Meditation. Every afternoon, I do a 10-minute meditation. I put on some meditation music, close my eyes, and sit still. During this short break, I am not using my phone, I am not in a meeting, and I am not talking to anyone. This provides me with peace, and it takes very little of my time. There are many ways to meditate. You might repeat a simple phrase (a mantra) or gaze at a single point (like a candle flame) or sit quietly and try to notice all immediate sensations around you or just sit and let your thoughts go without controlling them. You could take a meditation class or read about different techniques and try them. Whatever technique you choose, it will likely have a stress-reducing effect on your brain and a consequential beneficial effect on your microbiome. I recommend starting with just five minutes per day, and working up to more, as it is comfortable. Using a timer helps—there are apps that can track your meditation, starting and ending it with peaceful sounds like chimes or bells.

There are many studies demonstrating the stress-reducing effect of meditation; some of the studies even look at brain images during meditation and prove it changes the brain.[216] Through this effect, meditation changes the microbiome. It has been shown to improve functional gastrointestinal disorders like IBS, it shifts the microbial balance, and it improves immunity.[217] It has many other documented positive effects, too, from general improvement in quality of life to specific improvements in symptoms, from the gastrointestinal to the psychiatric.[218] While we need more research into the direct effects of both yoga and meditation on the microbiome, preliminary research seems to give both techniques a thumbs-up.

Walking. On top of all its other good effects, walking reduces stress. I take short walks at lunchtime (I especially enjoy this in the summer when I can walk outside). Sometimes I spend my lunch hour taking a short visit to the Cleveland Museum of Art, which is a nice way to take my mind off mundane things.

Accentuate the positive. I like to spend time with positive people because they energize me. I try to avoid people who are negative. I say hello, but I usually don't linger since they always want to talk about how difficult it is for researchers to get funding, and I don't find that to be a productive mindset. It just causes more stress!

Talk it out. I talk to my friends and family members when I have something on my mind. I find this to be a great stress reducer.

No news. I understand that it is important to know what is going on in the world, but the news has become stressful. When I used to live in England, I listened to the six o'clock BBC news every evening. It lasted for 15 minutes and that was enough to let me know what was happening in the world. Even when I was a student at the American University of Beirut, I took an English course and the professor said, "I want you to write an essay and then give a talk to the class, and it should not last more than five minutes. The BBC news gives you the World News in 15 minutes, so you should be able to tell us about your topic in 5." (Nowadays they call it an elevator pitch.) Those were the days! These days, it seems we are bombarded by news all day and night, and most of it isn't very informative. They also rarely tell you the good news.

Cultivate optimism and hope. I have an optimistic view of the world. I

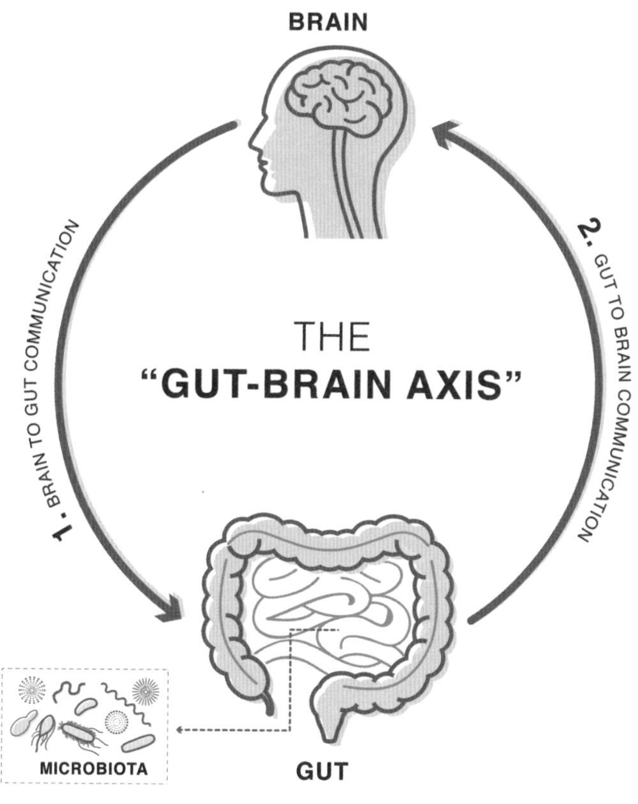

The gut-brain axis is critical in maintaining microbial balance in the gut. Disturbances in this balance may lead to dysbiosis, prompting a multitude of gastrointestinal disorders and mood-altering effects.

1.

Changes in the levels of cortisol affects the way our body responds to stress and can lead to gastrointestinal disturbances and subsequent disruption (dysbiosis) in the balance of the gut microbiota.

2.

Dysbiosis in the gut alters certain chemicals in the brain (e.g. serotonin and dopamine) that directly impact mood. These changes can lead to increased anxiety and depression, and may bring about a change in eating habits, causing further imbalance of the gut microbiota.

Summary of the gut-brain axis communication and the role it plays in keeping the microbiome in balance.

always have hope that things are going to be fine. What harm could this do? You know what they say—expect the best but prepare for the worst. I believe that how we view life is central to well-being. My mother used to tell me, "Without hope, you do not go to heaven." That was motivation enough for me, and maybe it can help to motivate you.

The Mycobiome Diet Stress Management Recommendation

Actively managing your stress is one of the best things you can do for your microbiome. Work purposefully to manage your stress for better life quality as well as better health and microbiome balance (with all its many benefits), via the gut-brain axis. Try to practice at least one stress management technique every day.

Although the main part of the Mycobiome Diet is the diet part, I hope you will take these additional recommendations into consideration. They are sure to boost your efforts and help your food choices make an even greater impact on your wellness.

8

Mycobiome Profiles

There are many ways to personalize this gut-friendly, fungi-balancing diet, but let's take it a step further by engaging in a little science-based profiling. Not of you—of your microbiome. It has been well demonstrated that certain types of lifestyles lead to certain types of microbiomes. I can't know the exact composition of your microbiome just by looking at you—especially since everybody's microbiome is as unique as a fingerprint—but with a few simple questions, I can get a pretty good idea of your microbiome's tendencies and some of the fungi and bacteria you are *likely to have*.

Understanding who may be hanging out in your gut is useful because there are some additional personalized things you can do on top of the Mycobiome Diet, such as taking certain supplements and adjusting certain lifestyle behaviors, to optimize your energy, weight, mood, and health.

If you want to know your *actual* microbiome configuration—the bacteria and fungi that are in there *for sure*—you could get a microbiome test, based on a stool sample. Testing a stool sample can accurately characterize the inhabitants of any person's microbiome, including the most prevalent bacterial and fungal phyla, genera, and species. If you are interested in doing this, you can learn more about that in the Appendix (with full disclosure that I cofounded a company that provides these tests—but of course, you don't have to use my company; it is not the only option).

However, testing is not necessary or required to get a good sense of an individual's microbiome. There has been some good research into the bacteria and fungi that tend to be most prevalent in people with different diets and health issues. I have done some work in this field myself. My aim has been to define microbiome composition inside individuals, in an attempt to classify you (to the extent possible) as a particular type of microbial ecosystem.

My team and I have been working very hard over the last decade to find a way to make more personalized dietary and lifestyle recommendations. The main question we wanted to answer is: What distinct profiles (also termed patterns or enterotypes) do healthy individuals share? My research informs us that microbiome profiling is complex, but it also suggests that some microbiomes tend to have certain characteristics that, while not necessarily mutually exclusive, are associated with certain types of health conditions, lifestyles, and dietary practices. Let's look at what I discovered when analyzing the thousands of people who have had their microbiomes tested through our company, BIOHM Health, in order to help you further refine and personalize your Mycobiome Diet.

WHAT WE KNOW ABOUT LIFESTYLES AND GUT BALANCE

To identify the distinct microbiome profiles that represent predominant microbiome enterotypes, we analyzed samples from thousands of people all across the United States.[219] Each person filled in a questionnaire about dietary habits, lifestyle, sleeping durations, stress levels, gastrointestinal symptoms (constipation, bloating, diarrhea, and the like), and weight gain or loss. For all medical conditions (current and previous) and medication usage, we also asked whether a doctor or health professional had ever diagnosed the individual with the condition.

In our analysis, we excluded those who reported serious chronic diseases (e.g., metabolic and gastrointestinal disorders, cardiovascular disease, immunodeficiency or autoimmune disorders, infectious diseases, and cancer). In addition, we excluded those with a BMI greater than 35 kg/m^2 as well as pregnant women and people on certain medications (antibiotics, antifungals, and acid reflux medications). This left us with 950 individuals ranging in age from 18 to 75, who had BMIs ranging from 18.6 to 34.9 kg/m^2. These criteria were in line with the guidelines for healthy individuals used by the Human Microbiome Project (HMP).

The Human Microbiome Project

The National Institutes of Health Human Microbiome Project was a massive project involving multiple institutions and researchers with the aim of investigating the nature and characteristics of the human microbiome. The project began in 2008 and ended in 2013 and is responsible for opening up vast new areas of knowledge about the microbial communities that call our bodies home.

Advanced DNA sequencing technologies have allowed researchers to discover and catalog many microbes that were previously unknown to us. Over 2,200 strains have been isolated and sequenced, based on 300 healthy adults between the ages of 18 and 40. Researchers took samples at five major body sites: the oral cavity, nasal cavity, skin, gastrointestinal tract, and urogenital tract, with 15 to 18 different sites within those areas sampled over one to three visits, for a total of over 11,000 samples.[220]

THE BACTERIOME PROFILES

Analysis of the microbiota of all 950 individuals showed that they could be grouped into three primary microbiome profiles or enterotypes: Group 1, Healthy Microbiome Profile (HMP); Group 2, Inflammatory Microbiome Profile (IMP); and Group 3, Obesity-Prone Microbiome Profile (OMP).

Group 1: Healthy Microbiome Profile (HMP). This group represented the healthiest population and was characterized by a high level (abundance) of Bacteroidetes, compared to the abundance of Firmicutes. This group most closely resembled the microbial profile of normal subjects reported in the Human Microbiome Project, which defines a healthy microbiome as having high levels of Bacteroidetes, moderate levels of Firmicutes, and low levels of Proteobacteria. Our analysis of the HMP group conforms to this model. This group was considered most healthy according to lifestyle reporting as well—they indicated the lowest levels of stress, the most restful sleep (defined by getting seven to nine hours of sleep per night), and the least amount of gastrointestinal issues.

Group 2: Inflammatory Microbiome Profile (IMP). This group was characterized as having the lowest levels of Bacteroidetes, moderate levels of Firmicutes, and high levels of Proteobacteria. High levels of Proteobacteria are associated with gut dysbiosis and inflammation.[221]

In a healthy gut, Proteobacteria should play no prominent role. It is considered a first-line responder, which means that it responds rapidly to certain environmental factors. This could mean changes in diet, stress, sleep, and existing inflammation elsewhere in the body. Elevated Proteobacteria often corresponds with inflammation, which could come from (or cause) digestive conditions or symptoms such as diarrhea, inflammatory bowel disease, irritable bowel syndrome, as well as stress, poor sleep, or consuming an inflammatory diet containing few vegetables and high amounts of sugar and animal fat. Regardless of the source, elevated Proteobacteria should be a red flag for inflammation and its related health issues.

Considering the link with inflammation, it is not surprising that IMP subjects tended to have lifestyles and health conditions typically linked with inflammation. They were more likely to:

- Report feeling extremely stressed
- Get inadequate sleep (less than four hours a night)
- Consume very low levels of vegetables (less than 1 cup per day)
- Consume very low levels of fruit (less than 1 cup per day)

The latter two points suggest their diets were probably mostly made up of starchy carbs, dairy products, meat, and sugar.

Group 3: Obesity-Prone Microbiome Profile (OMP). This group was characterized as having moderate levels of Bacteroidetes, high levels of Firmicutes, and the lowest levels of Proteobacteria. Excessive levels of Firmicutes are often associated with obesity[222] as well as sleep disorders,[223] jet lag,[224] and shift work.[225] Recent obesity research has focused on the Firmicutes to Bacteroidetes ratio, with particular interest in whether manipulation of this ratio could promote lasting weight loss and a healthy weight. We aren't there yet, but this is a fascinating area of gut health research and a promising focus for the future of personalized medicine.

Note that increased Firmicutes during pregnancy is considered a healthy, normal adaptation. During pregnancy, the mother requires more energy, which is provided by Firmicutes (they have the ability to break

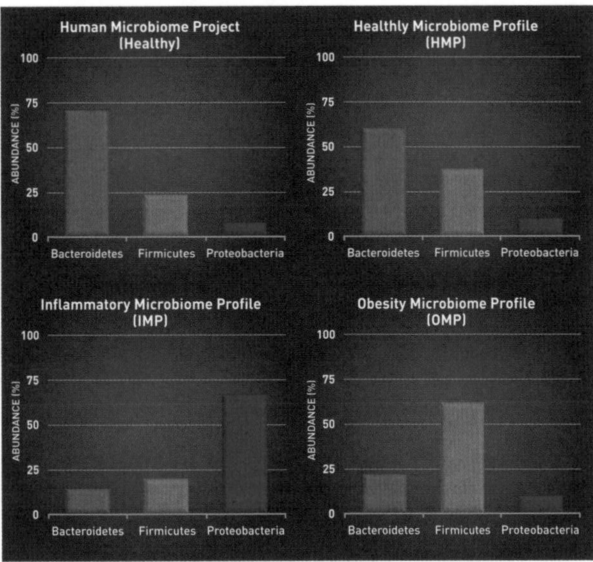

Different microbiome profiles of individuals tested, compared to the Human Microbiome Project (HMP) healthy profile. Note the similarity between the HMP profile and that of healthy participants in the project.

down food, resulting in a higher caloric output, which is subsequently used by the mother). However, studies indicate that it is desirable to promote higher levels of Bacteroidetes and encourage moderate Firmicute levels while maintaining the lowest levels of Proteobacteria, even during pregnancy.[226]

THE *CANDIDA* ADD-ON

But what about the mycobiome component of these microbiome groups? In our analysis, not surprisingly, *Candida* species were the key players. The presence of *Candida* did not appear to be associated more strongly with any of the three groups—some of the microbiomes in each of the groups had high levels of *Candida,* and some did not. Any subject might be HMP (Group 1), IMP (Group 2), OMP (Group 3), or the same group with elevated *Candida,* HMP+C, IMP+C, or OMP+C.

Remember that *Candida* species are normal inhabitants of the human gut—many people have *Candida albicans, Candida glabrata,* and sometimes *Candida tropicalis* and *Candida parapsilosis,* and these people can be perfectly healthy. However, when *Candida* was present and elevated relative to the average amount of *Candida* in the human gut (as often happens after a course of antibiotics, or with immune system problems or gut permeability issues), the subjects tended to have elevated stress levels, carbohydrate-rich (especially sugar-rich) diets, inadequate amounts of sleep, and vitamin deficiencies.

After you have determined which group you are likely to be in, you can also determine whether or not *Candida* is likely to be a problem for you, and if so, you can have additional "prescriptions" based on your probable *Candida* status.

YOUR MICROBIOME STATUS

How do you know which group you are likely to be in? Check the boxes that describe you, your lifestyle, or your health. The column with the most checkmarks will determine the group you would *probably* fall into, if you were to have your microbiome tested.

HMP (Group 1)	IMP (Group 2)	OMP (Group 3)	+C (elevated *Candida*)
☐ You eat a lot of vegetables and fruits, and/or you are a vegetarian or vegan. ☐ Most of your protein and fat come from whole food plant sources. ☐ You don't eat processed, packaged, or "fast" food very often. ☐ You usually get enough fiber and have "regular" digestion. ☐ You get 7 to 9 hours of sleep on most nights. ☐ You get some exercise on most days. ☐ You get stressed sometimes but don't feel stressed constantly. ☐ You are in normal weight range (BMI of 18 to 25). ☐ You usually enjoy your job and have generally healthy relationships. ☐ You consider yourself pretty healthy.	☐ You feel stressed a lot of the time or would describe yourself as "chronically stressed." ☐ You eat less than 1 cup of vegetables daily. ☐ You eat less than 1 cup of fruit daily. ☐ You tend to eat a lot of animal fat and animal protein. ☐ You eat high-fat dairy products like cheese, cream, and ice cream. ☐ Your weight fluctuates a lot, or you are a "yo-yo dieter," often gaining and losing the same 10 or 20 pounds. ☐ You don't often get enough sleep and feel tired during the day. ☐ You have frequent digestive problems like acid reflex, constipation, or IBS. ☐ You have been diagnosed with a health condition related to inflammation, such as an autoimmune disease like IBD or celiac disease. ☐ You have mood swings or suffer from depression and/or anxiety.	☐ You are overweight or obese or have a BMI higher than 27. ☐ You have trouble controlling your appetite or portion sizes. You know you probably eat more than you need, but you find it hard to stop. ☐ You regularly consume artificial sweeteners (such as diet soda). ☐ You don't exercise regularly. ☐ You spend most of your day sitting. ☐ You get tired during the day but have trouble falling asleep at night, or you have insomnia. ☐ You typically get 6 or fewer hours of sleep per night. ☐ You travel into different times zones frequently. ☐ You work the night shift and sleep during the day, or your job schedule changes frequently so you often change when you sleep and eat. Or, your schedule is just generally irregular. ☐ You have problems with your kidneys, or you have cystic fibrosis.	☐ You have a "sweet tooth" and often crave sweets. You generally eat sugary foods on most days. ☐ You eat a lot of processed, packaged, or "junk" foods. ☐ You drink a lot of fruit juice, and/or eat a lot of high-sugar fruits, like pineapple, watermelon, mango, bananas, or any dried fruit. ☐ When you eat foods high in sugar or starch, it just makes you feel hungrier. ☐ You drink alcohol on most nights, even if it's just a small glass of wine or one beer, or you regularly have 3 or more drinks in one day. ☐ You took antibiotics frequently as a child. ☐ You have taken antibiotics in the last year. ☐ You regularly take acid-reducing medication. ☐ You have a lot of digestive symptoms like indigestion, gas, bloating, cramping, diarrhea, constipation, vomiting, nausea, or abdominal pain. ☐ You have problems with blood sugar, such as metabolic syndrome, prediabetes, diabetes, or hypoglycemia.
TOTAL:	TOTAL:	TOTAL:	TOTAL:

Scoring

HMP: If you checked the most boxes in the HMP column, you probably have a healthy balance, with dominant Bacteroidetes. Congratulations! See the HMP prescription that follows this scoring list.

IMP: If you checked the most boxes in the IMP column, you probably have elevated Proteobacteria and inflammation (and all its health-related issues) may be a problem for you. You also probably suffer from digestive complaints, not to mention stress. See the IMP prescription that follows.

OMP: If you checked the most boxes in the OMP column, you may have a problem with weight gain, or you might be predisposed to this problem, even if it isn't a problem yet. You probably also have dysbiosis related to sleep disturbances and other lifestyle factors. See the OMP prescription that follows. (If you are pregnant, you don't have to worry about being in this group, as this may be temporary. You should follow the diet and lifestyle recommended by your doctor, or generally strive for the healthiest possible diet.)

+C: If you checked more than three items in the +C column, you probably have elevated *Candida* and should consider the +C prescription along with the prescription for your dominant group.

Now let's look at what you can do, on top of practicing the Mycobiome Diet, to customize your diet and lifestyle for maximum positive microbiome impact.

Should You Take a Multivitamin?

In general, I believe most people should get their nutrition from food.[227] However, not everyone always gets everything they need. Since daily multivitamins may be more beneficial than harmful, I recommend that anyone would be fine taking a daily multivitamin that meets the Recommended Daily Allowance (RDA) of nutrients for the majority of adults. For women who could become pregnant, the CDC recommends folic acid as a supplement to help prevent certain birth defects. For those who are pregnant, a prenatal vitamin is always a good idea.

But there is significant data supporting the idea that higher intakes of folic acid, vitamin B6, vitamin B12, and vitamin D will benefit many people.[228] I recommend that the following individuals will benefit from multivitamins and should take one daily:

- Women who might become pregnant.
- People who consume one or more alcoholic drinks per day on a regular basis.
- Individuals 65 years of age and older, due to a reduced ability to absorb vitamin B12 and vitamin D.
- People who don't eat any animal products (vegans), especially vitamin B12.
- People who are unable or unwilling to eat a variety of fruits and vegetables daily.

Caution: Although it is rare, there have been instances of serious complications in immunocompromised individuals who took dietary supplements. Be sure to tell your doctor about any supplements you are taking, even if it is just a multivitamin.

Also, it is important to realize that supplements are not meant to treat diseases. Doing so may cause health issues. Supplements support health. They are not curative.

HMP (GROUP 1) PRESCRIPTION: STAY THE COURSE

You probably have a generally healthy microbiome, so your prescription is to stay the course. Continue to support your healthy balance by eating lots of prebiotic foods rich in polyphenols and resistant starches, as recommended on the Mycobiome Diet to maintain. Strive for variety. If you do experience occasional digestive upset, or if you undergo a period of stress or sleep problems, don't lapse into bad habits. Keep up with a healthy diet, and your issues are likely to resolve quickly.

Supplement Recommendations

1. Consider taking a probiotic, especially if you have to take antibiotics or develop any digestive issues.[229] Probiotics can also help to maintain a healthy microbiome during periods of stress.[230] Look for varieties that contain these beneficial species:
   - *Lactobacillus*
   - *Bifidobacteria*
2. You may not need a multivitamin, but you can always take one for extra nutritional insurance, just in case. If you are a vegan, be sure to get enough vitamin B12.

What Are Probiotics?

Probiotics are live microorganisms, that when taken in adequate amounts, can provide a health benefit to both humans and animals.[231] Most probiotics in the market contain bacteria. The most widely used bacteria in probiotics belong to the genera *Lactobacillus* and *Bifidobacterium*. Other bacterial genera used as probiotics include *Escherichia, Enterococcus, Bacillus,* and *Propionibacterium.* Besides bacteria, the yeast *Saccharomyces boulardii* (a strain of *Saccharomyces cerevisiae*) is used as a probiotic also—it is particularly good at fighting off *Candida.*

Benefits of Probiotics

Research has demonstrated that probiotics contribute to health in the following ways:

- Improves digestive function
- Enhances immune function
- Reduces antibiotics-associated diarrhea
- Reduces the development of allergies
- Improves lactose intolerance
- Manages the relapse of some inflammatory bowel conditions
- Decreases *Helicobacter pylori* colonization of the stomach (the bacteria that can cause stomach ulcers)
- Helps reduce the risk of certain acute common infectious diseases (such as infections caused by *C. difficile*)
- Reduces crying time in colicky babies (talk to your pediatrician)

Probiotic products should be safe, effective, and should maintain their effectiveness and potency through the end of their product shelf life. Look for documentation from the manufacturer involving third-party testing. You can also call the manufacturer product line to ask questions. Some other ways to determine whether you are getting a quality probiotic are to look for:

- Containers guaranteed to keep microbial strains alive and maintain the product's potency.
- Clear instructions on how to store the product, such as whether the product should be kept at room temperature or refrigerated.
- Capsules or probiotic strains that are coated, so they can survive the acidic conditions of the stomach.
- Assurance that the product meets an acceptable level of safety and efficacy.
- A product with a minimum of two bacterial strains representing *Lactobacillus* and *Bifidobacterium,* although the product could contain more

strains of both bacteria and fungi that are proven to have an effect. Ideally you want a probiotic to have good bacteria and good yeast, so that you can address the total microbiota.

Disclaimer: My company, BIOHM Health, makes probiotics, but I am in no way requiring or suggesting that you should buy my product. If you are interested in the research behind our formulation, however, please see the Appendix.

IMP (GROUP 2) PRESCRIPTION: LOWER INFLAMMATION

Since most people tend to fall into this category, and this is also a category that can put people at risk for developing serious health issues, I'm going to give you a lot of recommendations. You don't have to take them all, but add the ones that fit into your life and budget.

The key here is to lower inflammation, and there are a lot of ways to do that. First, and most important, stick closely to the Mycobiome Diet for best results! High fiber and resistant starch foods have been shown to reduce Proteobacteria, and the diet's heavy reliance on polyphenol-rich plant foods will feed the beneficial microbes and discourage Proteobacteria.

Supplement Recommendations

If you have, or suspect you have, "leaky gut syndrome" or compromised intestinal barrier (common with inflammation), I recommend adding these supplements to your daily routine (you can knock out many of them with a good multivitamin):

- Collagen peptides
- Zinc
- Vitamin C
- Vitamin A
- Vitamin D3

Also, because Proteobacteria levels increase in response to inflammation in the body, you can reduce its abundance by reducing your inflammation through certain supplements. Try these (some are already incorporated into the Mycobiome Diet):

- Ginger—use it in the foods you prepare. It can help with digestive problems.
- Turmeric—use this in cooking as often as you can. It is a potent anti-inflammatory.
- Mucilage herbs like DGL (deglycyrrhizinated licorice) and marshmallow root. You can find these in tea form.
- Probiotics, which can help to reduce stress by lowering the levels of stress hormone.[232] (Stress is another hallmark of the IMP profile. Less stress can equal less inflammation.)

There are a few specific strains that target the typical complications of elevated Proteobacteria (inflammation, compromised mucosal barrier function or "leaky gut syndrome," and anxiety). Look for a probiotic that contains:

- *L. rhamnosus,*[233] which has been shown to have anti-inflammatory benefits and improve gut mucosal barrier function, as well as reduce anxiety.
- *S. boulardii,*[234] which has been shown to lower inflammation and is a promising therapy for digestive disorders.
- *B. breve,*[235] which has been shown to ease digestion, boost immunity, and play an important role in immune function and allergy response. It also can help with compromised mucosal barrier function and may reduce anxiety, too.

What Are Prebiotics?

You already know that many good foods are prebiotics—the ones containing fiber and resistant starch—and that your beneficial microbes consume them. But what about prebiotic supplements? In a world where people consume more sugar and less fiber, including a lot fewer vegetables and fruits than they should, prebiotic supplements have become an option.

I would *always* recommend food sources of prebiotics over supplements, but supplements are better than no prebiotics at all. For example, many children these days primarily eat food lacking in fiber, and many of them have constipation and other gastrointestinal issues at a young age. Over time, this could lead to infections and kidneys issues. I can tell you, my little grandchild is suffering from this as I write! The problem is that kids don't often eat vegetables and other healthy foods. They get stuck in a rut of a few high-fat, high-sugar, refined carbohydrate foods like macaroni and cheese, breaded fried chicken strips, and of course, sweet snacks and soda. Parents are busy, this kind of food is cheap, and although we all know kids should eat healthy food, the reality is that sometimes it doesn't happen. Prebiotics can help to circumvent health issues in both children and adults, as they work on improving their diets at a rate they can manage.

Prebiotic supplements (like prebiotic foods) contain nondigestible ingredients that selectively stimulate the growth and/or activity of the beneficial microorganisms that live in our guts. The most common prebiotics are oligosaccharides (carbs such as sucrose, maltose, trehalose, and lactose). Oligosaccharides are found in human milk. Inulin-type fructans and the galacto-oligosaccharides (GOS) are the two main chemical groups that have been extensively investigated to determine the effect of prebiotics on human health. Research into prebiotics has shown that they can selectively stimulate the growth of beneficial *Bifidobacteria* and, to a lesser extent, *Lactobacillus.* Increase in the growth of these good-guy microbes can lead to significant alteration in the composition of the gut microbiota.

There are a number of advantages for using prebiotics:

- They improve microbiome balance by feeding the beneficial microbes.
- They improve intestinal function and "regularity."
- They can increase mineral absorption, resulting in improved bone health with greater density and calcium content.
- They can increase satiety (feeling full after eating).
- They can improve energy metabolism.
- They can help to reduce "leaky gut syndrome" or compromised intestinal barrier.
- They can reduce the risk of gastrointestinal infections.
- They reduce the risk of obesity, metabolic syndrome, and type 2 diabetes.
- They can reduce intestinal inflammation.
- They may reduce the risk of colon cancer.
- Preliminary data suggest that prebiotics may positively influence overall immune function.

Although no serious adverse effects were reported with the use of prebiotics, it should be noted that prebiotics can cause some temporary stomach upset in people who aren't used to them (just as increasing foods with fiber and resistant starch can). Normally the body adjusts, but it's a good idea to start with a small amount and gradually increase to the recommended dosage, to avoid discomfort. **Disclaimer:** My company, BIOHM Health, makes prebiotics. But, as with probiotics, I am in no way requiring or suggesting that you should buy my products. If you are interested in the research behind our formulation, however, please see the Appendix.

OMP (GROUP 3) PRESCRIPTION: IMPROVE LIFESTYLE HABITS

If your Firmicutes levels are out of proportion to your Bacteroidetes levels, you can shift the balance back in your favor. My primary advice to start is to emphasize good plant-based protein and more fiber. Eat fewer animal products and more plants! If you've been considering going vegetarian, this could be a great reason to go for it. A diet heavy in plant foods and low (or absent) in animal foods can quickly reduce Firmicutes to more moderate, healthy levels.[236] Plus, Bacteroidetes love fiber,[237] and you can only get fiber from plant foods. Fiber especially nurtures beneficial *Bifidobacteria* and *Lactobacillus*.[238]

One of the Mycobiome Diet's most important recommendations for you is green tea. Green tea may assist in improving your metabolism and supporting weight balance.[239]

Supplement Recommendations

Consider taking a probiotic containing the beneficial microbes you are trying to increase. Look for one containing:

- *Bifidobacteria* and *Lactobacillus*
- *L. rhamnosus*,[240] to reduce inflammation and to help balance blood sugar, which is often a concern with elevated Firmicutes
- *B. breve*,[241] which is anti-inflammatory and also tends to be low in people who are carrying excess weight
- *S. boulardii*,[242] which also appears to positively affect inflammation, excess weight, and type 2 diabetes

Dietary Recommendations

Data suggest that elevated Firmicutes levels are associated with inadequate fiber and plant food in the diet, as well as with high animal fat intake and excessive calorie intake. For these reasons, a high-fiber vegetarian diet may be particularly therapeutic for people in the OMP group.

Lifestyle Recommendations

Another key for people in the OMP group is lifestyle modification. Here are the most important things to focus on:

- If you are overweight, losing weight can make a big difference in your microbiome balance, tipping you back into a more favorable ratio of Bacteroidetes to Firmicutes. The Mycobiome Diet and regular exercise could help you do this effectively.
- Work on improving your sleep patterns.
- If your blood sugar is abnormal, try reducing carbohydrate portions. Be sure to spread out small servings throughout the day, rather than eating larger amounts of carbohydrate-rich food all at once.
- Go vegetarian or vegan—or mostly. Emphasizing plants can help shift the balance back toward the normal by increasing Bacteroidetes.
- Get your protein and fat from fish (my favorite exception to the vegetarian rule), along with plant food sources like avocado, nuts, seeds, flax, and chia.
- Start exercising regularly, if you don't already. Regular exercise is proven to favorably shift microbiome balance and can also help with weight loss.

+C PRESCRIPTION

No matter your group, if you have elevated *Candida,* there are some additional things you can do to get that pesky sugar-loving group of fungi back under control. The Mycobiome Diet, of course, is an excellent start, especially due to the high level of polyphenols from vegetables, fruits, nuts, and seeds it contains. Polyphenols feed the bacteria that manage *Candida* levels. It's also important to increase good seafood- and plant-based proteins and fats, while reducing simple carbohydrates, especially sugar. These are powerful weapons against *Candida.*

Anti-inflammatory foods help, too, since *Candida* favors an inflammatory state.[243] Look for it in:

- Ginger
- Turmeric
- DGL (deglycyrrhizinated licorice)[244]
- Marshmallow root[245]

Healthy fats also contribute to a reduction in *Candida* growth, as does the quality protein found in collagen.[246] Bone broth is a great source for this (see Carley's Corner: Chicken Bone Broth, page 187).

Supplement Recommendations

Candida is often further exacerbated by vitamin inadequacies. You can discourage *Candida* with these additional supplements:

- A multivitamin. These supplements can provide the key nutrients related to *Candida* elevation (vitamins A, C, and B—especially B6), as well as those related to gut healing (zinc,[247] vitamin A,[248] and vitamin C[249]).
- A probiotic, especially containing *S. boulardii*. This beneficial fungal strain works to balance *Candida* levels and reduce biofilm development to support overall microbiome health.
- Anti-fungal supplements. Look especially to those containing garlic, polyphenols, and grapeseed extract.

Lifestyle Recommendations

- If you are able, avoid unnecessary antibiotics, which, as you know, open the door for *Candida* excess. Always check with your doctor about the necessity of your antibiotic prescription and do not go against your doctor's advice.

Stress encourages *Candida,* so stress reduction is important (Chapter 7). Stress reduction is also anti-inflammatory and is helpful for easing digestive upset.

9

The Mycobiome Diet Recipes

The best part about managing your mycobiome and feeding the superstars in your microbiome is that you get to do it with delicious food. These recipes were developed, written, tested, and photographed by food writer and photographer Rosie Hatch (find out more about her at rosiehatch.com) with extra nutrition information contributed by Certified Nutritional Therapy Practitioner Carley Smith (aka the Fairy Gutmother—find out more about her at fairygutmother.com). Every recipe highlights the natural foods that are beneficial to curating the mycobiome specifically and the microbiome generally. They are based on the principles scientifically proven to dissolve biofilms and balance the mycobiome. These foods favor beneficial bacteria and encourage outcomes such as better health, weight loss, and reduced inflammation. The recipes are also easily adaptable—every recipe can be made using 100% plant-based, gluten-free, or grain-free ingredients. Simply follow the variations at the end of each recipe. No matter your dietary preference or restrictions, you can still do what's best for your microbes so they can do what's best for you. These recipes are also so satisfying that you may forget how therapeutic they are. This is the best kind of "medicine" for your microbiome!

Note: Most but not all recipes serve two, so check the serving size. Any recipe can be halved or doubled.

RECIPES FOR THE MYCOBIOME DIET

Breakfasts

Lunches

Dinners

Smoothies and Other Snacks

BREAKFASTS

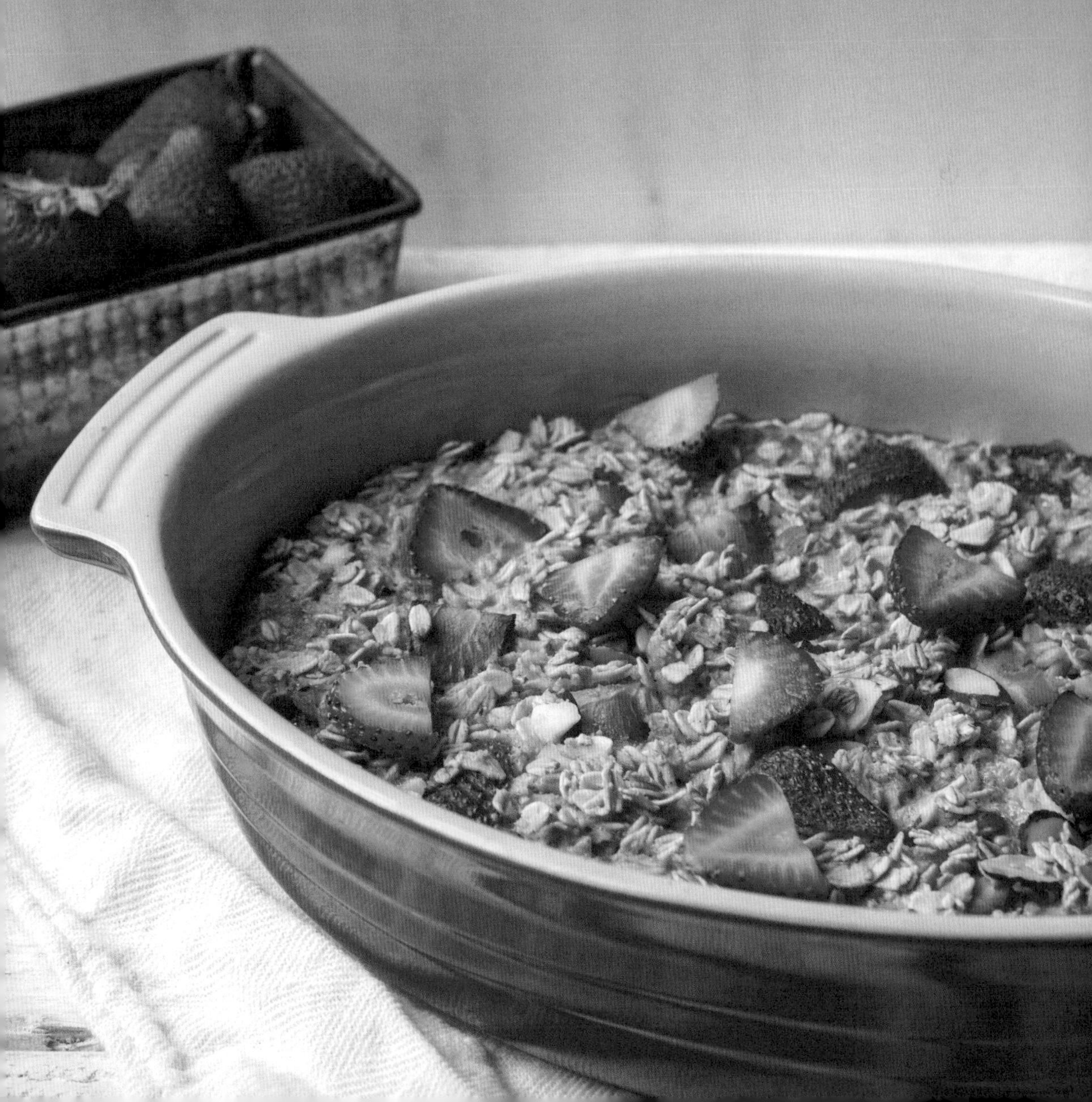

CACAO OATMEAL BOWLS

SERVES 2

TIME: 5 MINUTES PREP (8+ HOURS SOAK)

Overnight oats are perfect for busy mornings because you do almost all the work (and there isn't much) the night before. Let it sit in a jar overnight and in the morning you've got a creamy, chewy, delicious breakfast. This recipe adds more flavor and microbiome-friendliness to your oats by adding raw cacao powder (different from cocoa powder, although you can substitute cocoa powder if you can't find raw cacao powder). For a grain-free option, see the recipe note.

1 cup rolled oats
1 cup almond milk (unsweetened or homemade; recipe follows)
1 tablespoon cacao powder
Honey or maple syrup to taste (optional, 1 tablespoon max)
1 teaspoon cinnamon
Goji berries (as much as you want)
Cacao nibs (as much as you want)
1 strawberry, sliced

1. In a large jar with a lid, add the oats, almond milk, cacao powder, honey, and cinnamon. Mix thoroughly, cover, and refrigerate overnight.

2. The next day, pour the oats into two bowls and top with goji berries, cacao nibs, and strawberry slices. Or, add toppings and eat it right out of the jar.

Grain-free variation: Eliminate oats. Bake two sweet potatoes. Cut them open and sprinkle them with the cacao powder and cinnamon, then drizzle on the honey, and add the remaining toppings. Serve the almond milk on the side as a beverage, or omit it.

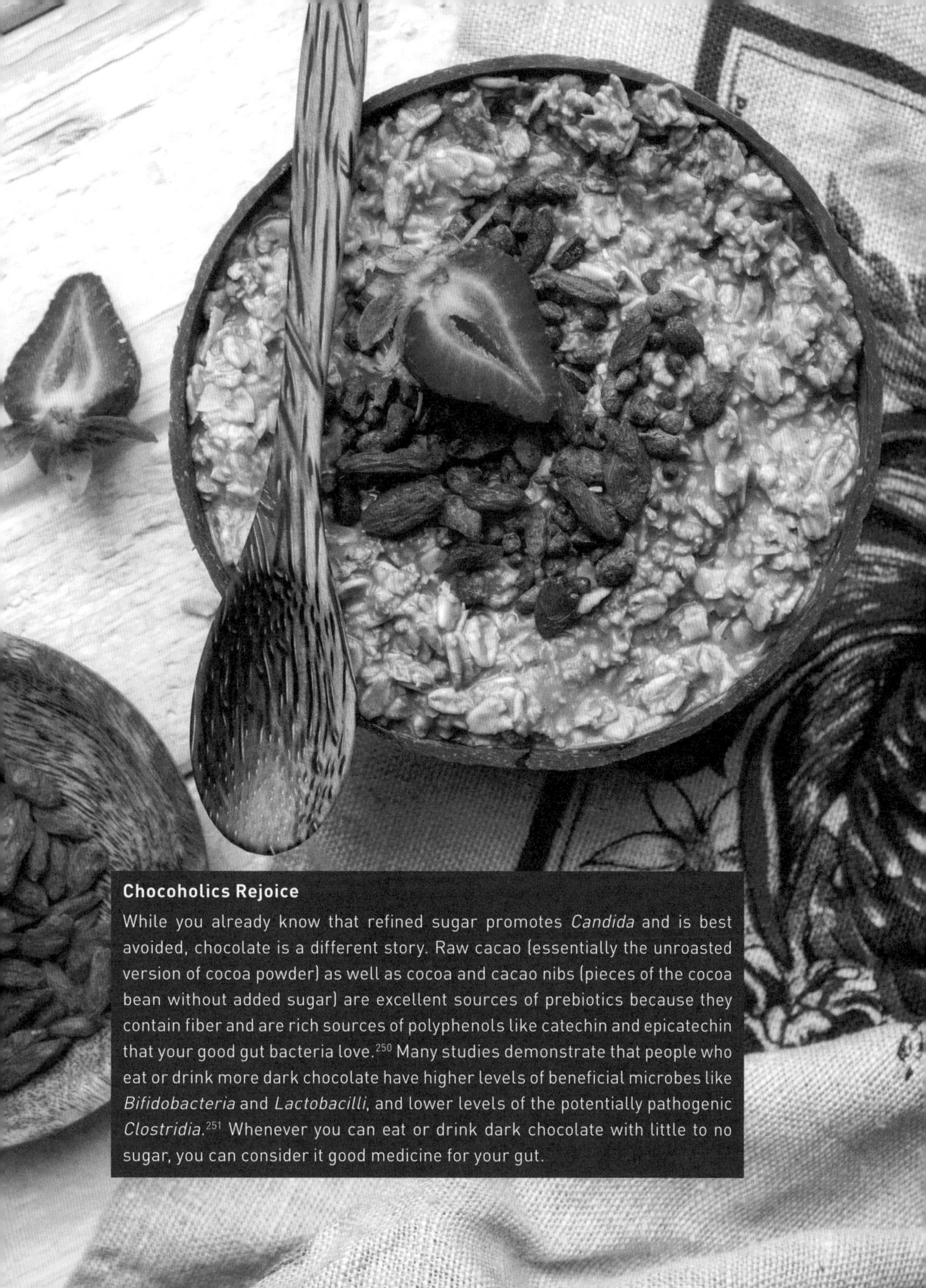

Chocoholics Rejoice

While you already know that refined sugar promotes *Candida* and is best avoided, chocolate is a different story. Raw cacao (essentially the unroasted version of cocoa powder) as well as cocoa and cacao nibs (pieces of the cocoa bean without added sugar) are excellent sources of prebiotics because they contain fiber and are rich sources of polyphenols like catechin and epicatechin that your good gut bacteria love.[250] Many studies demonstrate that people who eat or drink more dark chocolate have higher levels of beneficial microbes like *Bifidobacteria* and *Lactobacilli*, and lower levels of the potentially pathogenic *Clostridia*.[251] Whenever you can eat or drink dark chocolate with little to no sugar, you can consider it good medicine for your gut.

HOMEMADE ALMOND MILK

MAKES ABOUT 2 CUPS

TIME: 15 MINUTES (PLUS OVERNIGHT SOAK)

It's easy to find unsweetened almond milk in the store these days, but homemade almond milk is even better. It doesn't contain any binders or additives, it's fresh, and you know exactly what's in it—just almonds and water, plus a bit of salt and optional honey or maple syrup. This recipe uses cheesecloth and a fine mesh strainer, but you could also use mesh bags, sold in health food stores as "nut bags," to strain out the nut pulp.

1 cup raw almonds, preferably organic
2 cups water, plus more for soaking
¼ teaspoon sea salt
Honey or maple syrup, to taste (optional, 1 tablespoon max)

1. Place the almonds in a bowl and cover with water, to about an inch above the almonds. Cover with a loose cloth and soak the almonds overnight at room temperature or in the refrigerator.

2. The next day, drain the almonds from their soaking water and rinse them thoroughly under cool running water. Place the almonds in a food processor with 2 cups fresh water and salt. Blend at the highest speed for a few minutes.

3. Line a fine mesh strainer with cheesecloth, place the strainer over a bowl, and pour the blended mixture through it. Squeeze out any additional liquid. Sweeten to taste, if desired.

"Recycling" Almond Pulp

Homemade almond milk is a treat, but what about all that almond pulp? Are you just supposed to throw it away? Almonds are expensive and that may seem like a waste. I agree! Don't throw away that almond pulp. Here are some things to do with it:

- Add it to baked goods like muffin batter, your morning oatmeal, granola, or smoothies for extra fiber and nutrients.
- Use it instead of chickpeas for hummus. Just mix it with tahini and your other favorite hummus ingredients (see Hummus Plate, page 192).
- Toast it in the oven on a tray and use it like breadcrumbs (gluten-free and grain-free!).
- Stir it into almond butter for an extra-crunchy version.
- Mix it with a little water, sea salt, and grated low-fat cheese (like Parmesan) or nutritional yeast. Roll it out and cut it into squares. Bake into crackers.
- Compost it to feed the soil.

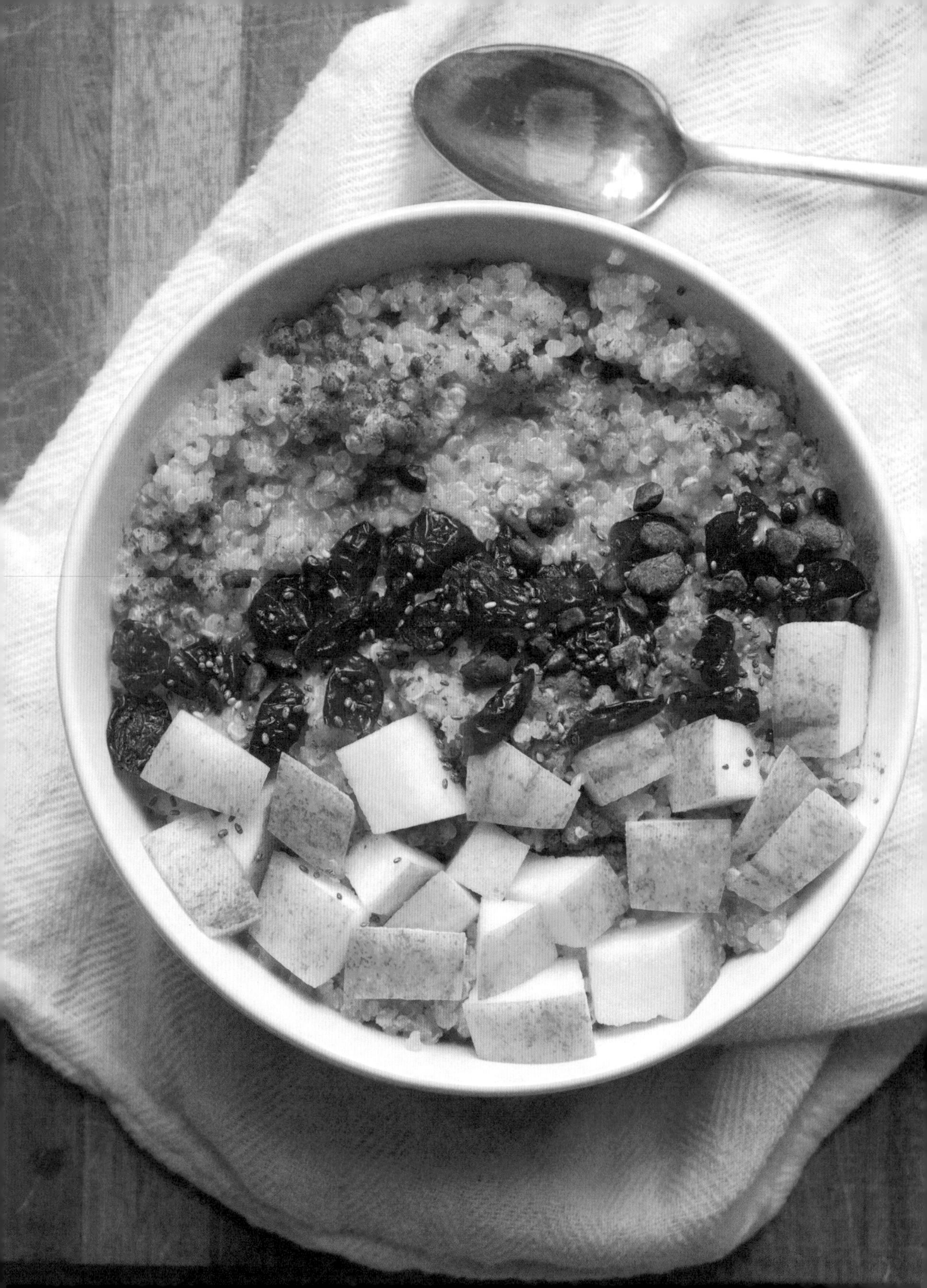

CINNAMON APPLE CRANBERRY QUINOA BOWL

SERVES 2

TIME: 20 MINUTES

Apple and cinnamon will forever be a breakfast favorite. Try these flavors with quinoa for a change. Cranberries, apples, cacao nibs, and chia seeds add more valuable prebiotics as well as flavor and texture you'll love. Raw cacao nibs and chia seeds are available in most health food stores and in health food aisles of regular grocery stores, as well as online. For grain-free variations, see the recipe notes.

1 cup quinoa
1 teaspoon cinnamon
1 teaspoon maple syrup (optional, 1 teaspoon max)
1 apple, cut into cubes
¼ cup dried cranberries (look for unsweetened)
1 tablespoon raw cacao nibs
1 teaspoon chia seeds

1. In a medium saucepan, bring 2 cups of water to a boil. Add quinoa then reduce heat to low and cover.

2. Once the quinoa has absorbed the water, about 15 minutes, add cinnamon and maple syrup. Divide the quinoa between two bowls. Top with cubed apples, cranberries, cacao nibs, and chia seeds.

Grain-free variation: Drain and rinse a can of chickpeas and put them in a food processor. Pulse the chickpeas a few times to chop them up. Use the chickpeas in place of the cooked quinoa, warmed in a saucepan with ¼ cup almond milk, low-fat or nonfat dairy milk, or apple juice before adding the other ingredients.

Another grain-free variation is to use about 3 cups of cauliflower "rice." Chop cauliflower in a food processor until it is rice-textured or buy fresh or frozen premade cauliflower "rice." Prepare as above, but cook the cauliflower rice in just ½ cup water until it is soft. (See page 202 for the full recipe.) This variation will take care of your cruciferous vegetable serving for the day, but you will need to add a resistant starch to this meal, such as a banana.

EGG BREAKFAST CUPS

SERVES 2

TIME: 20 MINUTES

These cute little breakfast cups combine greens, tomatoes, and eggs for a savory dish that takes minimal time out of your busy mornings. Serve them as a breakfast entrée for two or a side dish for brunch. For a vegan version, see the recipe note.

1½ cups raw baby spinach or artisan lettuce, coarsely chopped
½ cup pico de gallo or marinara sauce (store-bought or homemade; recipes follow)
4 eggs
1 teaspoon red pepper flakes
1 avocado, cubed
4 dashes sea salt

1. Preheat oven to 350°F. Grease four 6- to 8-ounce ramekins and divide one cup of the spinach or lettuce equally among them. Spoon the pico de gallo or marinara sauce on top of the greens, then sprinkle with remaining spinach or lettuce.

2. Crack one egg in each ramekin and sprinkle with red pepper flakes. Place on a baking sheet and bake for 10 to 12 minutes or until the egg white is cooked through.

3. Cool slightly and add avocado cubes to each ramekin along with a sprinkle of sea salt. Serve warm.

Plant-based variation: In place of the eggs, crumble or cube 8 ounces of firm or extra-firm tofu and divide it between the 4 ramekins. Continue with the rest of the recipe as written.

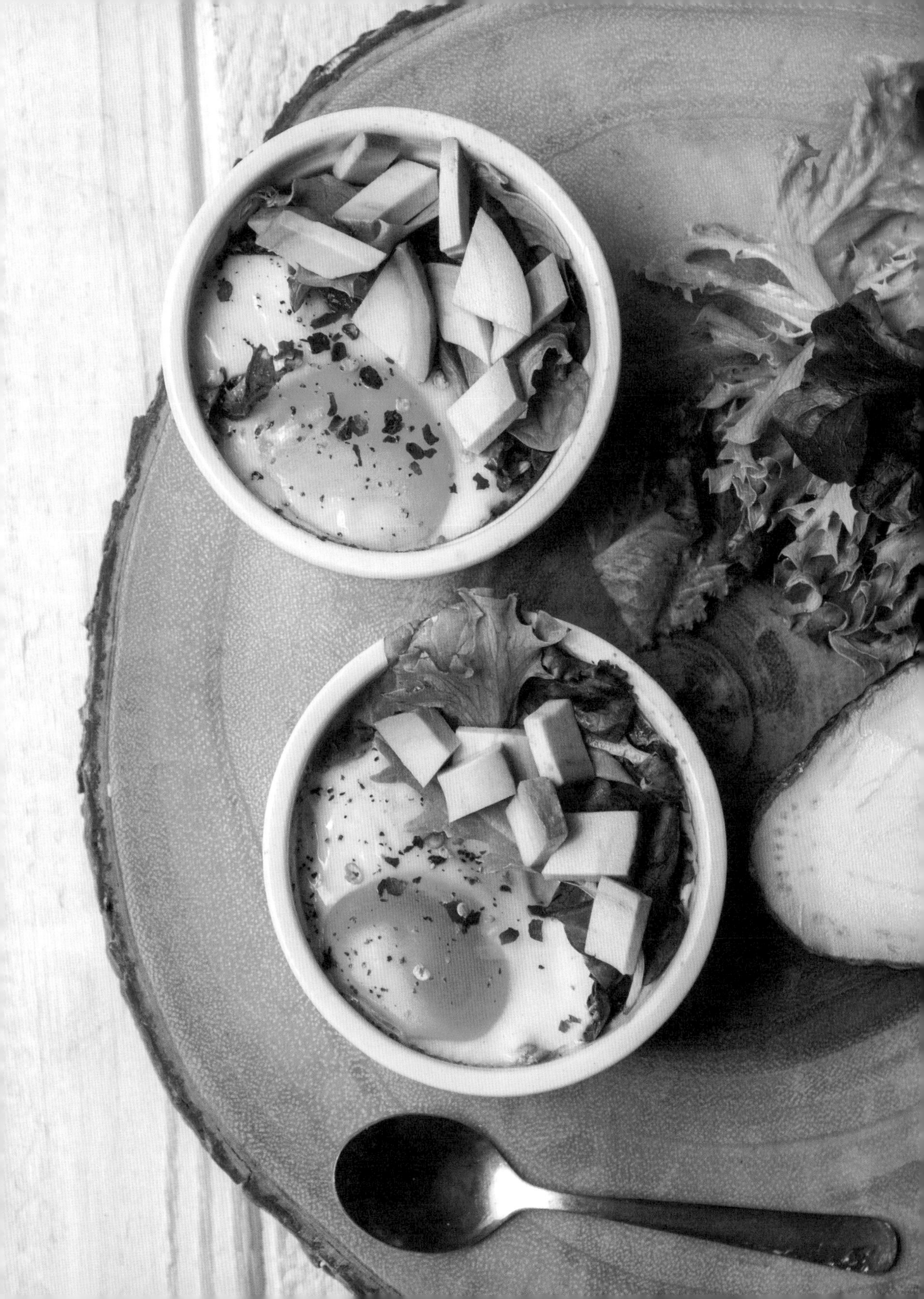

HOMEMADE PICO DE GALLO

MAKES ABOUT 2 CUPS

TIME: 10 MINUTES

Pico de gallo is best made fresh. Although you can purchase it, this made-to-order version is superior to anything that has been sitting in a store. It's especially good in the summer when tomatoes are at their most ripe and flavorful. This doesn't keep well for more than a day in the refrigerator, so ideally make just as much as you need. This recipe can easily be halved or doubled.

2 large or 3 medium fresh tomatoes, cut in half, seed pulp squeezed out, chopped (you don't need to remove the skin)
½ medium white onion, minced
1 small green pepper, finely chopped
1 jalapeño pepper (more or less depending on how hot you like it), seeded and minced
½ cup chopped cilantro leaves
1 lime, juiced
1 teaspoon sea salt

Combine all the ingredients in a bowl and stir. Let sit for about 10 minutes, then serve fresh.

Oregano and Your Microbiome

Several studies have demonstrated that oregano essential oil is good for the gut because of the anti-inflammatory, antioxidant, and antimicrobial properties of the volatile aromatic compounds it contains. When scientists looked more closely at this effect, they discovered that oregano essential oil actually improves the integrity of the intestinal barrier, which could guard against conditions like "leaky gut syndrome" or a compromised gut lining.[252] That's why I often include oregano in food. Of course, oregano is where oregano oil comes from, and even though the natural plant form doesn't have the highly concentrated oil you would get from an essential oil, it does have all the other plant properties that are "packaged" with that oil. Another study demonstrated that in the treatment of small intestinal bacterial overgrowth (SIBO), herbal remedies that included oregano oil, red thyme oil, and sage leaf extract were just as effective as the drug rifaximin (a prescription antibiotic), with virtually no side effects (the drug had many serious side effects).[253] Science is only beginning to understand the power and potency of herbal medicine, but in the meantime, using plenty of natural herbs and spices in your food couldn't hurt and might have real therapeutic value for the health of your microbiome.

HOMEMADE MARINARA SAUCE

MAKES ABOUT 3 CUPS

TIME: 30 MINUTES

Marinara sauce is another staple that you can buy in the store, but most packaged brands are filled with sugar. Marinara is so much better—more flavorful and fresh, not to mention sugar-free—if you make your own. And it's easy! Next time you need marinara, make this recipe and save any leftovers in the freezer.

1 teaspoon olive oil (not extra-virgin)
2 cloves garlic, peeled and smashed
One 28-ounce can crushed tomatoes (or fresh, peeled tomatoes, chopped, to make about 4 cups)
1 teaspoon dried oregano, crumbled
½ teaspoon sea salt
¼ teaspoon black pepper
2 tablespoons chopped fresh basil

Heat a large saucepan over medium heat and add the olive oil. When it's hot, add the garlic and sauté for just a minute. Stir in the tomatoes, oregano, and salt and pepper. Reduce the heat to medium low and simmer for an additional 15 to 20 minutes, stirring often to prevent sticking. Stir in the basil and serve warm.

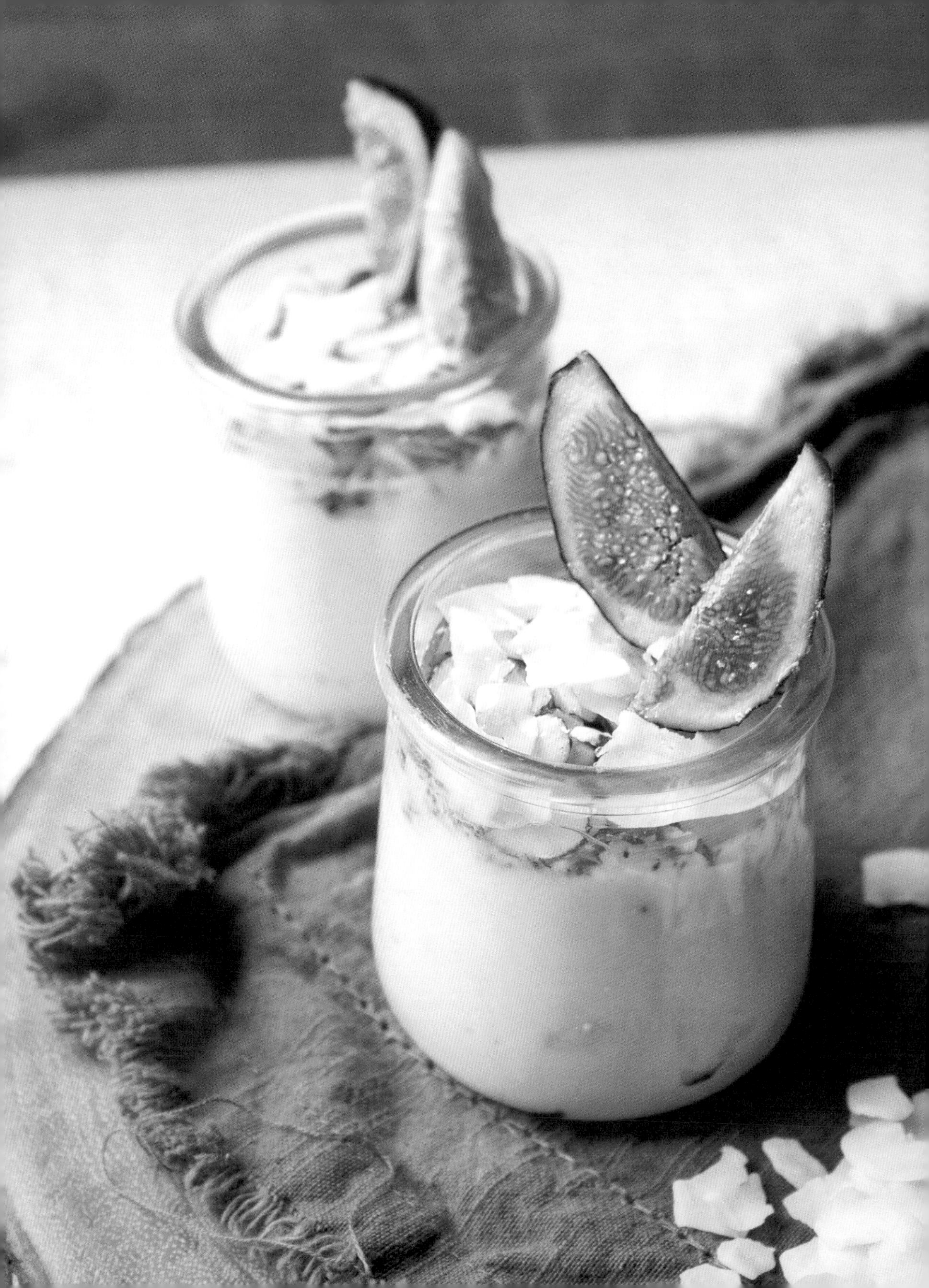

FRESH FIG YOGURT CUPS

SERVES 2

TIME: 10 MINUTES

This easy morning yogurt cup features Mediterranean flavors with a pleasing crunch from almonds, coconut, and chia seeds. Full of prebiotic-rich toppings and probiotic yogurt, it's a double dose of microbiome goodness.

1½ cups plain, unsweetened nonfat or low-fat dairy yogurt or plant-based yogurt
Honey or maple syrup to taste (optional, 1 tablespoon max)
2 fresh figs, cut in half or chopped
¼ cup sliced almonds
¼ cup toasted unsweetened shredded or flaked coconut (stir it in a dry pan over medium-low heat for a few minutes until it smells toasty, or purchase pretoasted)
1 teaspoon chia seeds

In a small bowl, combine the yogurt and honey, if using. Divide the yogurt between two serving cups. Top each cup with half of the figs, almonds, coconut, and chia seeds.

GOLDEN MILK YOGURT PARFAITS

SERVES 2

TIME: 10 MINUTES

Golden milk is a warm, immunity-boosting drink spiced with turmeric, cinnamon, and a touch of real maple syrup (see the recipe on page 255). While this recipe doesn't contain actual prepared golden milk, it is inspired by it, and contains those same flavors in a sweet treat using yogurt instead of milk. You'll get the anti-inflammatory benefits of turmeric along with all the benefits of probiotics in the yogurt.

1½ cups plain, unsweetened nonfat or low-fat dairy yogurt or plant-based yogurt
1 tablespoon turmeric powder
1 teaspoon cinnamon
Honey or maple syrup to taste (optional, 1 tablespoon max)
1 peach, cubed, for topping
¼ cup almond slices, for topping

In a small bowl, combine yogurt, turmeric powder, cinnamon, and honey (if using). Divide the yogurt between two small jars or cups and top with peaches and almonds.

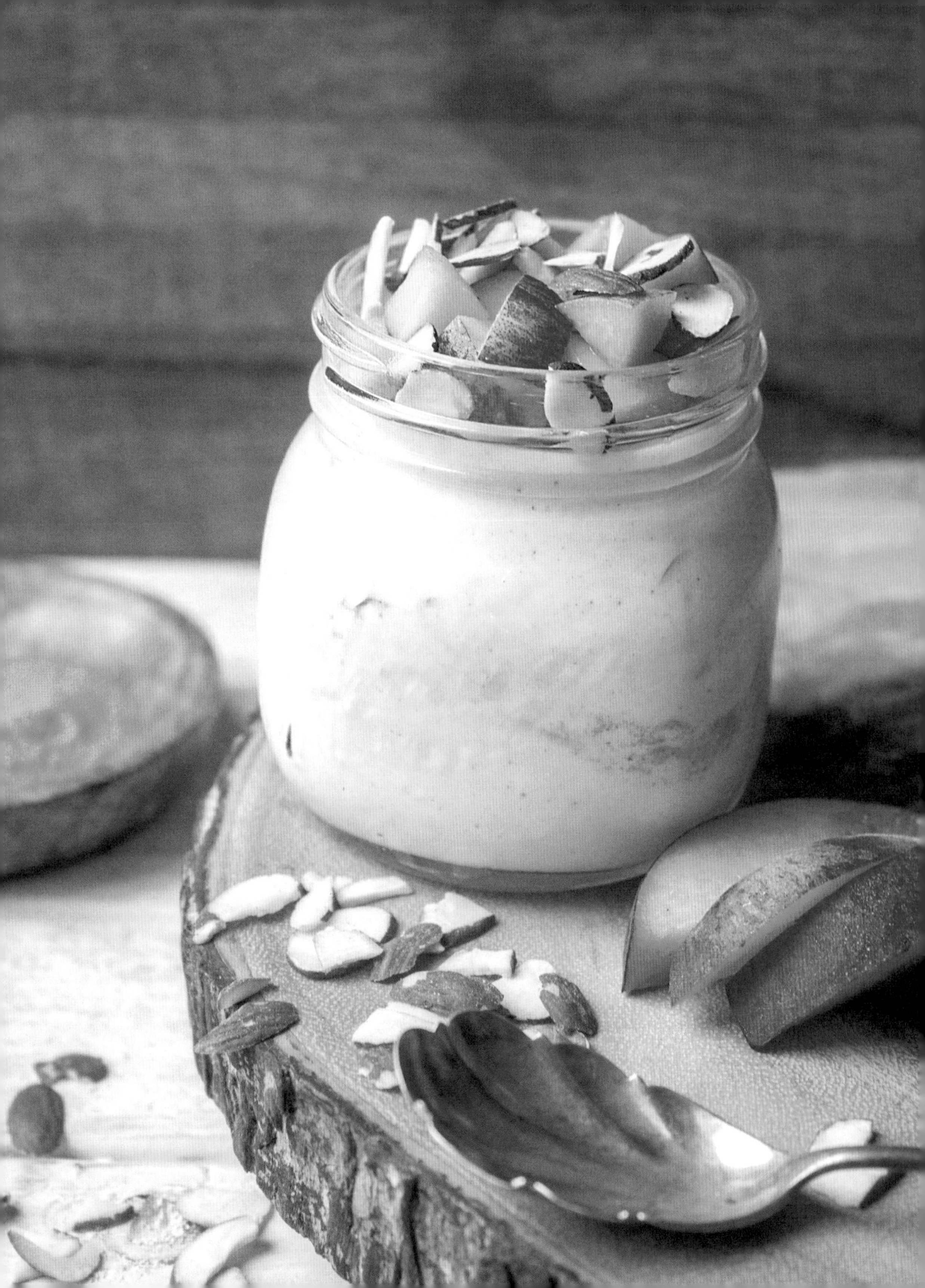

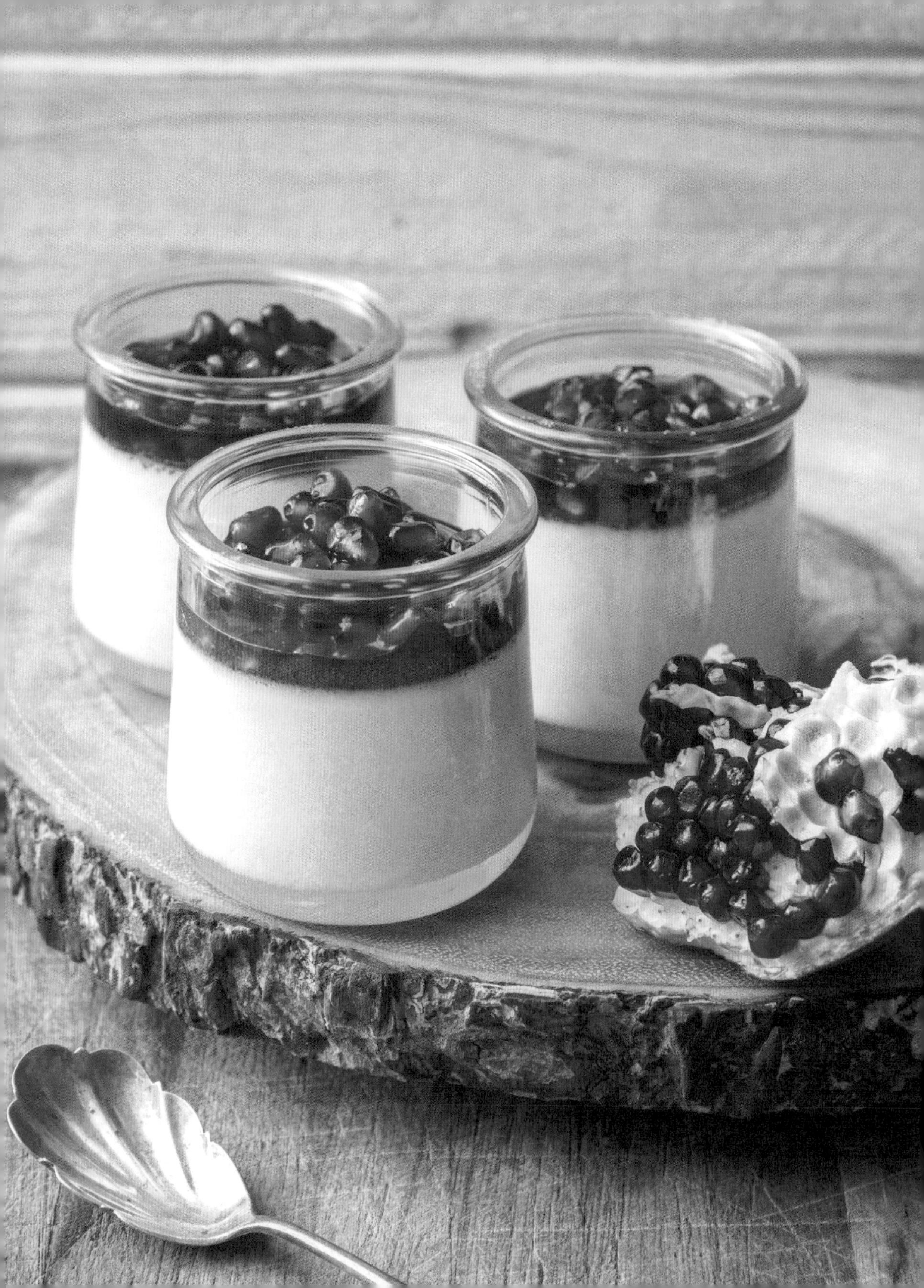

POMEGRANATE BREAKFAST PANNA COTTA

SERVES 2

TIME: 10 MINUTES (PLUS 2 HOURS TO CHILL)

Free of dairy and refined sugar, these panna cotta cups are the perfect make-ahead breakfast. Treat yourself for a refreshing and light breakfast on-the-go.

2 tablespoons water
1½ teaspoons gelatin (use 1½ teaspoons agar powder for a plant-based option)
One 13.5-ounce can coconut milk
Maple syrup to taste (optional, 1 tablespoon max)
½ cup pomegranate juice
1 cup pomegranate arils

1. In a small bowl, add the water. Sprinkle gelatin on top and let it sit for 5 minutes.

2. Add coconut milk and maple syrup, if using, to a medium saucepan over medium heat and whisk until the sweetener completely dissolves. Add the gelatin mixture and whisk until the gelatin dissolves.

3. Pour the mixture into ramekins or small cups and place in the refrigerator for at least two hours. Once the panna cotta is set, pour the pomegranate juice evenly on top and sprinkle on pomegranate arils.

ROASTED STRAWBERRY YOGURT CUP WITH PISTACHIOS

SERVES 2

TIME: 25 TO 30 MINUTES

With only four ingredients, this goes down as one of the easiest breakfasts ever, as long as you have a few extra minutes to roast the strawberries. Roasting brings out their natural, gooey sweetness. Crushed pistachios add a crunchy texture and a dose of microbiome food. Swirled together on top of yogurt, the result is sublime.

1 pint fresh strawberries
Honey or maple syrup to taste (optional, 1 tablespoon max)
1½ cups plain, unsweetened nonfat or low-fat dairy yogurt or plant-based yogurt
2 tablespoons crushed pistachios

1. Preheat the oven to 400°F. Remove the stems from the strawberries and slice them into halves. Put them in a baking dish and toss with honey, if using.

2. Bake the strawberries for 15 to 20 minutes or until they start to bubble and soften. Remove them from the oven and set them aside to cool. Spoon yogurt into two cups, then top with warm strawberries and crushed pistachios.

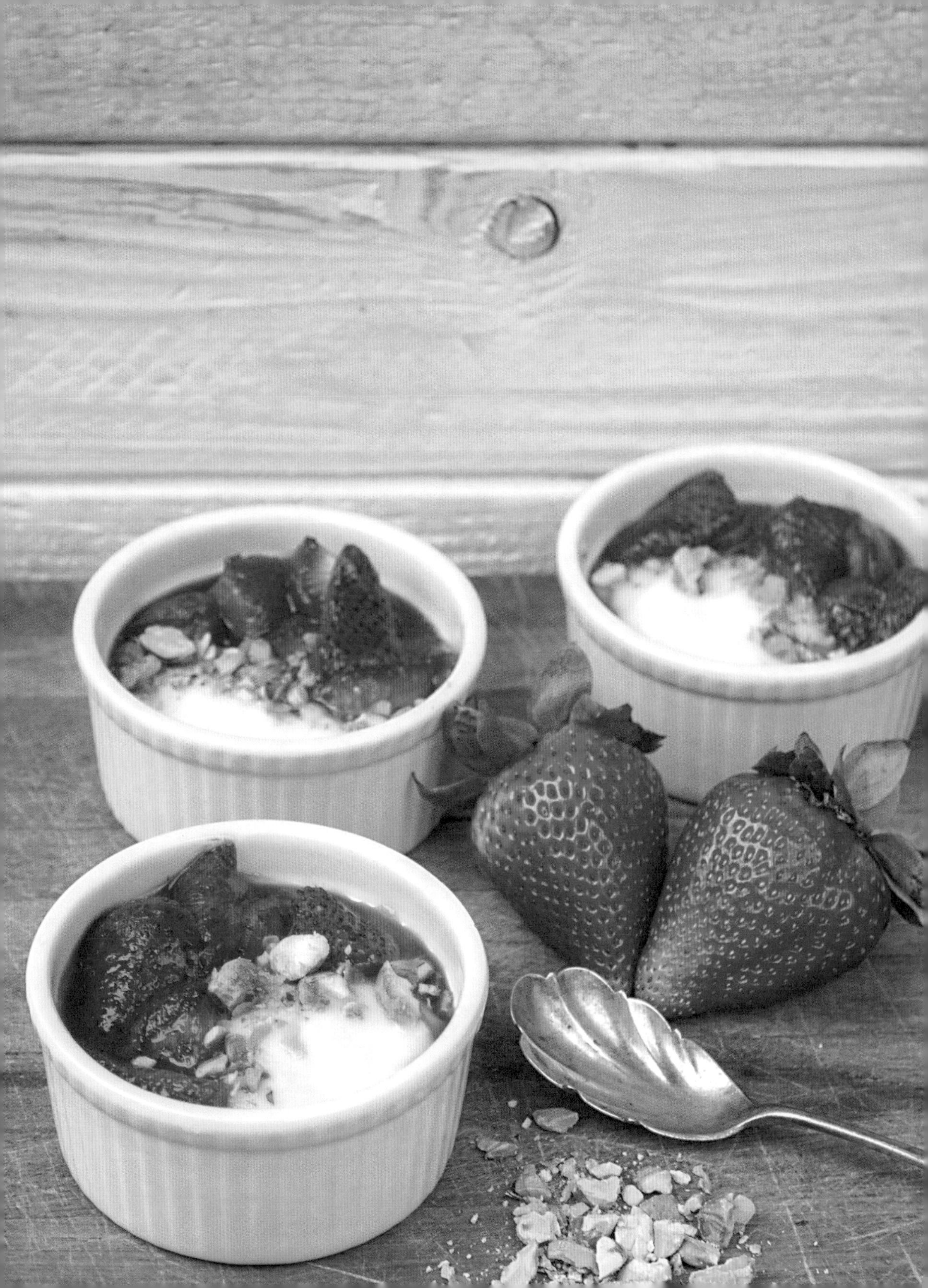

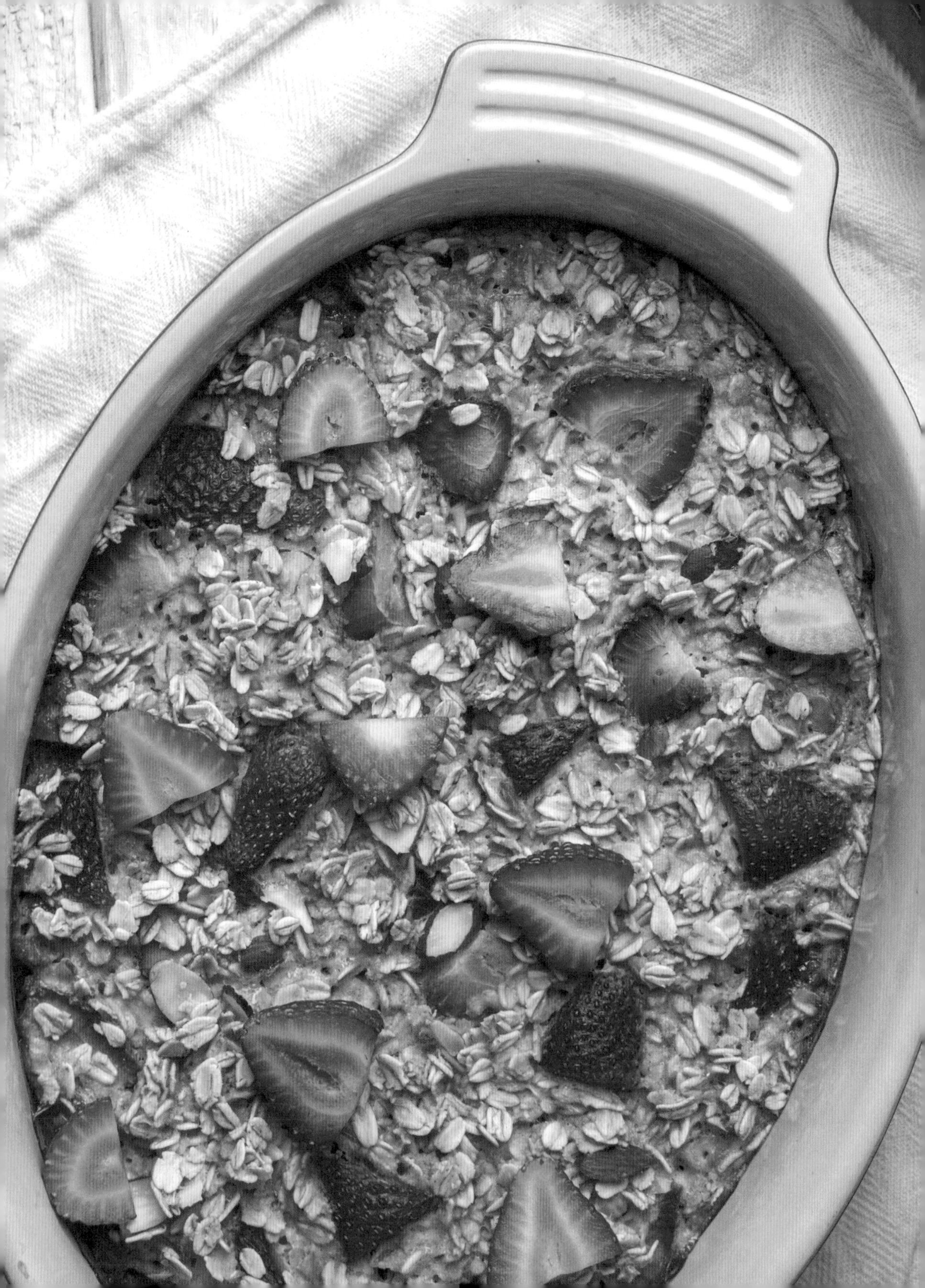

STRAWBERRY BREAKFAST BAKE

SERVES 2

TIME: 35 MINUTES

This strawberry granola bake tastes great on its own, or you can use it to top yogurt or smoothie bowls. It is subtly sweet without excess sugar and contains your daily dose of fiber and plenty of manganese to help you stay awake and alert in the mornings. For grain-free variations, see the recipe notes.

1 pint strawberries
2 cups old-fashioned oats
1 cup nonfat or low-fat dairy milk or unsweetened plant-based milk (see the recipe for Homemade Almond Milk, page 156)
1 egg (or ½ cup applesauce)
1 ripe banana, mashed
¼ cup sliced almonds
1 teaspoon baking powder
1 teaspoon cinnamon
1 teaspoon maple syrup (optional, 1 teaspoon max)
1 teaspoon sea salt

1. Preheat oven to 350°F and grease a medium baking pan.

2. Slice the strawberries into quarters or thin slices. Set aside half the strawberries.

3. Combine the other half of the strawberries and the rest of the ingredients in a bowl and then pour the mixture into the pan. Bake 30 minutes or until cooked through. Top with the remaining sliced strawberries. Serve warm.

Gluten-free variation: Use certified gluten-free oats.

Grain-free variation: In place of the oatmeal, increase the sliced almonds to ½ cup and add 1 additional egg. Also add 1 cup shredded apple and/or shredded sweet potato.

SWEET POTATO HASH AND FRIED EGGS

SERVES 2

TIME: 30 MINUTES

Some mornings call for a hearty breakfast, and for those mornings, try this sweet potato hash with fried eggs. It will give you that warm comfort-food feeling all day. For a plant-based version, see the recipe notes.

2 sweet potatoes or yams
2 tablespoons coconut oil, divided
2 eggs
½ teaspoon sea salt
¼ teaspoon black pepper
1 bunch cilantro, chopped

1. Peel and cube sweet potatoes. In a medium skillet or pan, heat one tablespoon of the coconut oil until melted. Add sweet potatoes, cook on medium until you can pierce them easily with a fork, about 10 minutes, stirring frequently. Set aside.

2. In a small skillet, add the other tablespoon of coconut oil on low heat. Once the oil is hot, crack eggs and cook until the whites are cooked through. Serve eggs over sweet potatoes and season with salt, pepper, and cilantro.

Plant-based variation: Substitute two slices of extra-firm tofu (about 3 ounces total) for the eggs. Cook them as you would cook the eggs. You can sprinkle them with nutritional yeast while frying for a more egg-y taste.

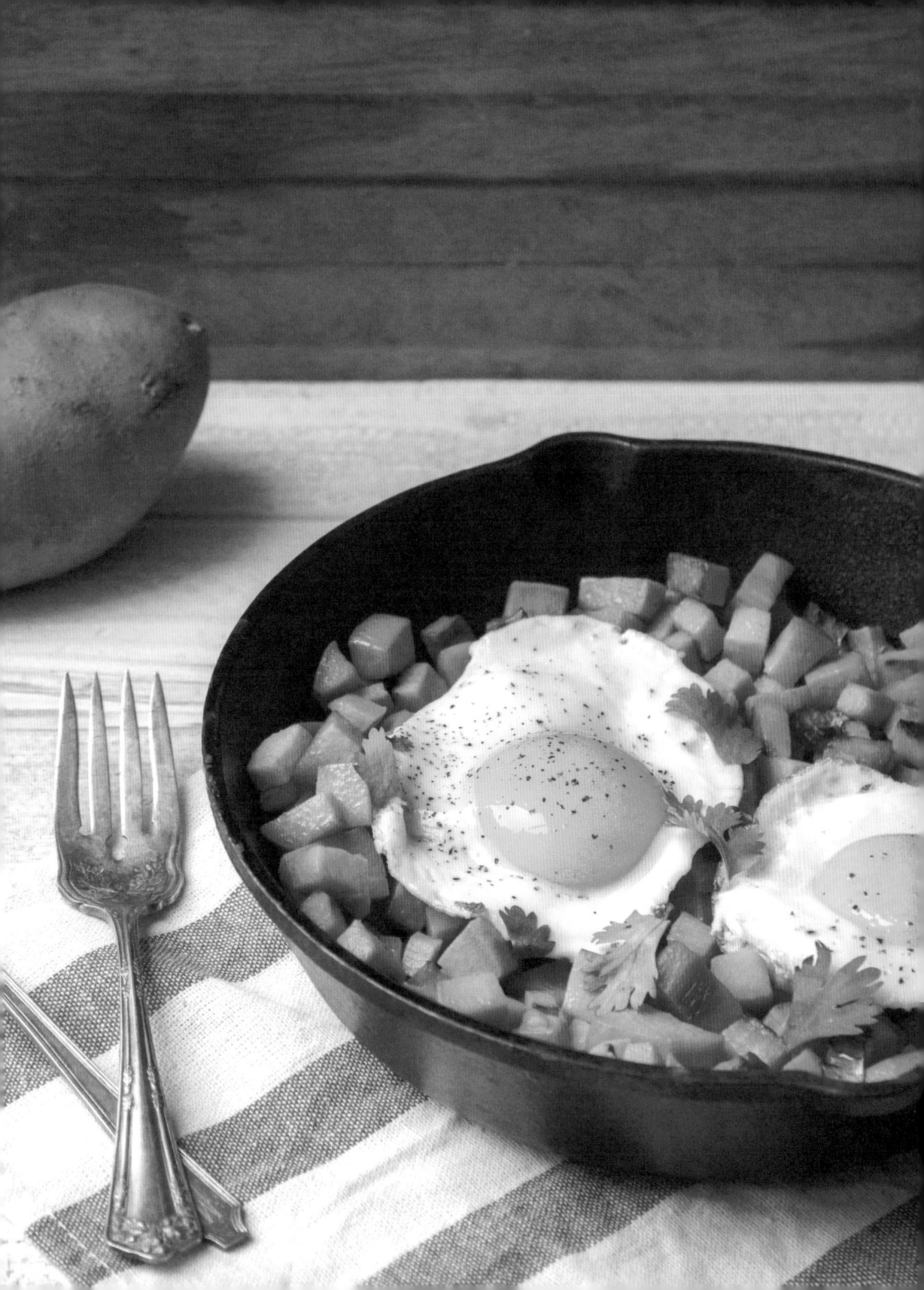

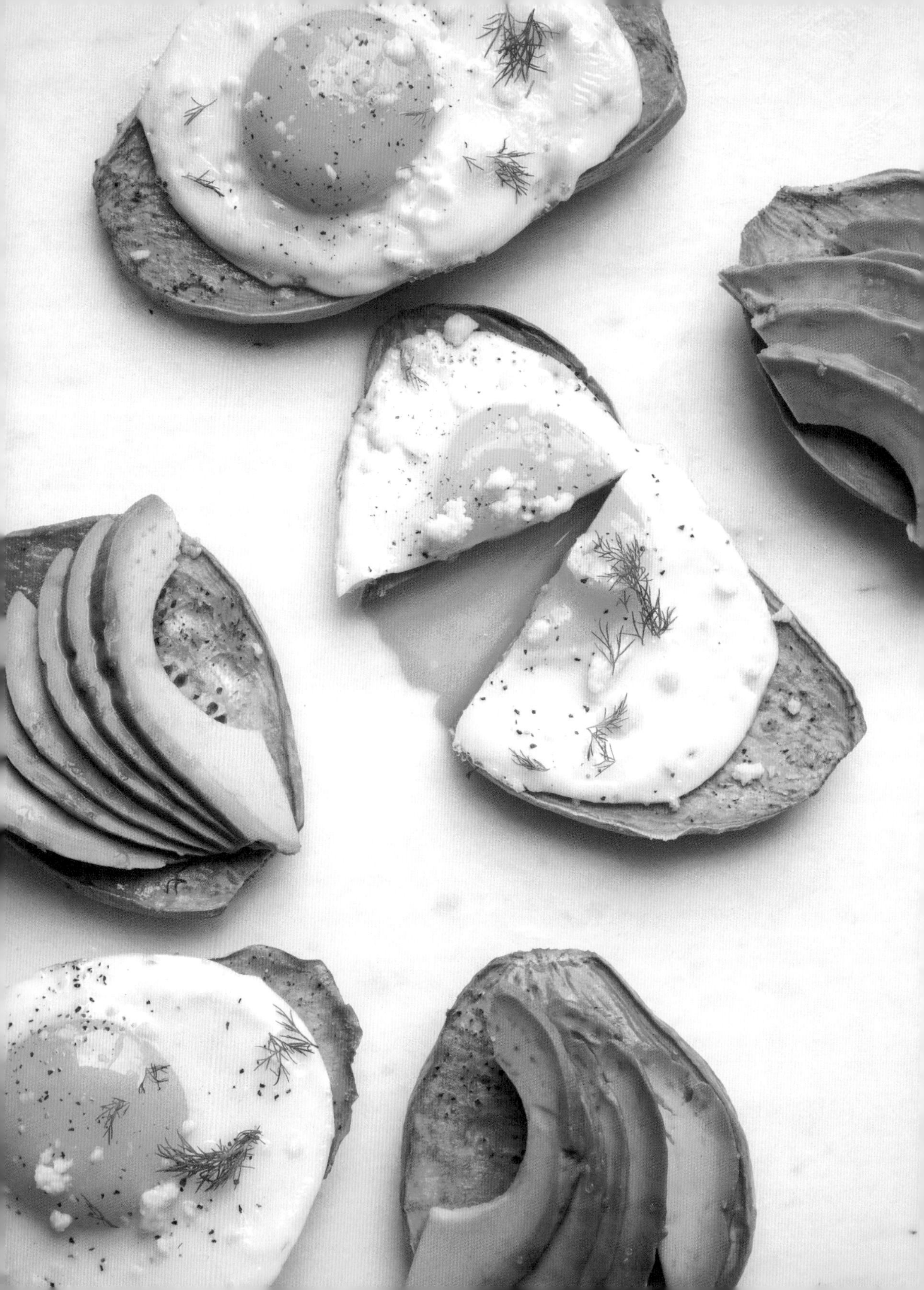

SWEET POTATO "TOAST"

SERVES 2

TIME: 30 MINUTES

Swap out bread for nutrient-richer sweet potatoes. They contain fiber, resistant starch, and magnesium, making them an excellent facilitator for healthy microbiome balance. Top them off with your choice of eggs or avocado (or both), sprinkle with low-fat or fat-free cheese, and you have a perfectly balanced breakfast. For more plant-based ideas, see the recipe note.

2 large sweet potatoes
1 tablespoon olive oil, divided
½ teaspoon sea salt
¼ teaspoon black pepper
3 eggs and/or 1 large avocado, pitted, peeled, and sliced
Nonfat cotija cheese (or other crumbly nonfat or low-fat cheese)
Fresh dill, chopped

1. Preheat oven to 375°F. Cut the sweet potato lengthwise into 1-inch-thick slices. Brush with some of the olive oil and salt and pepper. Place on a baking sheet and bake for 15 to 20 minutes or until soft.

2. In a pan over low heat, add the rest of the oil and fry the eggs (if using) until the white is cooked through. Top each sweet potato slice with eggs and/or avocado slices. Sprinkle with cheese, salt and pepper, and dill.

Plant-based variations: You can leave out the egg and just use avocado, or you can substitute three 1-ounce slices of extra-firm tofu for the eggs. Use vegan "Parmesan" or nutritional yeast in place of the cheese.

LUNCHES

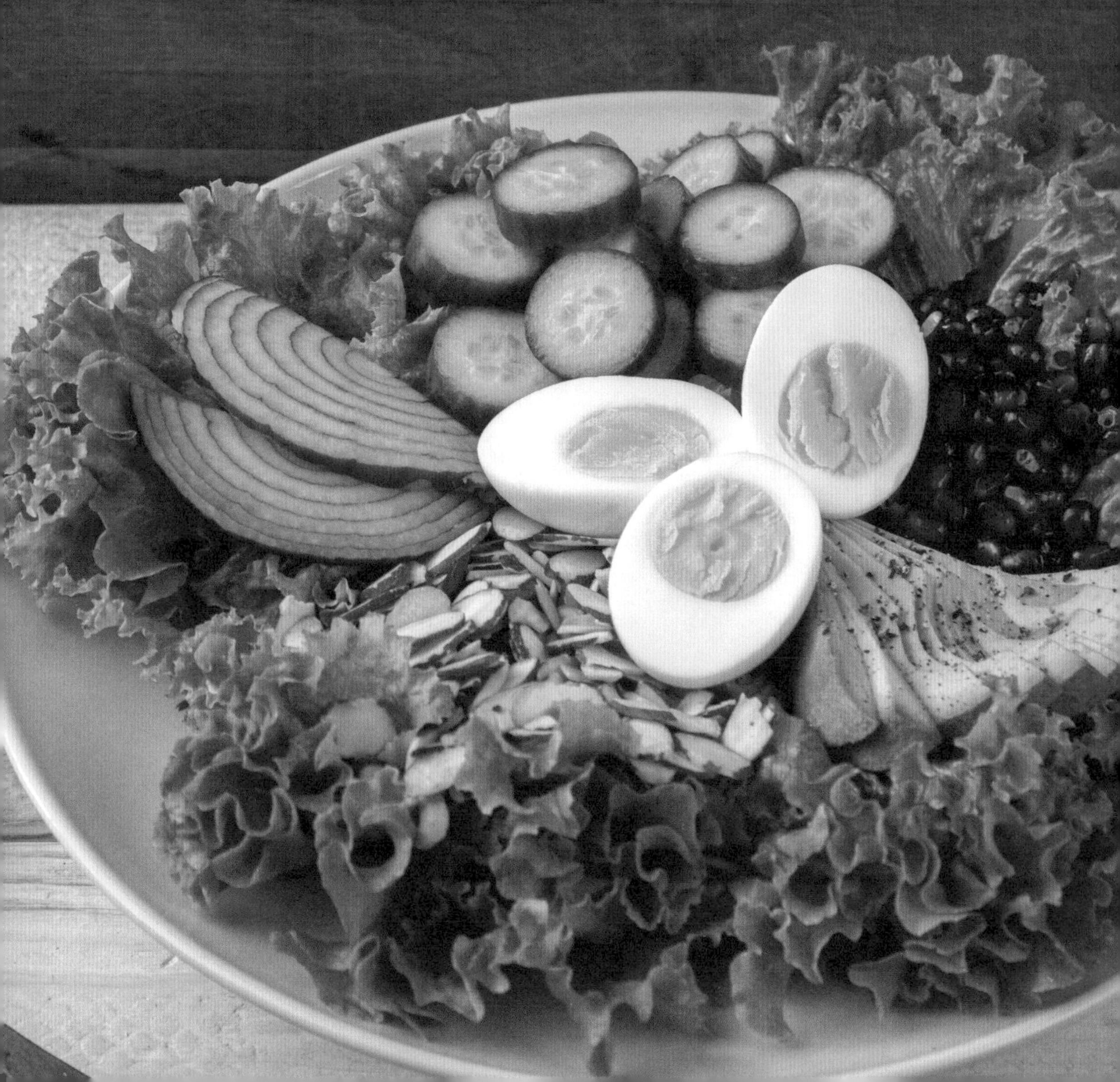

AVOCADO AND GREEN TOMATO SALAD

SERVES 2

TIME: 15 MINUTES

Here's a lunch salad perfect for the tomato lover—heirloom varieties make this even more special. This salad is full of vibrant, green watercress, avocado, and snap peas, and is sprinkled with lemon juice and sesame seeds.

1 cup watercress
3 green heirloom tomatoes, sliced
8 to 10 cherry tomatoes
1 avocado, sliced
5 snap pea pods
1 lemon, juiced
1 tablespoon sesame seeds
½ teaspoon sea salt

Put the watercress on a plate. Next, layer tomatoes, avocado, and peas on top of the watercress. Squeeze lemon juice on top, then sprinkle with sesame seeds and salt.

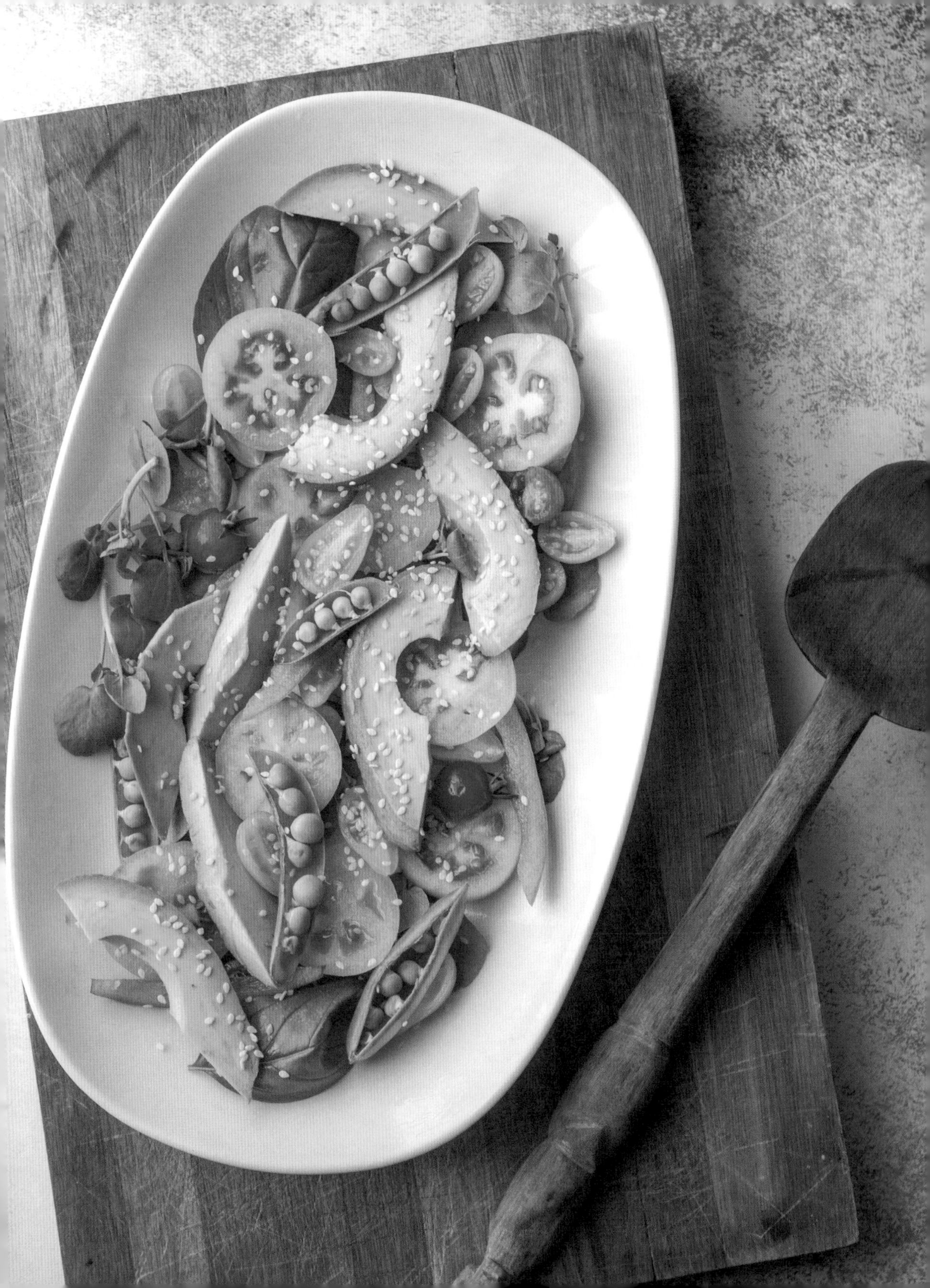

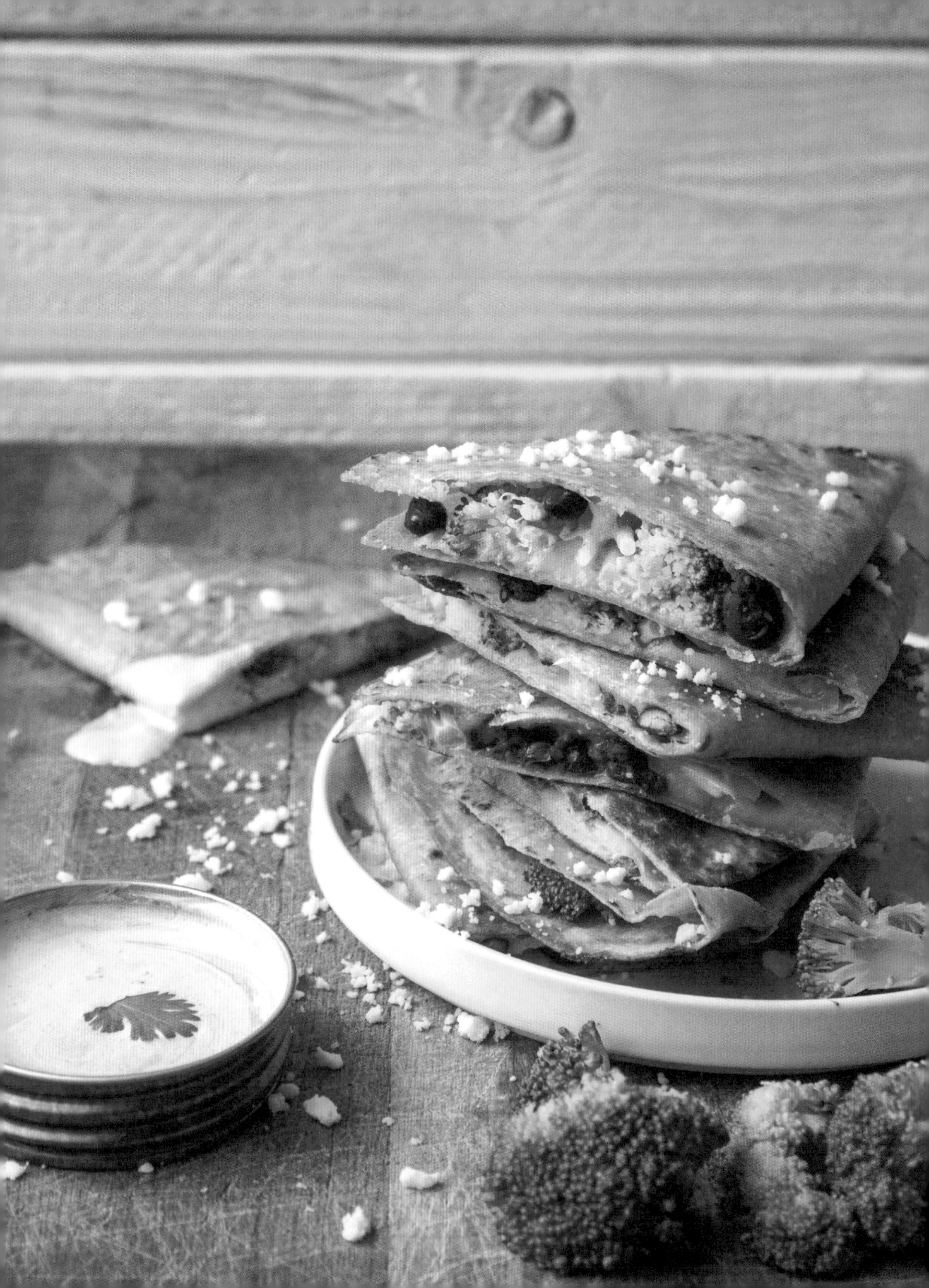

BROCCOLI BLACK BEAN QUESADILLAS

SERVES 2

TIME: 35 MINUTES

Take this Mexican favorite to a healthier level by filling it with broccoli, black beans, and melted mozzarella. Heat it with coconut oil and serve with a yummy spicy yogurt sauce that's perfect for dipping.

1 head broccoli, washed and cut into florets
1 teaspoon sea salt
One 15-ounce can black beans
1 tablespoon coconut oil
Two 10- to 12-inch whole wheat, sprouted grain, gluten-free, or grain-free tortillas
1 cup nonfat mozzarella cheese, shredded (or use shredded nondairy cheese or ½ cup hummus)
Feta cheese, optional
Spicy Yogurt Dipping Sauce (recipe follows)

1. Fill a large saucepan with water and bring it to a boil. Add the broccoli and salt. Reduce the heat to a simmer. Cook until the broccoli is tender and bright green, about 5 minutes. Drain and chop the florets coarsely. Set aside.

2. Drain and rinse the beans. Set aside.

3. In a large skillet, heat the coconut oil over medium heat. Add one tortilla. Quickly add half the cheese (or hummus), broccoli pieces, and black beans to one side of a tortilla. Fold over the other side. Repeat with the other tortilla and fillings.

CONTINUED

4. When one side is golden-brown, about 3 minutes, carefully flip the quesadillas over and brown the other side, then remove them to a plate to cool slightly. Top them with the feta cheese, if you are using it. Serve with the Spicy Yogurt Dipping Sauce.

SPICY YOGURT DIPPING SAUCE

MAKES ABOUT ½ CUP

TIME: 2 MINUTES

½ cup plain, unsweetened nonfat or low-fat dairy yogurt
or plant-based yogurt
1 teaspoon chipotle powder
1 tablespoon lime juice
1 teaspoon sea salt

In a small bowl, add all the ingredients and mix until fully combined. Serve it with the quesadillas, for dipping.

CHICKEN QUINOA SOUP

SERVES 2

TIME: 35 MINUTES

It's chicken noodle soup without so many starchy carbs. Quinoa stands in for the noodles, so you get more iron and protein as well as hearty texture and rich flavor. The precooked chicken makes prepping this soup a breeze, so you spend more time eating and less time in the kitchen. For grain-free and plant-based variations, see the recipe notes.

1 tablespoon olive oil
3 carrots, diced
3 stalks celery, diced
½ onion, diced
2 cloves garlic, minced
3 tablespoons whole wheat flour
4 cups chicken or vegetable broth
1 cup water
⅔ cup uncooked quinoa
1 rotisserie chicken, shredded
1 teaspoon sea salt
1 teaspoon paprika

1. Heat the oil in a large soup pot over medium-high heat. Add carrots, celery, onions, and garlic. Sauté until the vegetables start to soften, about 3 minutes. Stir in flour, and completely coat the vegetables with it. Slowly whisk in broth and water. Make sure the flour is mixed in and no lumps remain.

2. Reduce heat to medium-low and stir in the quinoa. Cover and simmer for 15 minutes, stirring occasionally. Add the chicken and seasonings, and simmer for another 10 minutes on low heat.

Grain-free variation: Replace the flour with cassava or almond flour, or any finely ground nuts or seeds, and use coarsely chopped chickpeas in place of the quinoa.
Plant-based variation: Instead of chicken, crumble an 8-ounce block of tempeh into the soup.

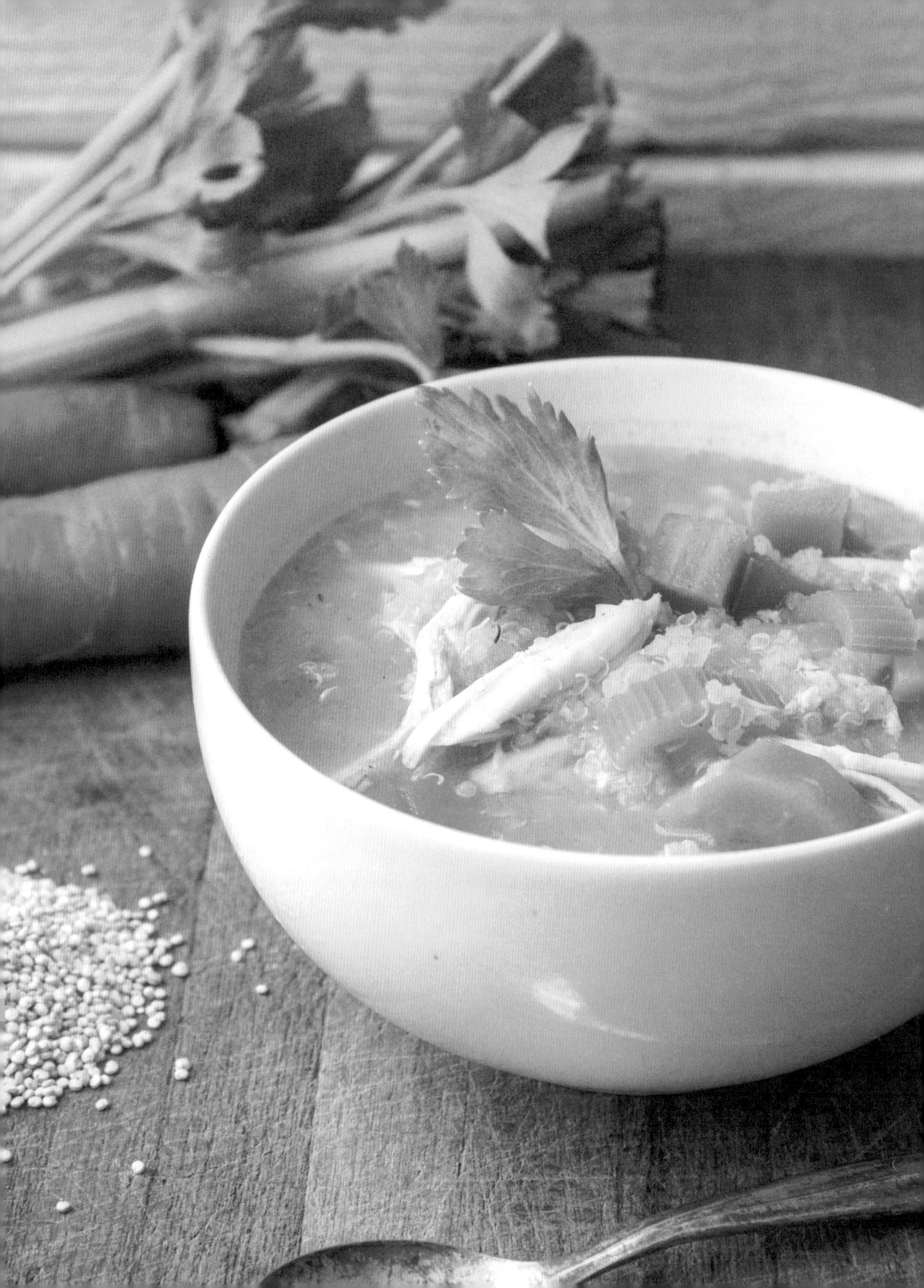

Carley's Corner: Chicken Bone Broth

Bone broth is an incredible superfood full of nutrients that help support the body's immune system. For one, broth is high in L-glutamine, an amino acid that is a building block of protein. As well, the collagen and cartilage (the connective tissues) in the broth are helpful in rebuilding gut lining. It is also full of vitamins and minerals, so it is great for hydration and replenishing your body's nutrients. Bone broth is recently widely available in most stores, but it can be pricey. I recommend making this recipe at home, which is best made in a slow cooker, or quickly in a pressure cooker. Sip it throughout the day or add to any soup for a nourishing and nutrient-dense meal. Plus, you can use it in almost any recipe like Beet Hummus (see page 262) or Cauliflower Rice (see page 202), salad dressings, marinades, and so much more.

1 chicken carcass or whole chicken (thawed or frozen)
6 carrots, chopped
4 celery stalks, chopped
1 yellow onion, chopped, skin on
1 small sweet potato, chopped
6 black peppercorns
3 bay leaves
1 teaspoon sea salt
A splash of apple cider vinegar (optional, to extract more nutrients from the bones)

Place all the ingredients in a slow cooker or in a pressure cooker. Cover the bones with filtered water and cook in the slow cooker on low 8 to 24 hours, or in the pressure cooker according to the instructions for bone broth or soup (or for about one hour on high). Strain and store in air-tight containers or Mason jars in the refrigerator. Broth generally stays fresh for approximately one week in the fridge or frozen for a year. You could also freeze it in ice cube trays and pop out a few whenever you need them.

CHICKPEA VEGETABLE WRAP

SERVES 2

TIME: 15 MINUTES

Wrapping raw vegetables, chickpeas, and hummus inside a whole-wheat tortilla is so simple that it makes lunch prep a breeze. Make these a few days ahead so that there's no temptation to go through the drive-thru.

2 carrots, trimmed and scraped or peeled
1 cucumber, optionally peeled
¼ red cabbage
½ cup hummus (store-bought or make Beet Hummus, page 262)
Two 10-inch whole wheat, gluten-free, or grain-free tortillas
1 cup cooked chickpeas

Slice the carrots and cucumber into long, thin slices and then chop the cabbage. Add hummus to each tortilla then pile the vegetables and chickpeas in the center. Roll them up and slice in half.

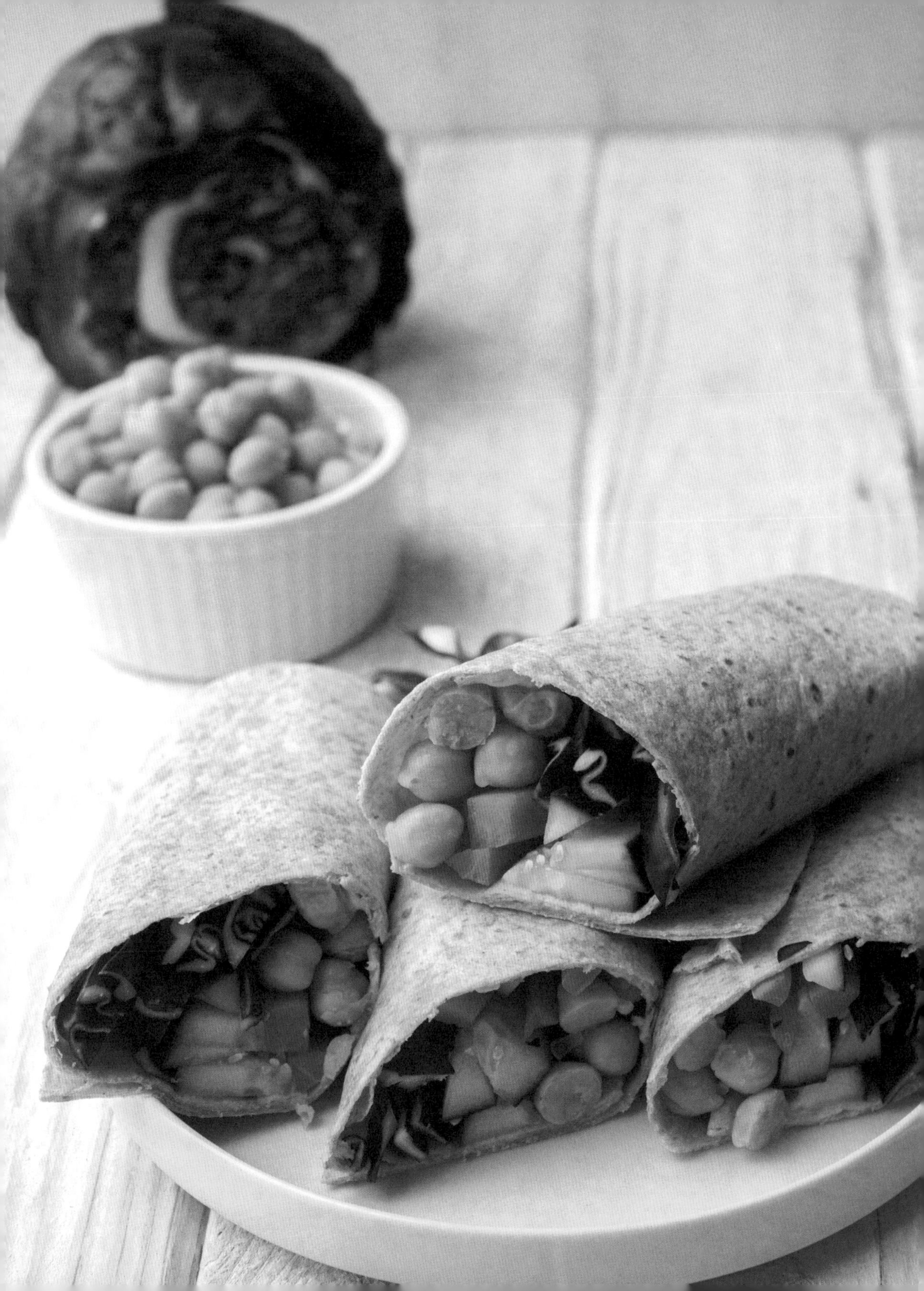

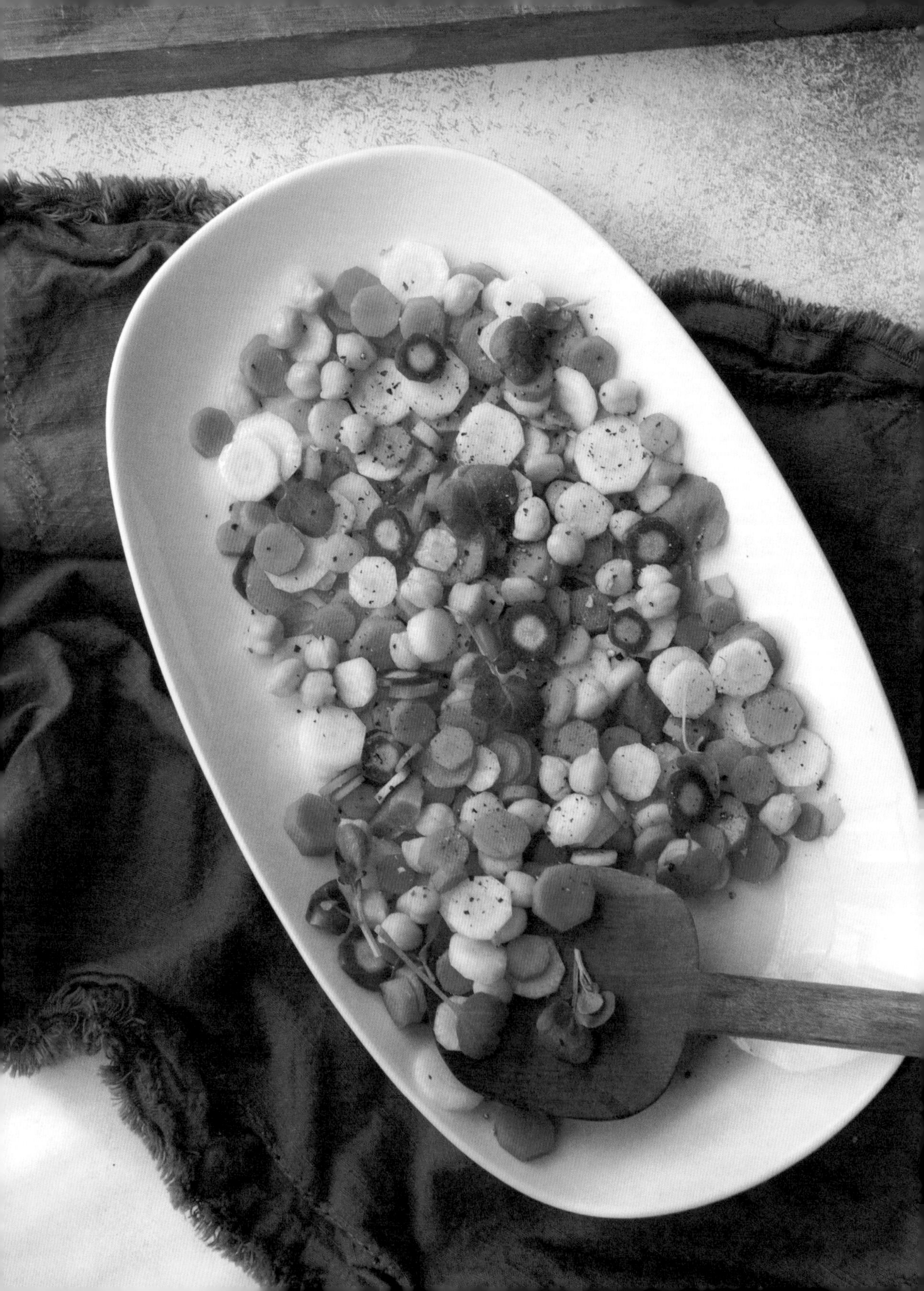

HERITAGE CARROT SALAD

SERVES 2

TIME: 10 MINUTES

With beta carotene, fiber, and vitamin A, carrots make an obvious choice to add to your salad. Not only are they nutritionally dense, but heritage or heirloom varieties taste amazing, especially when drizzled with this savory vinaigrette and sprinkled with lemon pepper.

6 heritage carrots, peeled
½ cup watercress
1 tablespoon lemon pepper
Homemade Vinaigrette Dressing (recipe follows)

Thinly slice carrots and arrange the slices on a large plate with watercress. Season with lemon pepper and drizzle with Homemade Vinaigrette Dressing.

HOMEMADE VINAIGRETTE DRESSING

MAKES ABOUT ¾ CUP

TIME: 5 MINUTES

½ cup extra-virgin olive oil
¼ cup raw apple cider vinegar
½ lemon, juiced
1 teaspoon brown or Dijon mustard
½ teaspoon dried oregano, crumbled
½ teaspoon sea salt
¼ teaspoon dried thyme, crumbled
Dash of black pepper

In a small bowl, whisk together all dressing ingredients until fully combined and creamy-looking. Use immediately.

HUMMUS PLATE

SERVES 2

TIME: 10 MINUTES

The Mediterranean diet always seems to get it right when it comes to balancing flavor with nutrition. Hummus, vegetables, and olives make an excellent snack to share or a meal all its own.

1 cup hummus (store-bought or make Beet Hummus, page 262)
Lettuce, for garnish
6 ounces kalamata olives
10 cherry tomatoes, cut in half
1 Persian cucumber, sliced
¼ cup nonfat feta cheese (optional)
½ teaspoon lemon pepper
1 tablespoon extra-virgin olive oil
Sprinkle of regular or smoked paprika

1. Spoon the hummus on half the plate. On the other side, lay down pieces of lettuce, then scatter olives, tomatoes, sliced cucumber, and feta (if you are using it) on the top.

2. Top the veggies with lemon pepper and the hummus with olive oil and paprika. Enjoy!

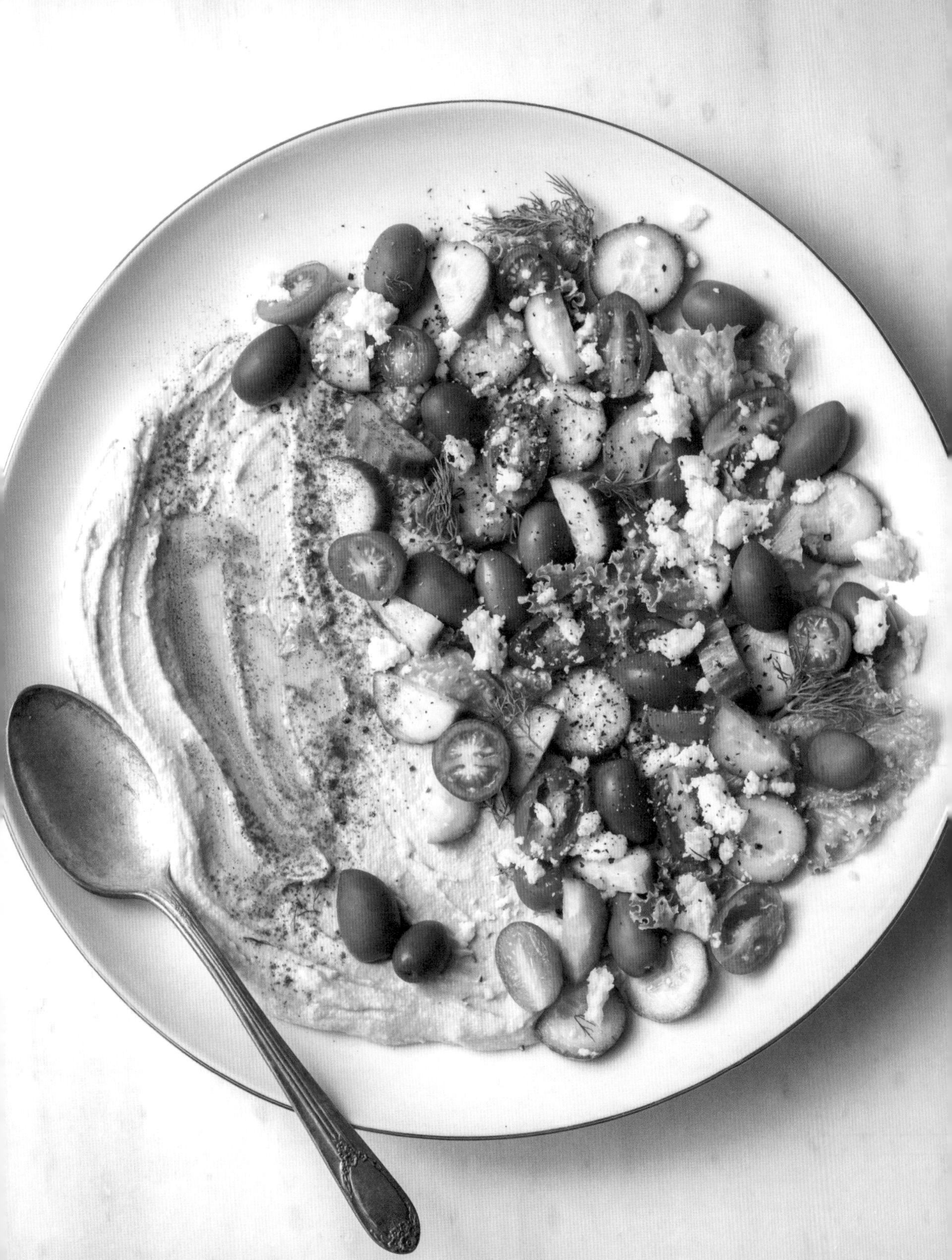

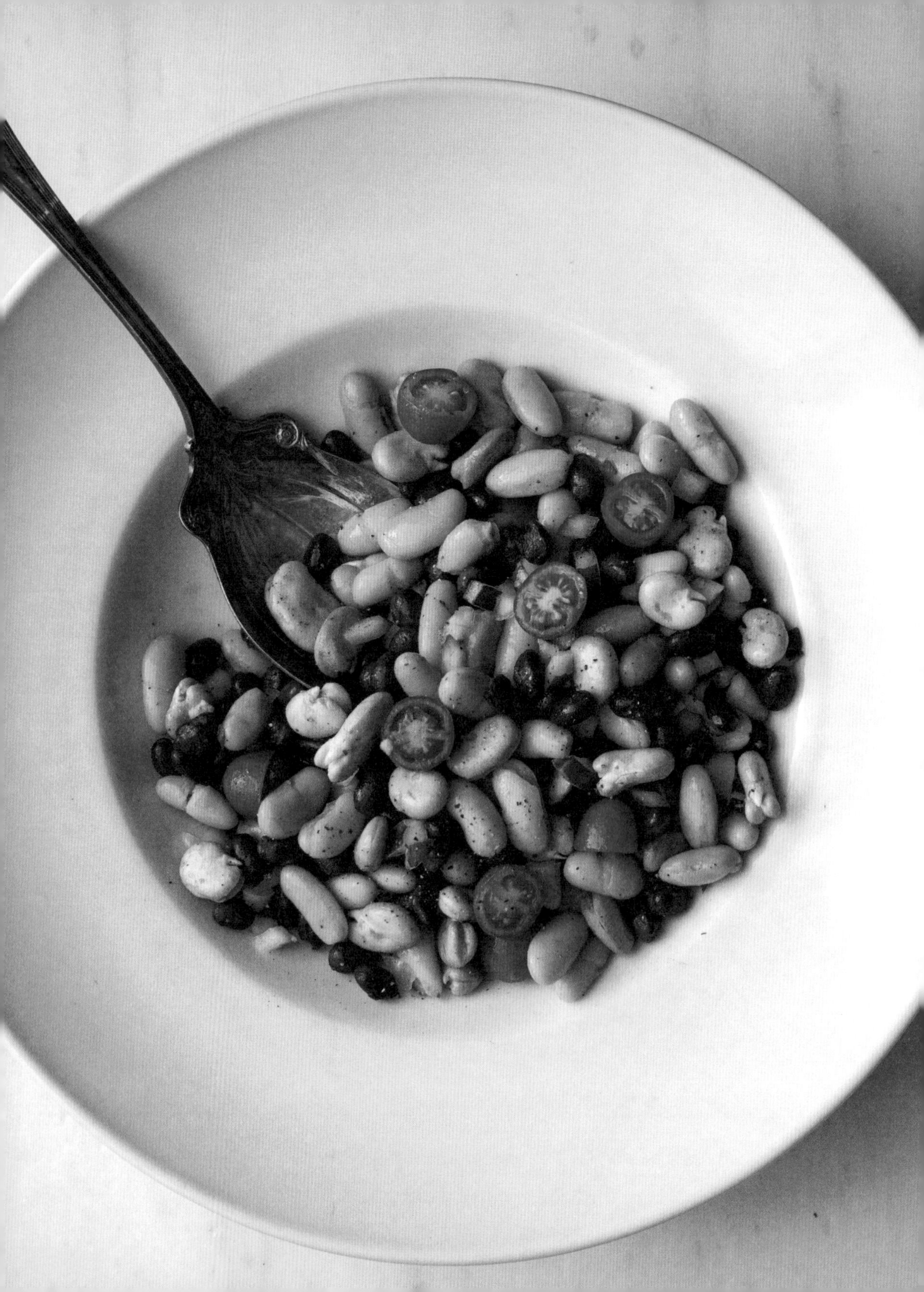

LUSCIOUS LEGUME SALAD

SERVES 2

TIME: 15 MINUTES

This salad is protein rich with good resistant starch, no meat required. It's easy to put together with canned legumes, but if you feel ambitious or have dried, soaked, and cooked legumes in your refrigerator, you can use those. You can also vary the legumes you use in this salad, according to what you have or prefer. If you can't find fava beans, you could substitute lima beans.

8 to 10 fava bean pods, seeds removed and peeled
One 15-ounce can black beans, rinsed and drained
One 15-ounce can white beans (great northern or cannellini), rinsed and drained
¼ red onion, minced
½ cup halved cherry tomatoes
½ cup freshly squeezed lemon juice
1 teaspoon sea salt
1 teaspoon black pepper

In a large saucepan, warm the fava bean pods, black beans, and white beans for at least 10 minutes, adding a little water to prevent sticking. Remove from the heat and let them cool. Combine beans, minced onions, and cherry tomatoes. Toss with lemon juice, salt, and pepper.

PEA AND RADISH SALAD

SERVES 2

TIME: 10 MINUTES

This salad is the perfect balance between sweet and savory. It features peas, radishes, cucumbers, and avocado, so you can knock out some of your daily requirements for resistant starch (peas), other MF veggies (radishes and cucumbers), and fat (avocado). Serve on a bed of artisan lettuce. For more color and texture, combine different types of lettuce.

2 cups artisan or butter lettuce
3 radishes, sliced
1 cucumber, diced
1 avocado, cubed
½ cup fresh peas
1 teaspoon sea salt
Homemade Vinaigrette Dressing (page 191) or Homemade Ranch Dressing (page 211)

Arrange lettuce on a plate. Add the rest of vegetables on top of the lettuce and season with salt. Drizzle with Homemade Vinaigrette Dressing or Homemade Ranch Dressing.

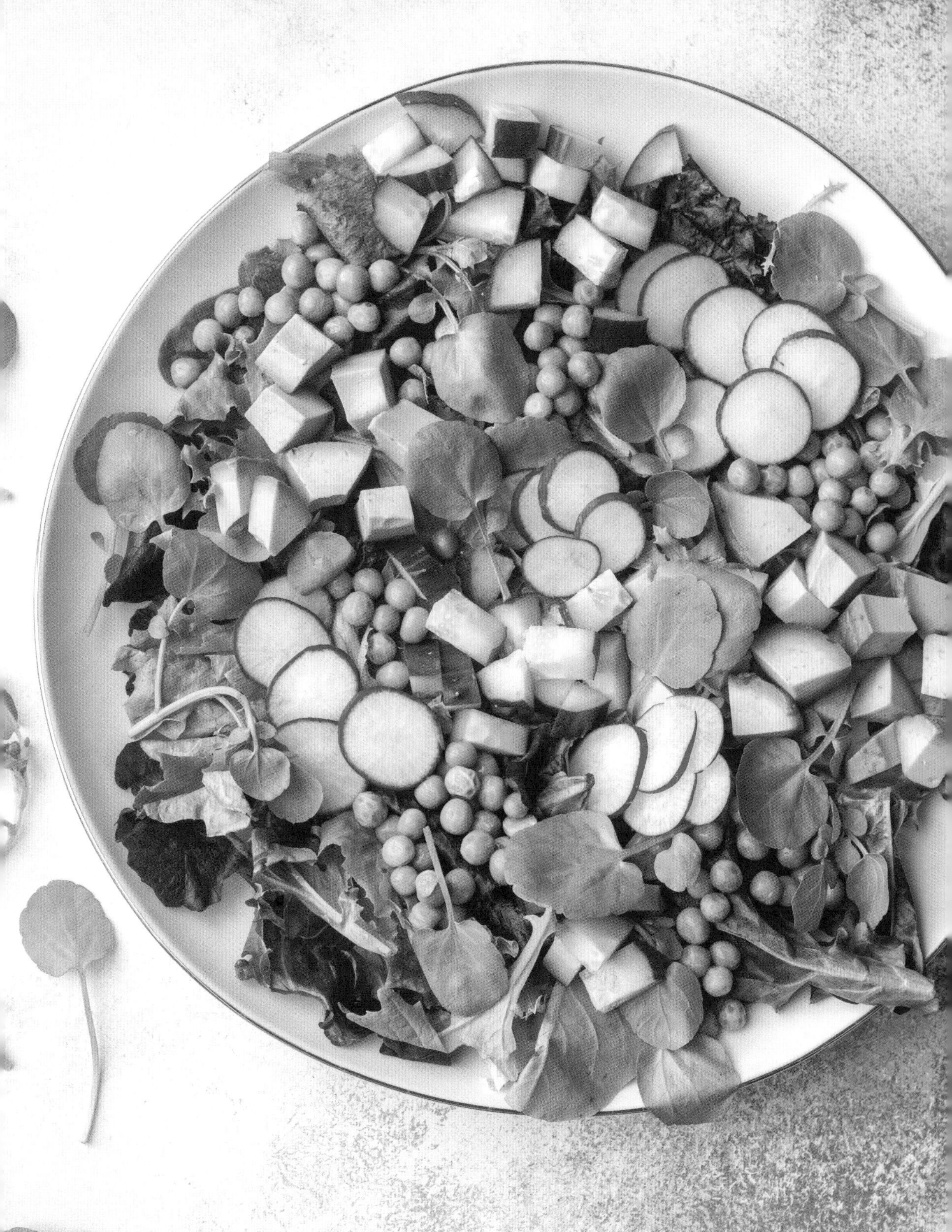

SUMMER SALAD

SERVES 2

TIME: 10 MINUTES

You can't call this colorful salad "boring," thanks to its filling eggs, almonds, a variety of vegetables, and brilliant red pomegranate arils (seed pods). Serve it up with your favorite homemade dressing and save the rest for an easy side dish for dinner that night.

1 head green leaf lettuce, washed
1 red onion, sliced
1 avocado, sliced
2 Persian cucumbers, sliced
2 hard-boiled eggs, cut in half
¼ cup sliced almonds
¼ cup pomegranate arils
1 teaspoon sea salt
1 teaspoon pepper
Homemade Vinaigrette Dressing (page 191) or Homemade Ranch Dressing (page 211)

Arrange the lettuce leaves on a plate. Arrange the onion, avocado, cucumber, eggs, almonds, and pomegranate arils over the lettuce. Season with salt and pepper. Serve with your choice of dressing, such as Homemade Vinaigrette Dressing or Homemade Ranch Dressing.

Carley's Corner: Coconut Aminos vs. Soy Sauce

Many soy sauces contain high amounts of sodium and other additives and preservatives. The good news is that you can easily substitute more natural coconut aminos to get that familiar, sweet-and-salty flavor. Derived from coconut sap, coconut aminos contain nutrients and antioxidants. Plus, they have a low glycemic index, so they shouldn't negatively impact your blood sugar. You can use this tasty sauce as a substitute for soy sauce in dressings and marinades. Sprinkle it over fish, tofu, or veggies for an added savory flavor.

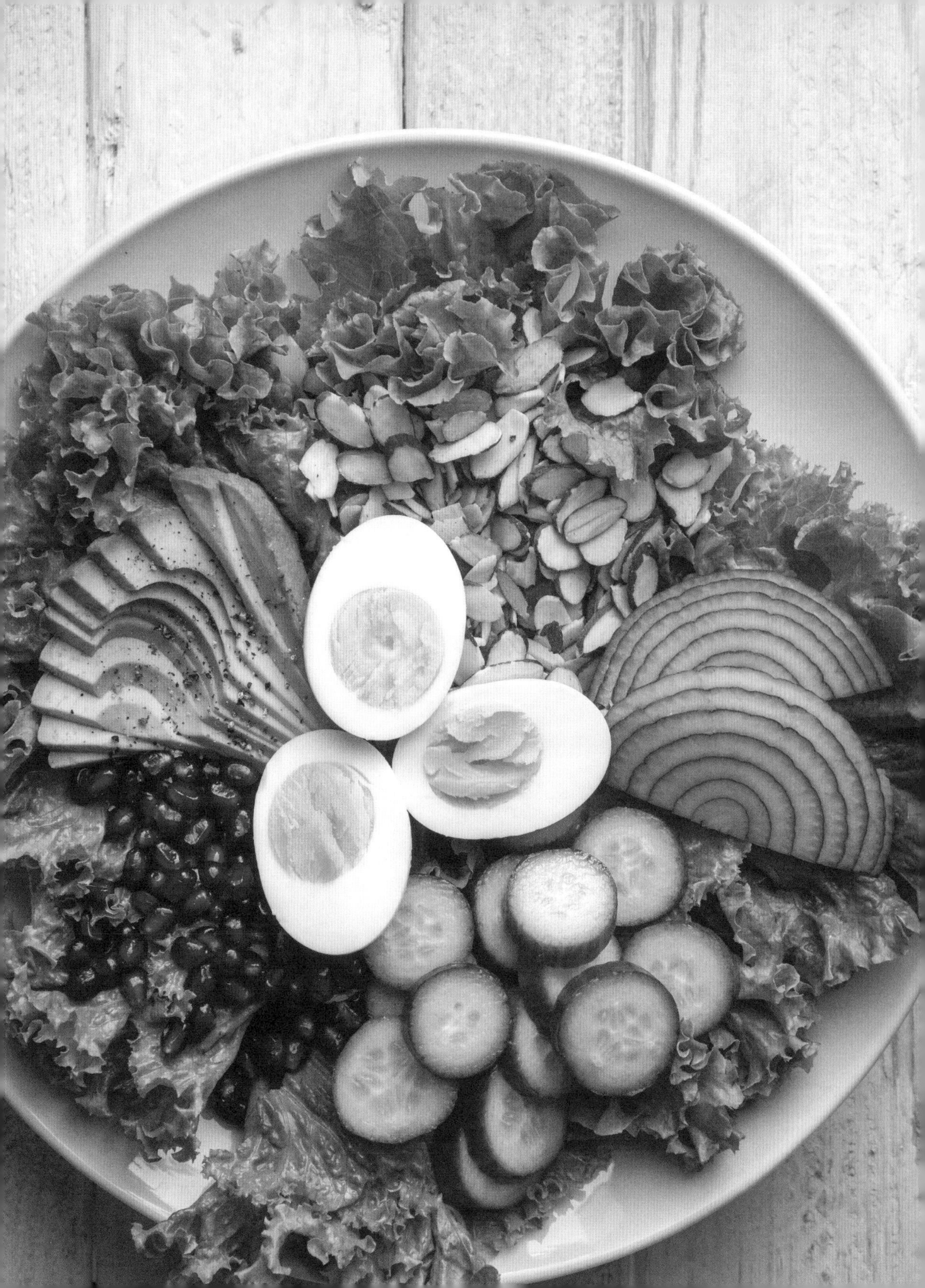

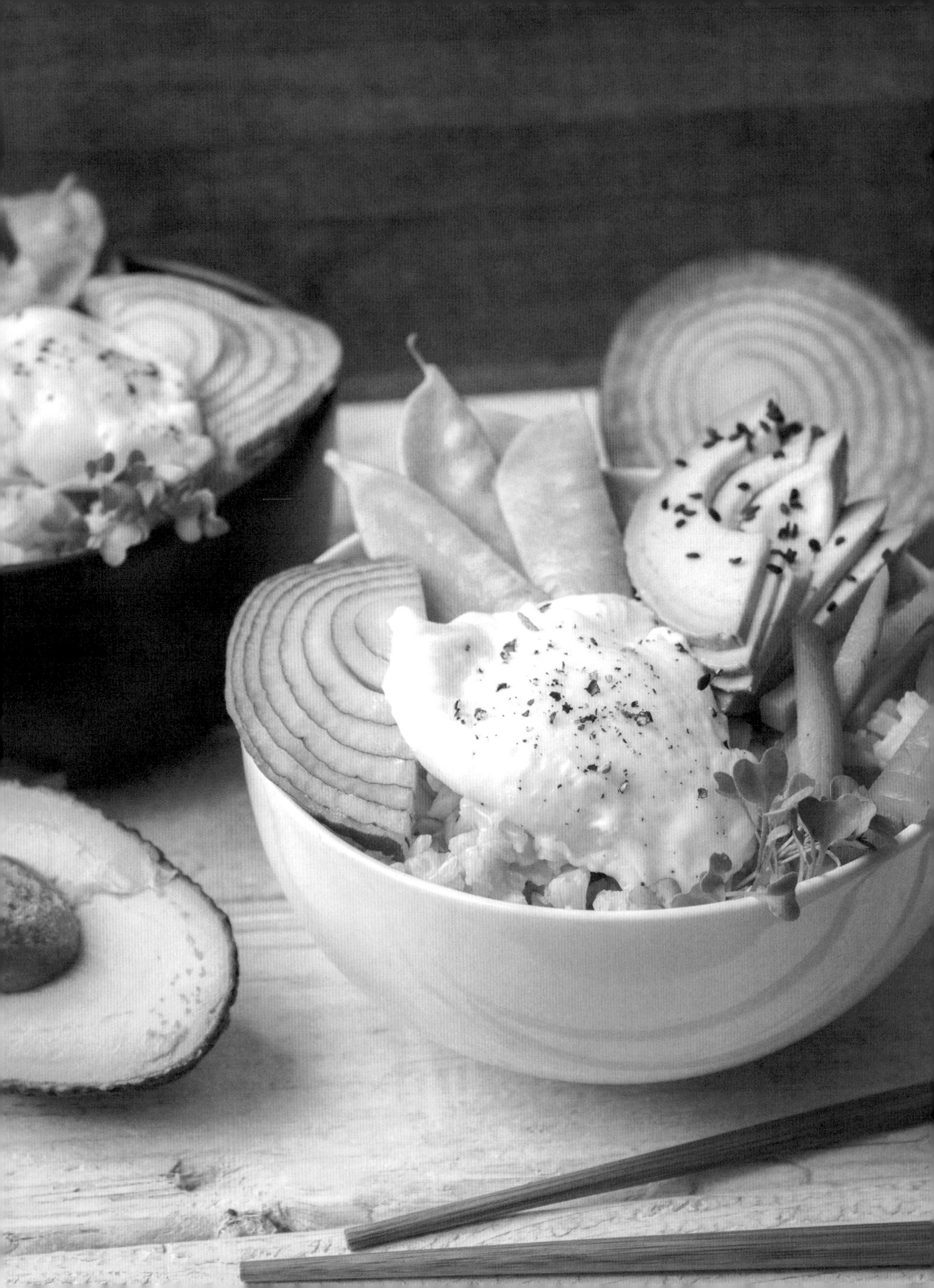

VEGGIE BUDDHA BOWL

SERVES 2

TIME: 45 MINUTES

There's no doubt Buddha bowls are what lunch dreams are made of. Fill yours with brown rice, vibrant vegetables, and a seasoned poached egg for protein. Use your favorite sauce as a drizzle on top or serve with low-sodium soy sauce or coconut aminos. For grain-free and plant-based variations, see the recipe notes.

1 cup brown rice
2 eggs
2 teaspoons white vinegar
1 teaspoon sea salt
1 teaspoon black pepper
1 avocado, sliced
Black sesame seeds (optional)
1 large carrot, peeled and sliced thinly
1 handful snow peas
¼ red onion, chopped
1 pinch broccoli microgreens

1. Cook brown rice according to the package directions. Fill each bowl with half of the cooked rice and set aside.

2. To poach eggs, heat a medium pot of water over medium heat until barely bubbling. Add the vinegar to the water. Crack one egg onto a small plate. Using a spoon, create a whirlpool in the boiling water. Slide the egg into the center of the pot and allow the egg whites to cook through. Remove the egg with a slotted spoon and set it onto a separate plate. Repeat with the second egg, then season eggs with salt and pepper and add to the bowl. Alternatively, you can cook the eggs any way you desire (fried, scrambled, hard boiled) and serve on top of the bowl.

CONTINUED

3. Add half of the avocado to each bowl and sprinkle it with sesame seeds. Add sliced carrots, snow peas, onions, and microgreens to each bowl.

Grain-free variation: Use "riced" cauliflower or broccoli in place of the brown rice (pulse the florets in a food processor until they are rice-sized). If you do this, be sure to substitute another resistant starch into this recipe from the list on page 98. Or serve this over a baked potato or sweet potato instead of rice.

Plant-based variation: Substitute 4 ounces extra-firm tofu, cut into cubes and tossed with 1 teaspoon sesame oil and 1 teaspoon soy sauce or coconut aminos. Sauté lightly on the stove over medium heat until golden-brown or bake in the oven at 375°F for about 30 minutes or until golden and crispy.

Carley's Corner: Cauliflower Rice

Cauliflower rice is a great substitute for most grains like rice or pasta. It's also an excellent source of fiber, so it's great for gut health! This recipe is perfect for meal prepping because you can make large quantities to have on hand throughout the week or to freeze for easy meal assembly. Strapped for time? Just grab some cauliflower rice, sauté with mixed veggies, add your protein of choice, top with coconut aminos or extra-virgin olive oil, and you have a gut-healthy meal in no time! (Keep in mind that if you substitute cauliflower rice for regular rice in a meal, you may need to add a different resistant starch.)

1 head cauliflower
1 tablespoon ghee butter (or coconut oil)
½ cup bone broth
½ tablespoon garlic seasoning
⅓ cup chopped parsley, for garnish

Chop the cauliflower into big pieces, removing any greens. Place the cauliflower into a food processor or Vitamix and gently pulse it until the cauliflower has a fine or grain-like texture. Melt the ghee in a pan over medium heat and add bone broth. Once combined, add cauliflower and garlic seasoning and cook until the cauliflower softens. Serve garnished with parsley and more seasoning.

DINNERS

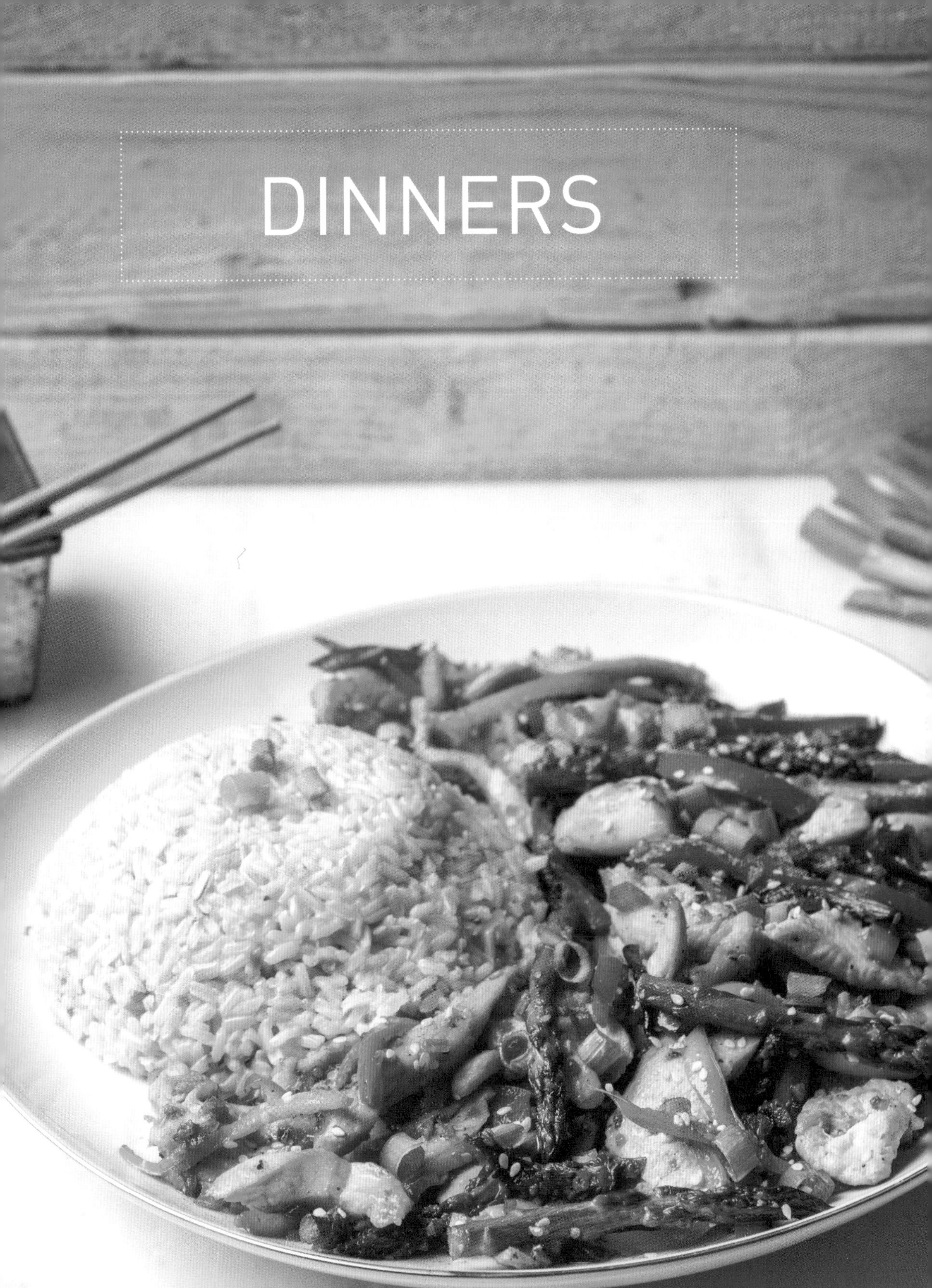

BROCCOLINI, POTATO, AND MUSHROOM SAUTÉ

SERVES 4

TIME: 25 MINUTES

For a light and vegetarian-friendly dinner, try this trifecta of flavors. The broccolini is loaded with vitamins like A, C, and K, and the mushrooms are proven prebiotics.

4 to 5 small potatoes, quartered
1 tablespoon coconut or olive oil
2 large bunches broccolini, chopped
5 cremini mushrooms, sliced
1 teaspoon sea salt
½ teaspoon black pepper
¼ cup chopped green onions

1. Add water to a large saucepan and bring it to a boil. Add the potatoes and cook until they are easily pierced with a fork, about 10 minutes (depending on how big your potatoes are).

2. Meanwhile, in a large pan or skillet over medium heat, heat the oil. Add broccolini to the pan and sauté, stirring often, until it starts to wilt and soften, about 3 minutes. Add mushrooms and continue to sauté and stir until the mushrooms shrink down and get tender, about 5 minutes.

3. Drain the potatoes and add them to the pan. Stir to combine everything, then remove from the heat. Season with salt and pepper, then top with the green onions.

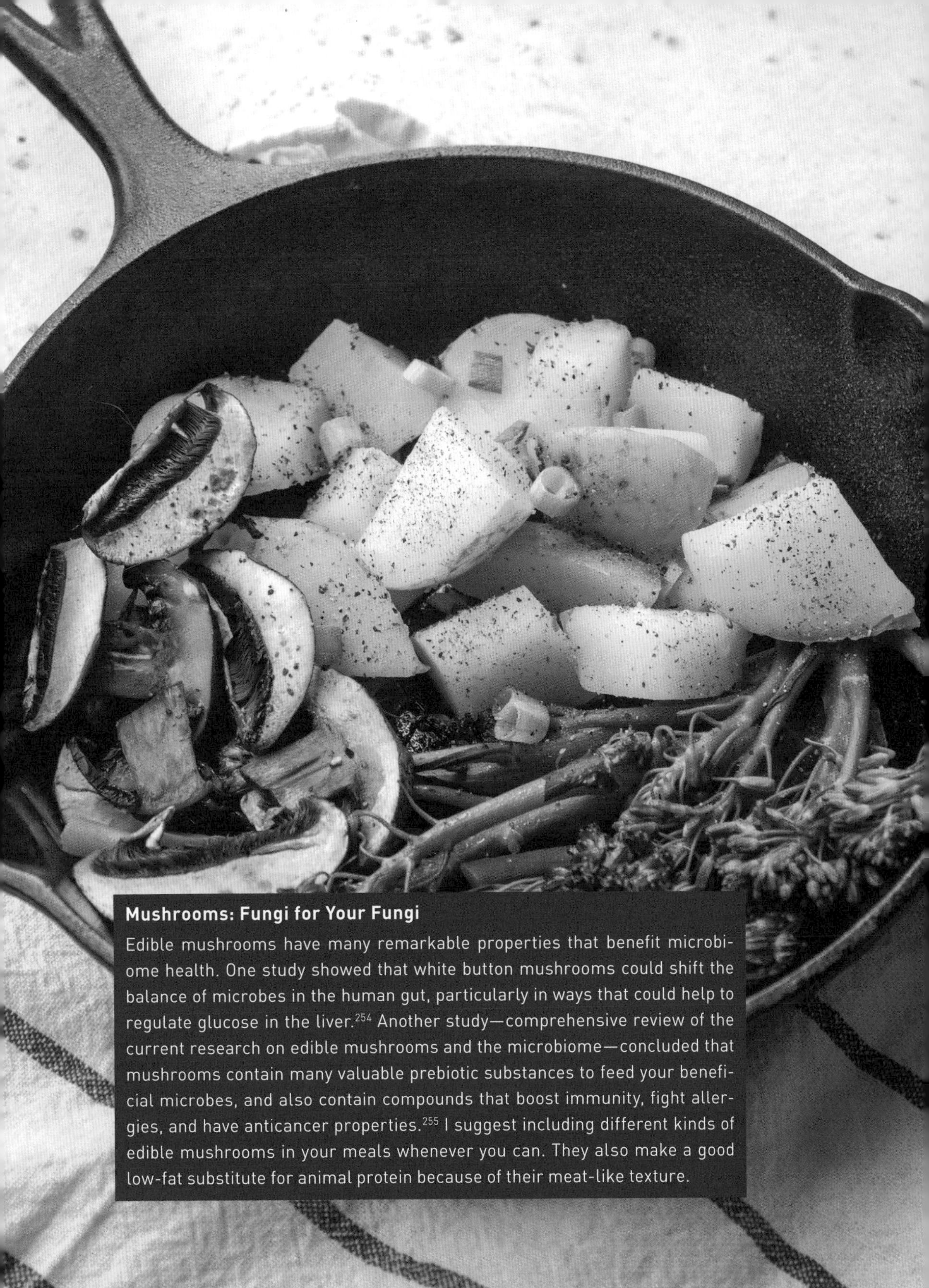

Mushrooms: Fungi for Your Fungi

Edible mushrooms have many remarkable properties that benefit microbiome health. One study showed that white button mushrooms could shift the balance of microbes in the human gut, particularly in ways that could help to regulate glucose in the liver.[254] Another study—comprehensive review of the current research on edible mushrooms and the microbiome—concluded that mushrooms contain many valuable prebiotic substances to feed your beneficial microbes, and also contain compounds that boost immunity, fight allergies, and have anticancer properties.[255] I suggest including different kinds of edible mushrooms in your meals whenever you can. They also make a good low-fat substitute for animal protein because of their meat-like texture.

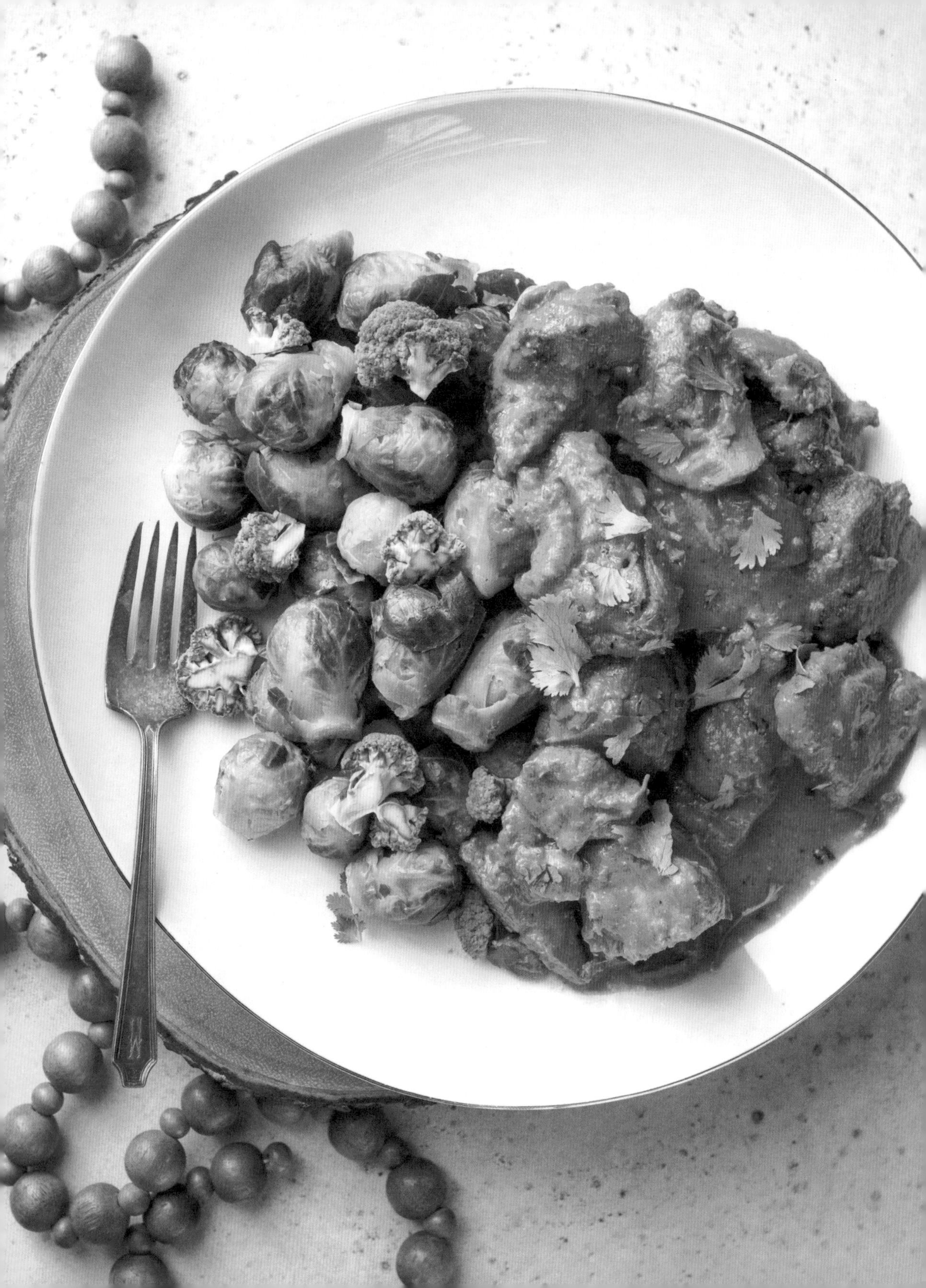

CAULI-BRUSSELS CHICKEN TIKKA MASALA

SERVES 4

TIME: 1 HOUR 30 MINUTES

You don't need to go out for Indian food if you make this savory dish at home. Brussels sprouts make an interesting and flavorful substitution for white rice. For plant-based options, see the recipe note.

1¼ cups plain, unsweetened nonfat or low-fat dairy yogurt or plant-based yogurt
2 teaspoons black pepper
2 teaspoons cayenne pepper
2 teaspoons ground cumin
1 teaspoon ground cinnamon
2 teaspoons sea salt, plus additional for seasoning
1½ pounds chicken breasts, cut into cubes
2 tablespoons olive oil (not extra-virgin) or coconut oil
1 clove garlic, minced
One 8-ounce can tomato sauce (or use Homemade Marinara Sauce, page 163)
2 cups fresh or frozen Brussels sprouts
½ purple cauliflower, cut into florets
¼ cup chopped cilantro, for garnish

1. In a large bowl, combine 1 cup of the yogurt with the black pepper, cayenne pepper, cumin, cinnamon, and 1 teaspoon of the salt. Add the chicken and toss to coat. Cover the bowl and refrigerate for 30 to 60 minutes.

2. Add 1 tablespoon of the oil to a skillet and place over medium heat. Remove the chicken from the marinade and cook it in the skillet until cooked through (no longer pink in the middle—about 10 minutes, depending on how big your cubes are). Put the chicken in a bowl or on a plate and set it aside.

CONTINUED

3. Add the remaining oil to the skillet. Sauté the garlic until it is golden brown (be careful not to burn it). Add tomato sauce, the remaining yogurt, and 1 teaspoon of salt. Cook for 20 minutes or until the sauce thickens. Add the chicken and simmer for another 10 minutes.

4. While the chicken is simmering, bring a large pot of water to a boil. Add the Brussels sprouts and cauliflower and boil for 10 to 15 minutes or until tender.

5. Put the Brussels sprouts and cauliflower on plates and top with the chicken and sauce. Garnish with cilantro and season with more salt if necessary.

Plant-based variation: Cube four large portobello mushroom caps or 1½ pounds of extra-firm tofu in place of the chicken. Prepare the same way as in the recipe.

CAULIFLOWER STEAK SALAD

SERVES 4

TIME: 20 MINUTES

This light and simple plant-based entrée takes just a short time to prepare and is surprisingly filling. Serve your cauliflower steaks on a bed of spinach and drizzle with Homemade Ranch Dressing.

1 large or two small heads cauliflower (purple or white)
1 tablespoon olive oil
1½ cups spinach
Homemade Ranch Dressing (recipe follows)
1 teaspoon sea salt
1 teaspoon pepper

1. Cut four to eight (depending on cauliflower size) 1-inch-thick slices from the center of a head (or two) of cauliflower to make four large or eight smaller "steaks." (Reserve the remaining cauliflower for another use.)

2. Heat oil in a large skillet over medium heat. Add the cauliflower steaks. Cook without moving the steaks until they begin to turn golden brown, about 5 minutes. Flip to brown the other sides. If the steaks are too big to fit in the skillet all at once, you can cook them in multiple batches. Add more oil as needed.

3. Arrange spinach on a large platter and then top with cooked cauliflower. Drizzle with Homemade Ranch Dressing and season with salt and pepper.

CONTINUED

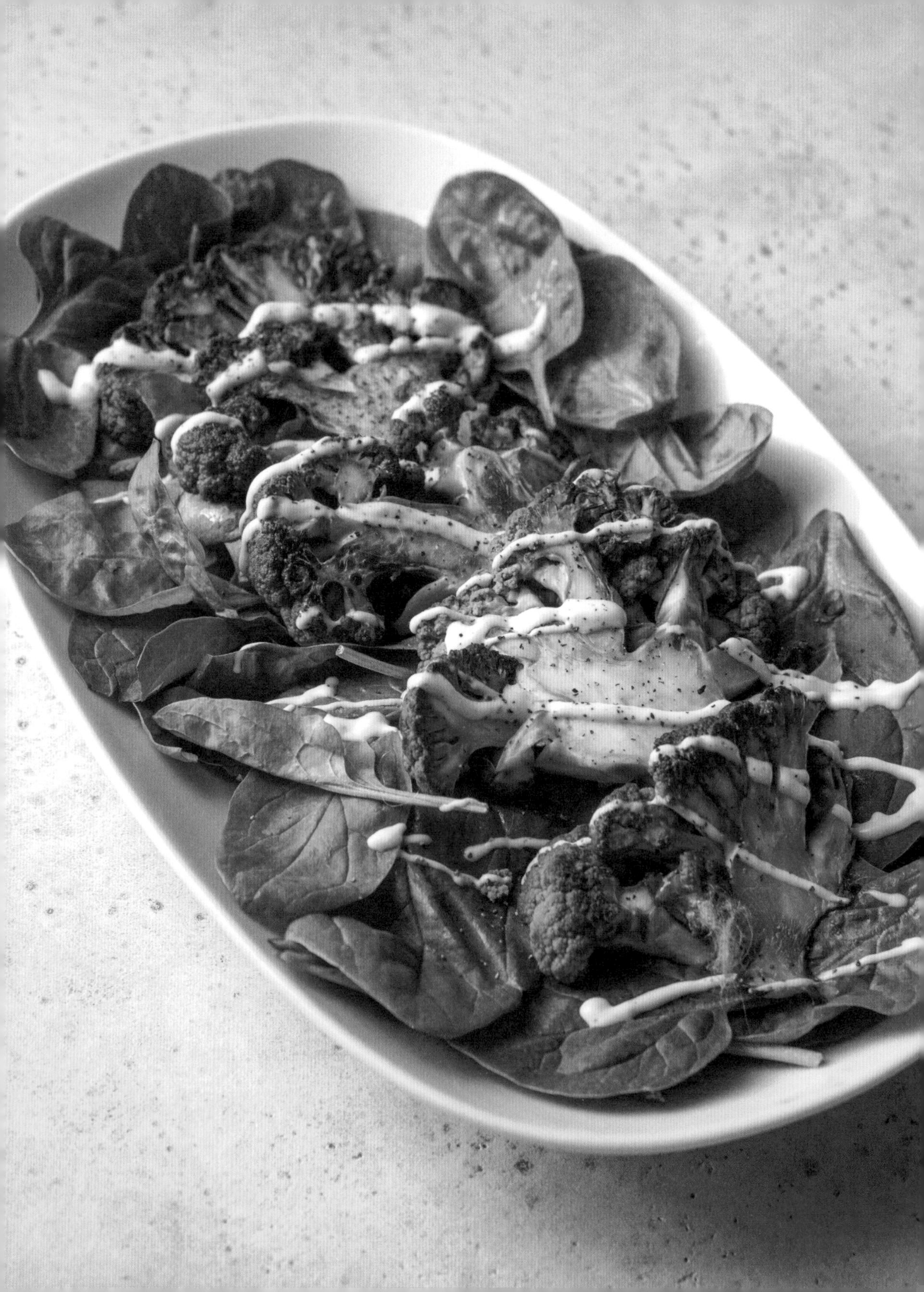

HOMEMADE RANCH DRESSING

MAKES ABOUT 2 CUPS

TIME: 5 MINUTES

Bottled dressings contain huge amounts of sodium and many preservatives as well as low-grade oils. Why buy them when you can easily make delicious, fresh salad dressing at home? You'll probably want to keep this dressing in your refrigerator at all times.

1 can coconut cream (or 2 cans coconut milk—skim off the solid cream and save the liquid for another use; see recipe note)
1 clove garlic, minced
3 tablespoons chopped chives
2 tablespoons apple cider vinegar
1 lime, juiced
1 teaspoon salt

Add coconut cream to a bowl. Stir in garlic, chives, vinegar, lime juice, and salt. Whisk to combine. Add a little bit of coconut milk or water if it's too thick.

Note: If you don't want to or can't use coconut cream because of the high fat content or because you don't like the taste, you can substitute low-fat or nonfat dairy milk or plain unsweetened plant milk like soy, almond, or cashew. The dressing will definitely be thinner, but it will still taste delicious.

CHICKEN AND POTATOES WITH ROSEMARY

SERVES 4

TIME: 45 TO 60 MINUTES

There's nothing quite like a simple chicken and potatoes meal. Use this as your go-to dinner when you're craving a filling comfort food with minimal meal prep. For a plant-based version, see the recipe note.

8 chicken drumsticks
3 tablespoons olive oil (not extra-virgin) or grapeseed oil
4 to 5 small potatoes, quartered
4 cloves garlic
1 onion, chopped
1 tablespoon dried or fresh rosemary
1 teaspoon sea salt
½ teaspoon black pepper
Chopped cilantro, for garnish

1. Preheat the oven to 375°F and add ¼ cup of water to the bottom of a large baking dish. Arrange chicken in the middle of the dish and top with 1 tablespoon of oil evenly distributed. Spread the potatoes, whole garlic, and chopped onions around the outside of the chicken. Drizzle the remaining oil over the top. Season the entire dish with rosemary, salt, and pepper.

2. Bake for 45 minutes to an hour, or until chicken and potatoes are cooked through. Add additional water to the bottom if the liquid cooks away and the pan gets dry. Remove from the oven and garnish with cilantro before serving.

Plant-based variation: Use two 8-ounce packages of tempeh in place of the chicken. Cut each block in half and then cut into triangles, for a total of eight pieces. For more flavor, you can marinate the tempeh first in a shallow dish with ¼ cup soy sauce or coconut aminos (see page 198 for more information), 1 tablespoon sesame oil, 1 teaspoon liquid smoke (optional), and two crushed garlic cloves. Let it sit for at least one hour or overnight in the refrigerator. Bake as you would the chicken.

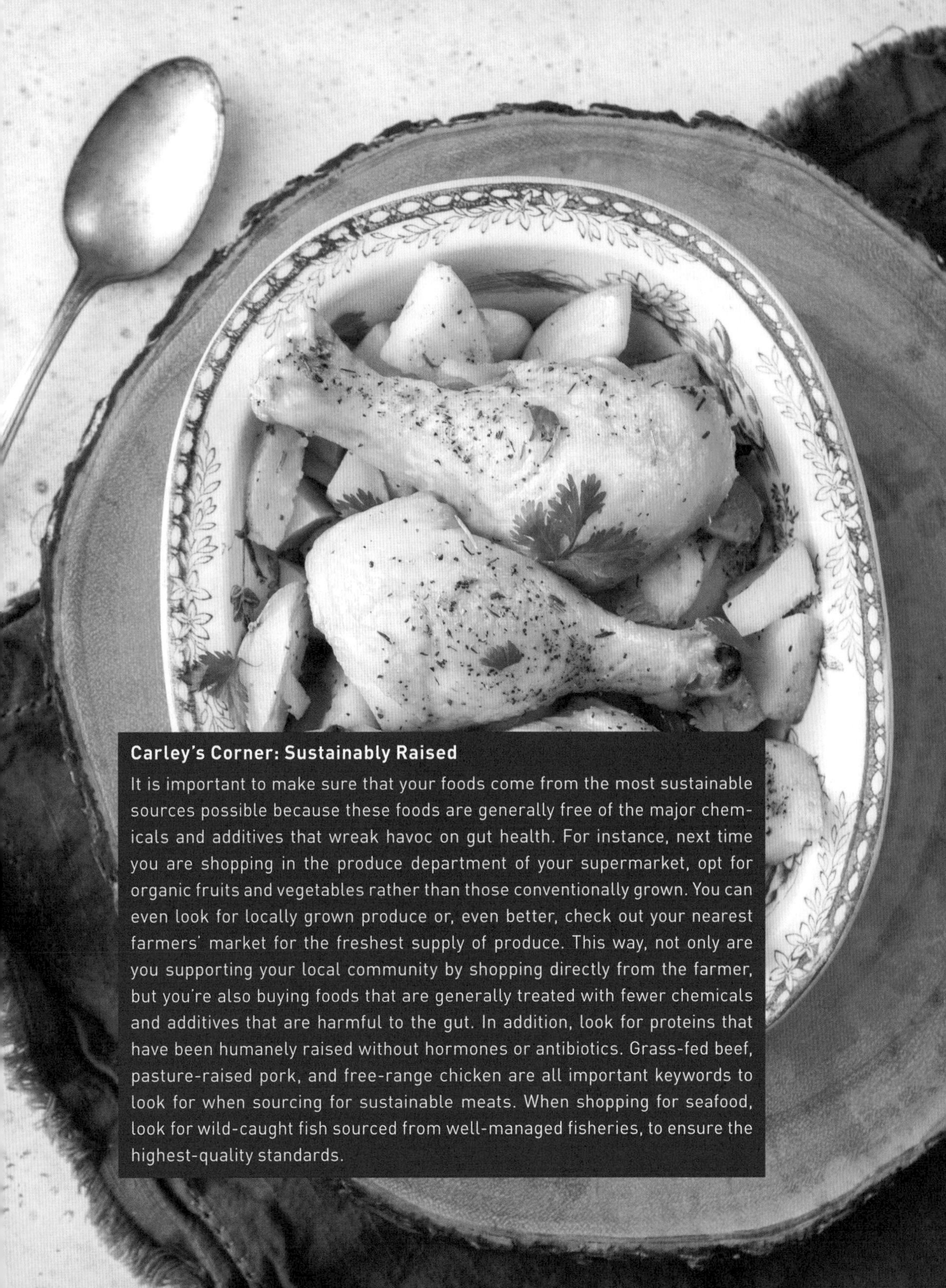

Carley's Corner: Sustainably Raised

It is important to make sure that your foods come from the most sustainable sources possible because these foods are generally free of the major chemicals and additives that wreak havoc on gut health. For instance, next time you are shopping in the produce department of your supermarket, opt for organic fruits and vegetables rather than those conventionally grown. You can even look for locally grown produce or, even better, check out your nearest farmers' market for the freshest supply of produce. This way, not only are you supporting your local community by shopping directly from the farmer, but you're also buying foods that are generally treated with fewer chemicals and additives that are harmful to the gut. In addition, look for proteins that have been humanely raised without hormones or antibiotics. Grass-fed beef, pasture-raised pork, and free-range chicken are all important keywords to look for when sourcing for sustainable meats. When shopping for seafood, look for wild-caught fish sourced from well-managed fisheries, to ensure the highest-quality standards.

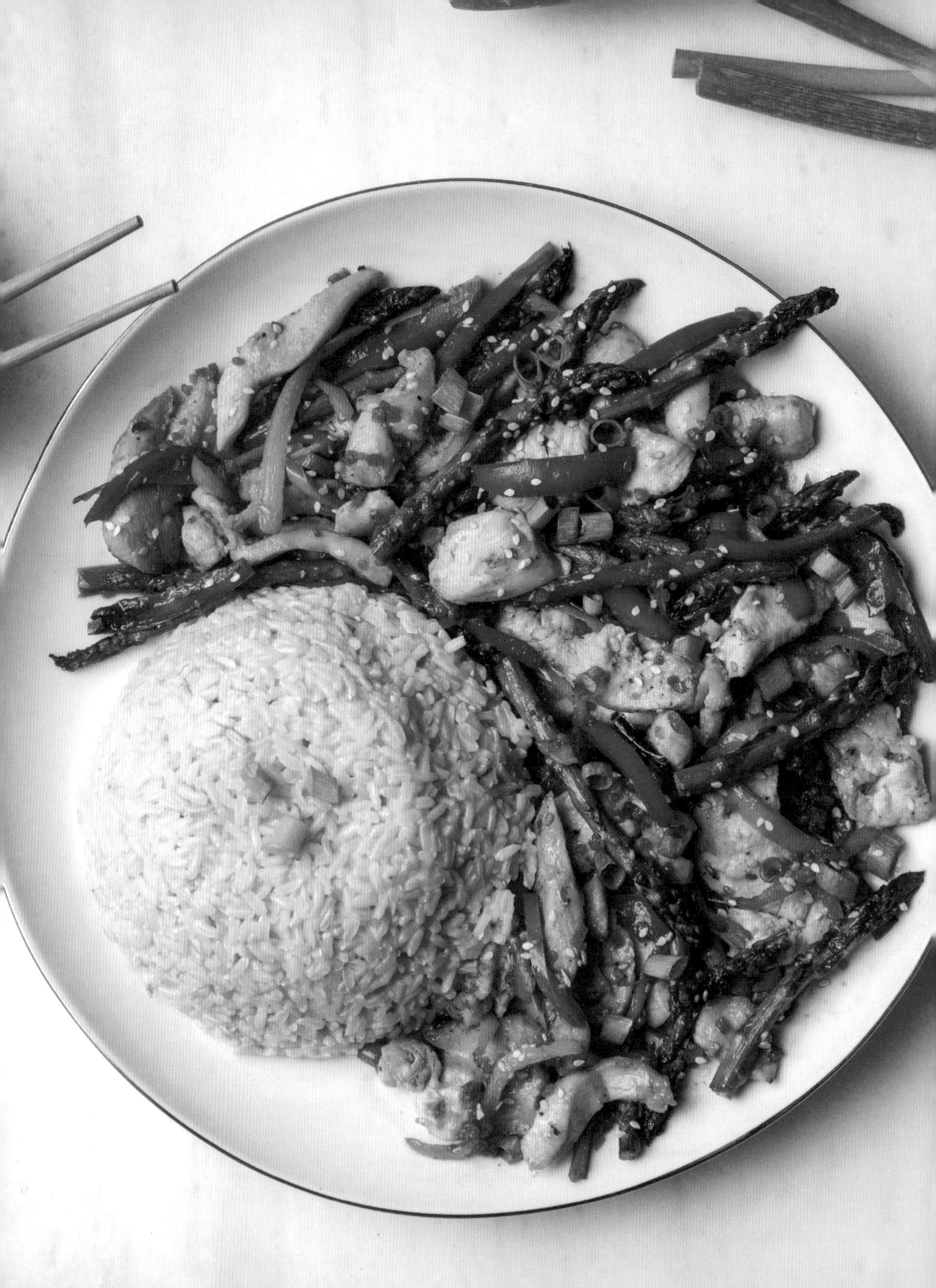

CHICKEN AND VEGETABLE TERIYAKI

SERVES 4

TIME: 30 MINUTES

A favorite at Asian restaurants but loaded with salt and preservatives, chicken teriyaki is much better made fresh at home—although it is okay to use a low-sodium bottled teriyaki sauce (look for one without MSG, or just substitute low-sodium soy sauce or coconut aminos). This recipe includes microbiome-feeding asparagus and colorful peppers. For grain-free and plant-based variations, see the recipe notes.

10 asparagus shoots
1 orange pepper
1 red pepper
½ yellow onion
1 tablespoon coconut or peanut oil
1 pound boneless chicken breasts, sliced into strips
¼ cup plus 1 tablespoon teriyaki sauce
¼ cup chopped green onions, for garnish
1 teaspoon sesame seeds, for garnish
2 cups cooked brown rice

1. Remove the ends from the asparagus stalks and cut them into 2-inch pieces. Chop the peppers into long thin strips and the onion into small cubes.

2. Heat half the oil in a large skillet or wok over medium to low heat. Add the chicken and cook until no longer pink on the inside and slightly brown on the outside, about 10 minutes. Remove the chicken, place on a plate, and set aside. Add the remaining oil and the vegetables and cook them until they are tender but still brightly colored. Add the chicken back into the mixture and drizzle teriyaki sauce over everything. Toss to coat. Top with green onions and sesame seeds. Serve with rice.

Grain-free variation: Serve without rice, or substitute cauliflower rice, mashed potatoes. or sweet potatoes.

Plant-based variation: Use 1 pound of extra-firm tofu, sliced into strips instead of chicken.

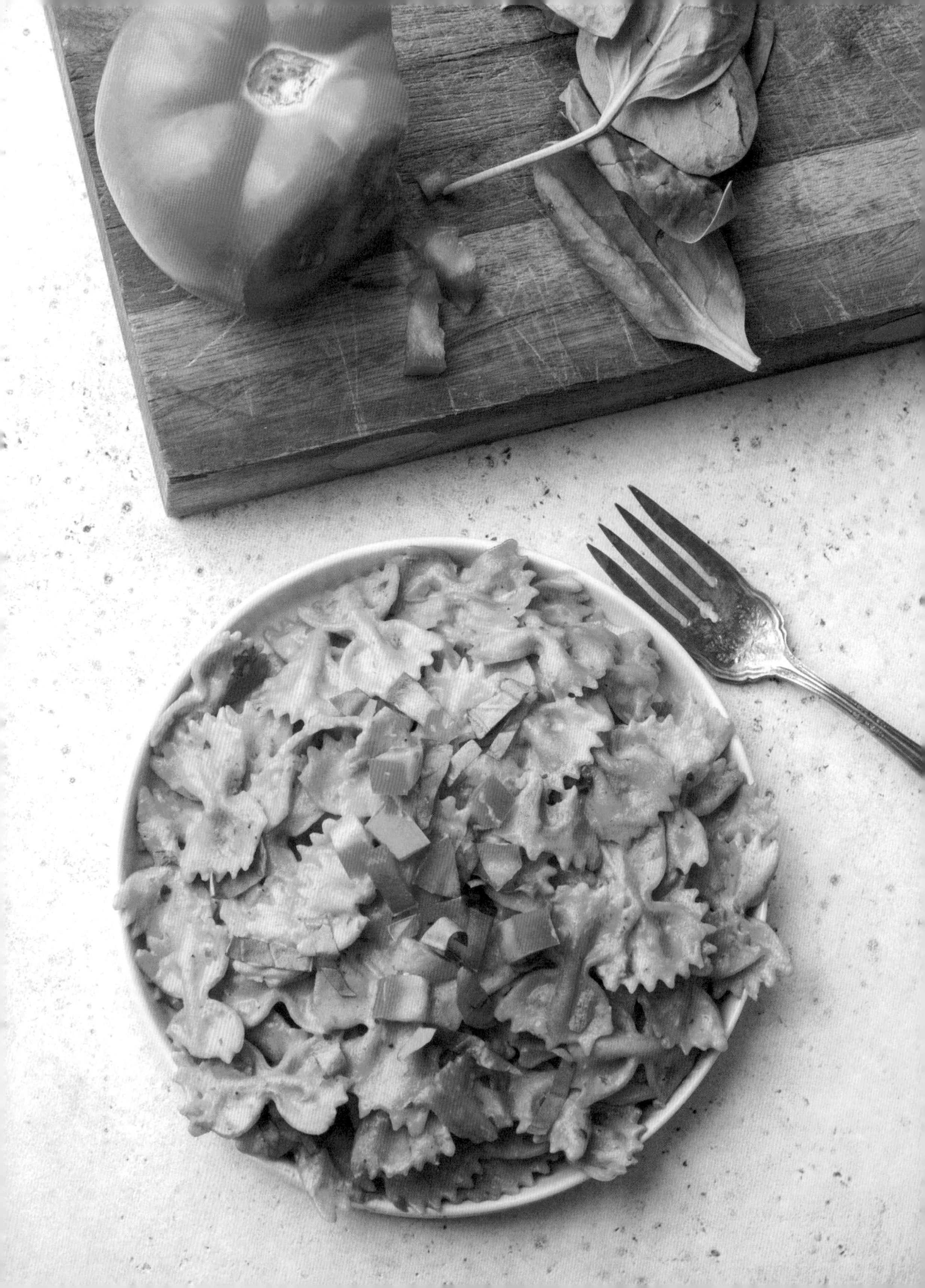

CREAMY WHOLE WHEAT PASTA WITH SPINACH

SERVES 4

TIME: 30 MINUTES

What is pasta without a great sauce? This sauce is nothing short of heavenly. Creamy tomato and spinach are the perfect pair for this whole wheat farfalle pasta.

½ cup fresh spinach
1 medium fresh tomato
1 pound 100% whole wheat farfalle pasta or whole-grain gluten-free or grain-free pasta
1 cup Homemade Marinara Sauce (page 163, or store-bought with no sugar)
¼ cup plain, unsweetened nonfat or low-fat dairy yogurt or plant-based yogurt
1 teaspoon sea salt

1. Bring a large pot of water to a boil. While the water is heating up, chop the spinach and tomato into small pieces. Add farfalle to the boiling water and cook until al dente, per package instructions. Drain and set aside.

2. In a medium saucepan, stir together the marinara sauce, yogurt, spinach, and tomatoes (reserve some for topping, if desired) and cook over medium heat until hot.

3. Add sauce to pasta and toss to coat. Sprinkle additional spinach and tomatoes on top and add salt.

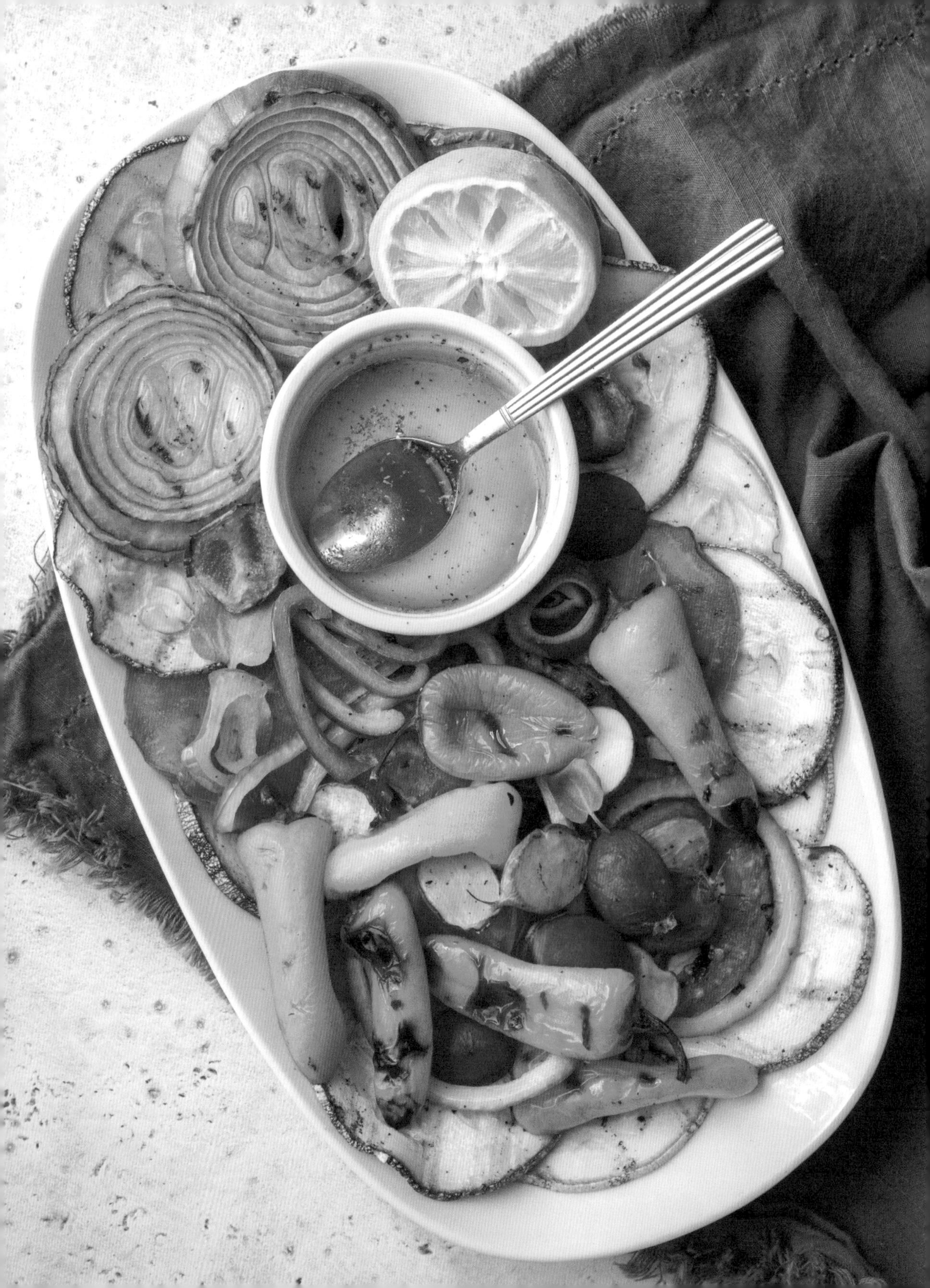

GRILLED VEGGIE DINNER

SERVES 4

TIME: 30 MINUTES

Seeing the rainbow on your plate never looked so beautiful, and eating it never tasted so good. Simply throw these vegetables on the grill, drizzle with a simple vinaigrette, and enjoy! If it's not grilling weather, you can also make this recipe using your oven's broiler function.

5 radishes, cut in half
4 to 5 small bell peppers in various colors, stemmed and seeded
1 red onion, sliced
1 tomato, sliced
1 zucchini, sliced
1 teaspoon sea salt
Simple Vinaigrette (recipe follows)

1. Fire up the grill (or your broiler). Brush the grill plates or broiler pan with a little oil or put the veggies in a grilling basket. Cook vegetables on both sides until tender; each vegetable may take different times—remove them as they become tender. Arrange them on a large plate. Sprinkle with salt and serve with Simple Vinaigrette.

SIMPLE VINAIGRETTE

MAKES ABOUT ½ CUP

TIME: 2 MINUTES

¼ cup olive oil
2 tablespoons red wine vinegar
1 teaspoon black pepper

In a small bowl, whisk together all the ingredients. Drizzle on top of the vegetables.

PISTACHIO-CRUSTED SALMON WITH ASPARAGUS

SERVES 4

TIME: 30 MINUTES

Add healthy fats to every bite with this fancy take on salmon. Pair your fish with simply cooked asparagus for a hearty, healthy dinner. For a plant-based variation, see the recipe note.

2 salmon fillets
1 tablespoon olive oil
One 7-ounce bag pistachios, shelled and crushed
2 teaspoons sea salt
10 ounces fresh asparagus spears

1. Preheat oven to 375°F. Brush the salmon fillets with olive oil. Add crushed pistachios to the top of each fillet, then sprinkle with 1 teaspoon of the salt. Bake on a foil-lined baking sheet for 15 to 20 minutes or until cooked through. Remove the fillets from the pan carefully to keep the nut crust on the top. (If some falls off, you can sprinkle it back on.)

2. Boil water in a large saucepan. Trim off the tough, lower stems from the asparagus, then add them to the boiling water. Reduce the heat to medium and simmer until the stalks are easily pierced with a fork but still bright green, about 5 minutes. Season with the remaining salt and serve next to the salmon fillets.

Plant-based variation: Cut an 8-ounce block of tofu into two slices. Marinate the slices in the juice of one lemon with ½ teaspoon of Old Bay Seasoning and a sprinkle of kelp flakes for 15 to 30 minutes. Prepare as you would the salmon, but sprinkle a little more Old Bay or kelp on the slices before adding the pistachios.

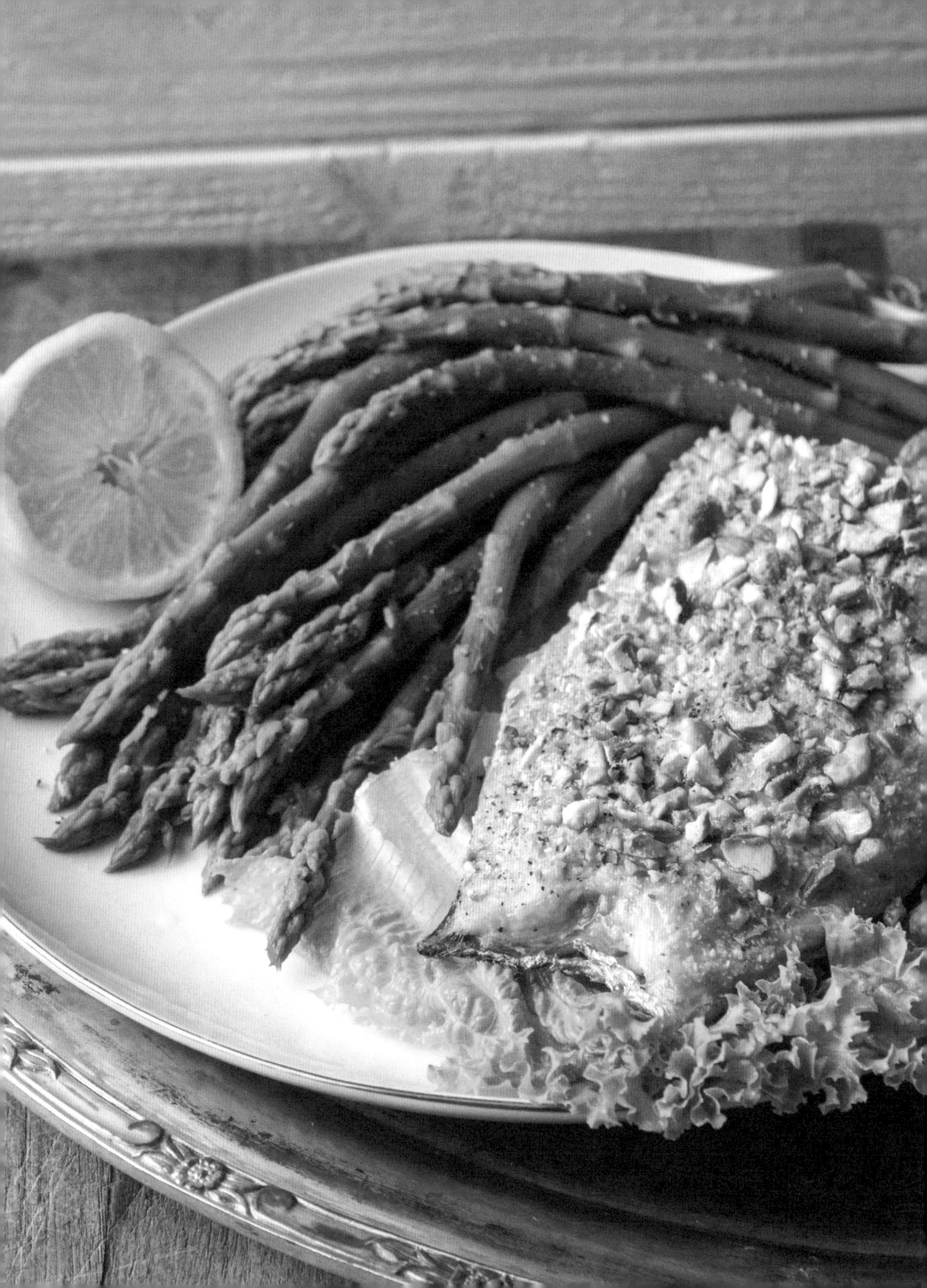

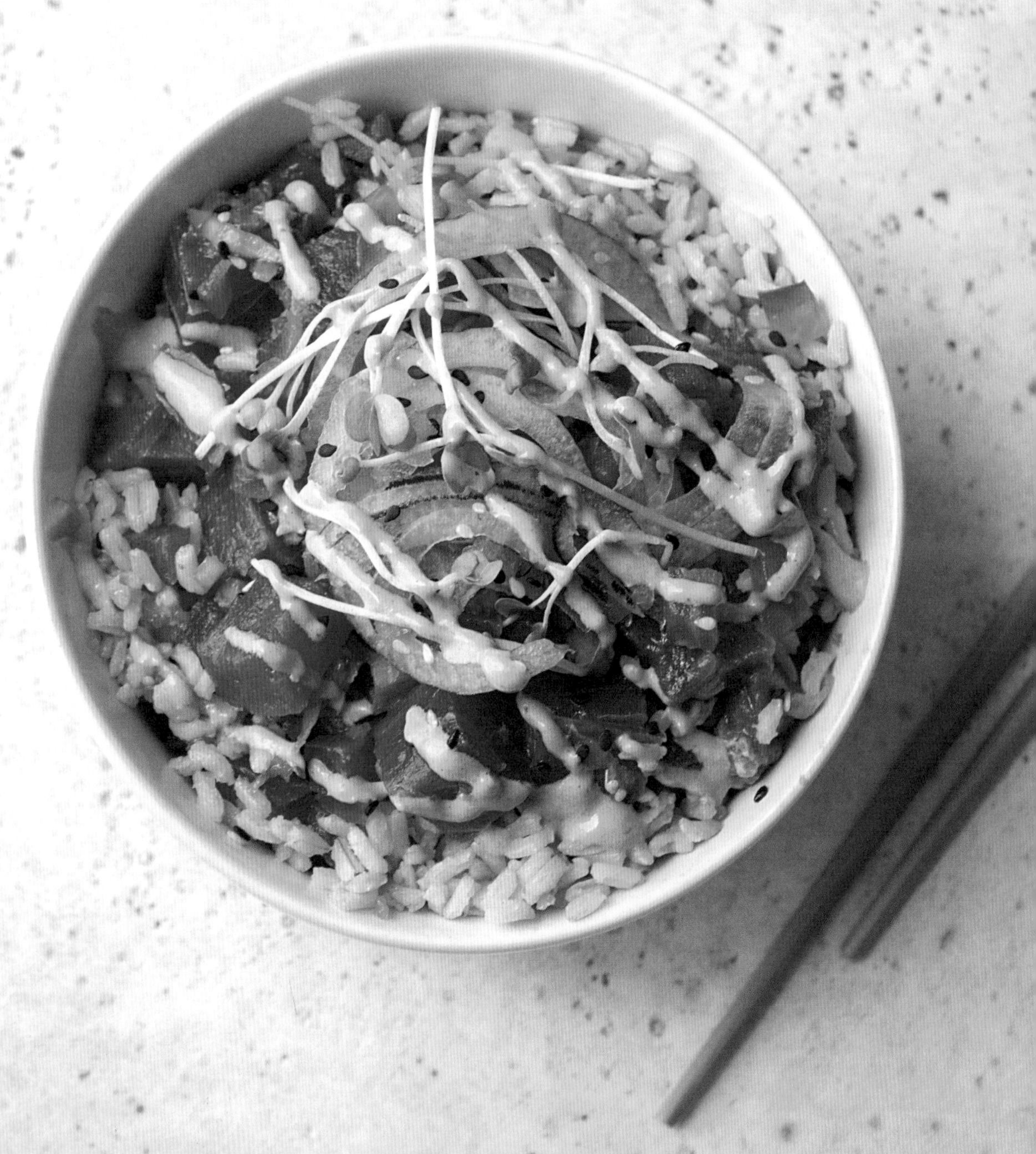

POKE BOWL WITH CREAMY CILANTRO DRESSING

SERVES 4

TIME: 45 MINUTES

It's possible to have an omega-3-rich poke bowl right at home with just a few easy steps. The key is to purchase sushi-grade ahi tuna and drizzle the final product with a yummy cilantro dressing. For grain-free and plant-based options, see the recipe notes.

2 cups cooked brown rice
1 pound sushi-grade ahi tuna, cut into cubes
1 tomato, cut into cubes
1 tablespoon low-sodium soy sauce or coconut aminos (see page 198 for more information)
1 teaspoon sea salt
¼ red onion, cut into thin slices
Black sesame seeds, for garnish
Broccoli microgreens, for garnish
Creamy Cilantro Dressing (recipe follows)

1. Divide the brown rice equally between 4 bowls.

2. Toss the ahi tuna and tomatoes in the soy sauce and salt. Add the mixture to the rice bowls. Top with red onion, sesame seeds, and microgreens. Drizzle with the Creamy Cilantro Dressing.

CONTINUED

CREAMY CILANTRO DRESSING

MAKES 1 CUP

TIME: 5 MINUTES

8 ounces plain, unsweetened nonfat or low-fat dairy yogurt or plant-based yogurt
1 bunch cilantro, stems removed, coarsely chopped
1 lime, juiced
Sea salt

In a blender, add the yogurt, cilantro, lime juice, and salt. Blend until creamy. Taste and add more salt or lime juice, if needed. Drizzle on top of poke bowls.

Grain-free variation: You can serve this on a bowl of steamed, finely chopped (or "riced") cauliflower or broccoli instead of rice. Or you can serve it on chopped salad greens. To get your resistant starch, you could also cube and bake a sweet potato to use in place of the rice. (Use approximately one medium sweet potato per person.)

Plant-based variation: Cube 1 pound of extra-firm tofu and toss with the juice of one lemon, ½ teaspoon of Old Bay Seasoning, and a sheet of nori (what you would use to wrap sushi), cut into very thin slices (chiffonade). Continue as you would with the tuna.

Carley's Corner: Digestive Support

Making sure that you are properly digesting your foods is a key component of optimal gut health. If you are not properly digesting your foods, your body may not be fully absorbing all the nutrients they contain, meaning you will not receive as many of the gut-healing (and other) benefits as you could. The body digests food in a few ways, but primarily through digestive enzymes and proper chewing.

Digestive enzymes are secreted proteins that are naturally released by the body to help break down fats, proteins, and carbohydrates, as well as eradicate any pathogens or harmful bacteria lurking in our food. If we have too little stomach acid, we may notice undigested food in stools or perhaps even immediate bloating or discomfort after eating.

One way to remedy this is by supplementing with digestive enzymes that help boost stomach acid levels like hydrochloric acid and pepsin. Another way to help stimulate digestive juices is through bitters, which is essentially a natural blend of herbs that help the body to release more enzymes. Finally, as simple as it sounds, you should make sure you are properly chewing your food. This can have a tremendous impact on digestion. The gut does not have teeth, so it is extra important to take time to completely chew your food, slowly, and thoroughly, so that everything can be easily absorbed by the gut.

It is also important to note that the body needs to be in a parasympathetic state in order to fully release digestive enzymes. In other words: Don't eat when you are stressed! Think of it this way: You have to rest in order to digest, meaning you need to take time to sit down for your meals, take a few deep breaths, and enjoy the nutrient-dense, nourishing, and gut-healing foods. This also means it's best to avoid eating on the go, in the car, at your desk, or in any other environment where you are thinking of a lot of things at once and can't fully relax and pay attention to your food. Otherwise, you will impair your body's ability to fully digest and absorb nutrients.

Another important way your body digests food is through probiotics, the beneficial bacteria and fungi that reside in the gut. Not only are probiotics important for maintaining a healthy balance of bacteria and fungi for optimal immune health, but these microorganisms are also responsible for helping break down resistant starches and fiber in the gut. Since beneficial bacteria help break down resistant starches and fiber, bringing in additional support through a probiotic supplement can be helpful in reducing the symptoms you may experience when you first switch to the Mycobiome Diet, like bloating and excess gas. Also know that as your body adjusts to the increased fiber and resistant starch in the Mycobiome Diet, you will likely find that these symptoms go away. In the meantime, however, a probiotic, as well as digestive enzymes, may help.

SCALLOPS WITH PEA PUREE

SERVES 4

TIME: 30 MINUTES

Scallops are incredibly high in protein and they help naturally lower cholesterol. Serve them on a bed of pea puree for a touch of sweetness, and finish it all off with freshly chopped chives for an elegant presentation. For a plant-based version, see the recipe notes.

1 tablespoon olive oil (not extra-virgin) or grapeseed oil
1 pound scallops (any size you prefer)
¼ cup chopped fresh chives for garnish

PEA PUREE

2 cups frozen green peas
½ avocado
2 tablespoons water
1 teaspoon sea salt

1. Heat a medium saucepan over medium heat and add the oil. Add the scallops. Don't move them until they are a golden brown on the bottom, about 5 minutes. Flip them once and cook until the other side is also golden-brown, about 3 minutes. Remove from the heat and set aside.

2. Boil water in a large saucepan. Add the frozen peas and blanch them for 3 minutes. Drain and add the peas to a food processor along with the avocado, water, and salt. Pulse until the mixture is thick and creamy (add more water if it is too thick).

3. Divide the puree between four shallow bowls. Top with the scallops and garnish with chives.

Plant-based variation: In place of the scallops, cut extra-firm tofu into scallop-sized circles or use canned sliced hearts of palm (if you use hearts of palm, add an additional protein to your meal). Toss either with the juice from one fresh lime and a sprinkle of kelp flakes. Cook the tofu as you would the scallops. For the hearts of palm, just arrange the marinated slices over the pea puree. (The hearts of palm version will not be warm—the final dish will be more like a salad.)

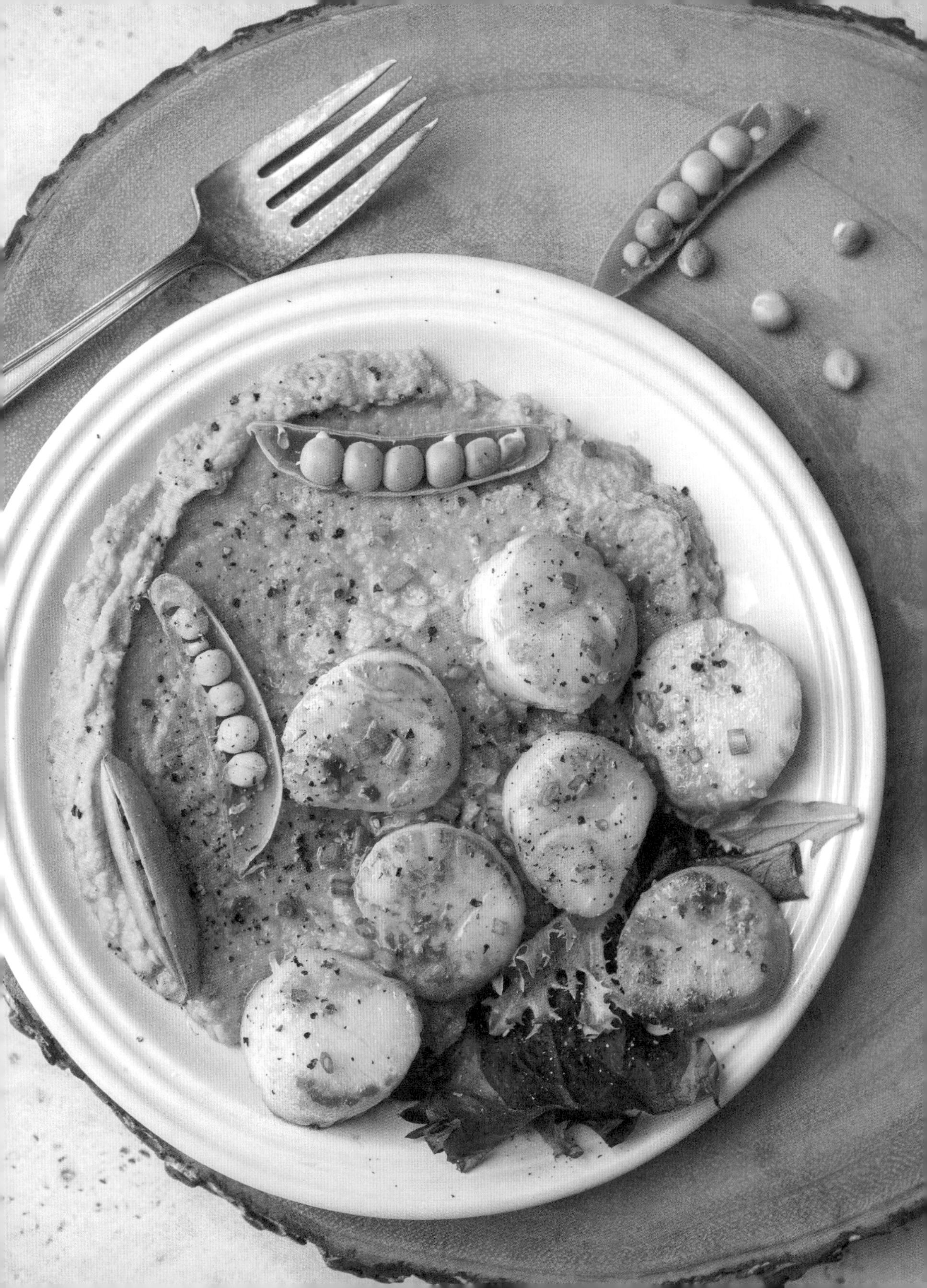

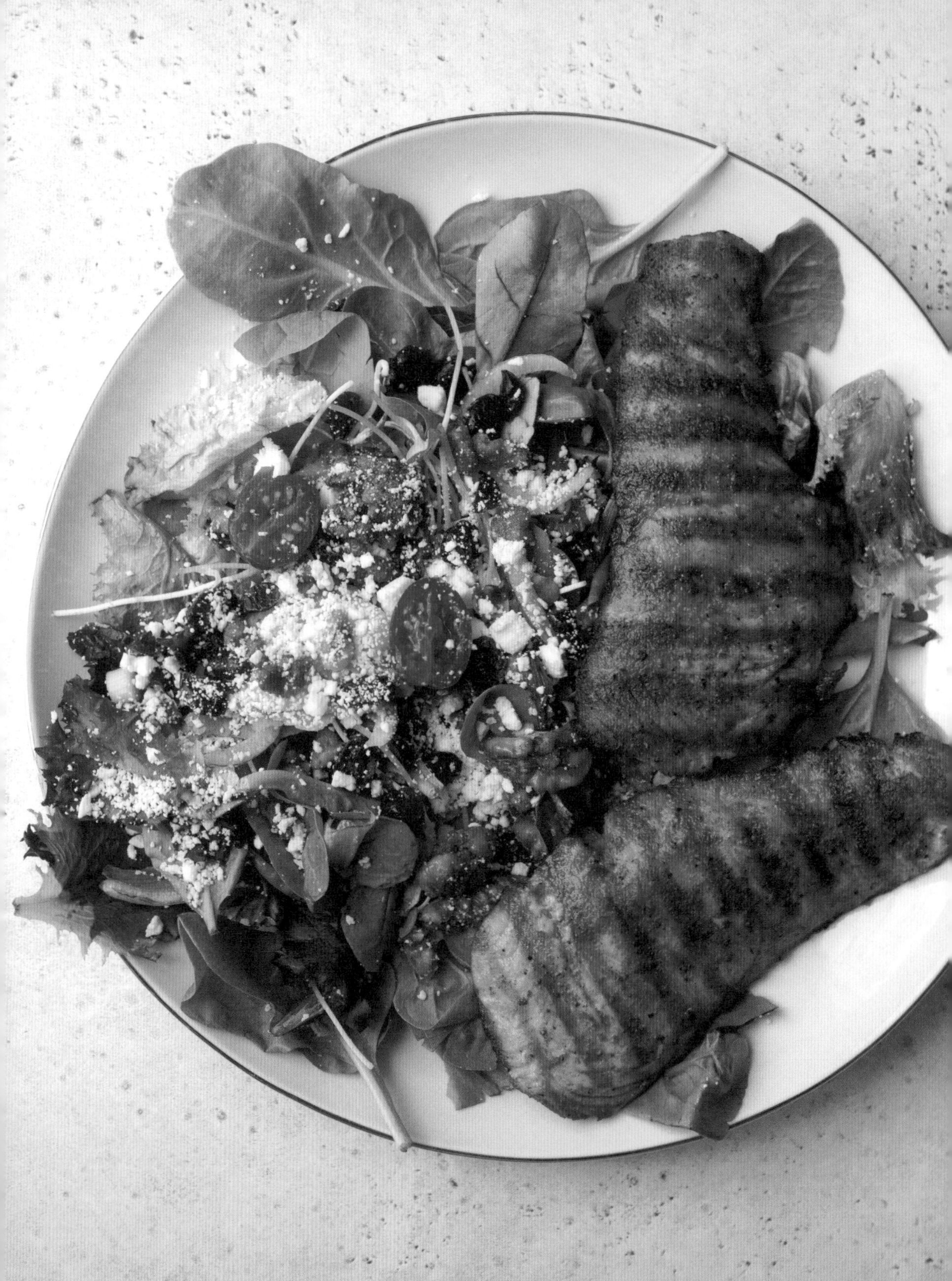

SPICY SALMON SALAD

SERVES 4

TIME: 30 MINUTES

This zingy dish contains omega-3-rich salmon with a medley of spices, along with crunchy walnuts, chewy dried cranberries, and fresh veggies. Feta cheese or hummus adds pleasing tanginess. For a plant-based version, see the recipe notes.

4 salmon fillets
1 tablespoon olive oil (not extra-virgin) or grapeseed oil
1 tablespoon ground cumin
1 teaspoon chili powder
1 teaspoon paprika
1 teaspoon sea salt
1 teaspoon black pepper
2 cups fresh spinach or artisan lettuce
½ cup walnuts
¼ cup dried cranberries
5 or 6 cherry tomatoes, sliced in half
¼ red onion, thinly sliced
½ cup nonfat feta cheese or hummus
Homemade Vinaigrette Dressing (page 191)

1. Fire up the grill or preheat the oven to 375°F. Brush each salmon fillet with oil. In a small bowl, mix the cumin, chili powder, paprika, salt, and pepper. Pat or sprinkle the seasoning mixture onto each salmon fillet. Place on the grill or on a baking pan and grill or bake until the salmon is cooked through, about 15 minutes, depending on the thickness of your fillets.

2. Arrange the greens on four plates. Sprinkle with the walnuts, cranberries, tomatoes, red onion, and feta cheese (if using hummus, add 2 tablespoons to the middle of each salad). Add salmon on top of the salad. Serve with Homemade Vinaigrette Dressing (page 191).

Plant-based variation: Cut a 1-pound block of tofu into four slices. Prepare as you would the salmon, but add 1 teaspoon of Old Bay Seasoning into your seasoning mix.

SWEET & SOUR SHRIMP BOWL

SERVES 4

TIME: 30 MINUTES

Honey, paprika, and red onion come together to make the tastiest flavor-packed shrimp you've ever tried. If you are avoiding honey, just leave it out. It won't exactly be "sweet and sour," but it will still be delicious. For grain-free and plant-based variations, see the recipe notes.

1 cup brown rice
1 pound raw shrimp, medium to large size, tails removed
¼ cup minced red onion
Honey to taste (optional, 1 tablespoon max)
1 tablespoon lime juice
1 teaspoon paprika
1 teaspoon coconut or grapeseed oil
½ cup chopped cabbage
1 handful mung bean sprouts
1 green onion, chopped
4 lime wedges for garnish

1. Cook brown rice according to the package directions and set aside.
2. In a bag or bowl with a lid, add the shrimp, red onion, optional honey, lime juice, and paprika. Toss to coat.
3. Heat a medium saucepan over medium heat. Add the oil. Add the shrimp mixture and sauté, stirring frequently, until the shrimp turns pink.
4. Divide the brown rice between four bowls. Top each with the shrimp, cabbage, mung bean sprouts, and green onions, and garnish each bowl with a lime wedge.

Grain-free variation: In place of the rice, steam or microwave frozen butternut squash cubes (you can puree the cooked squash cubes, if you prefer) and serve the shrimp over the squash.
Plant-based variation: Slice 1 pound of oyster mushrooms (remove the tough parts of stems) and prepare as you would the shrimp.

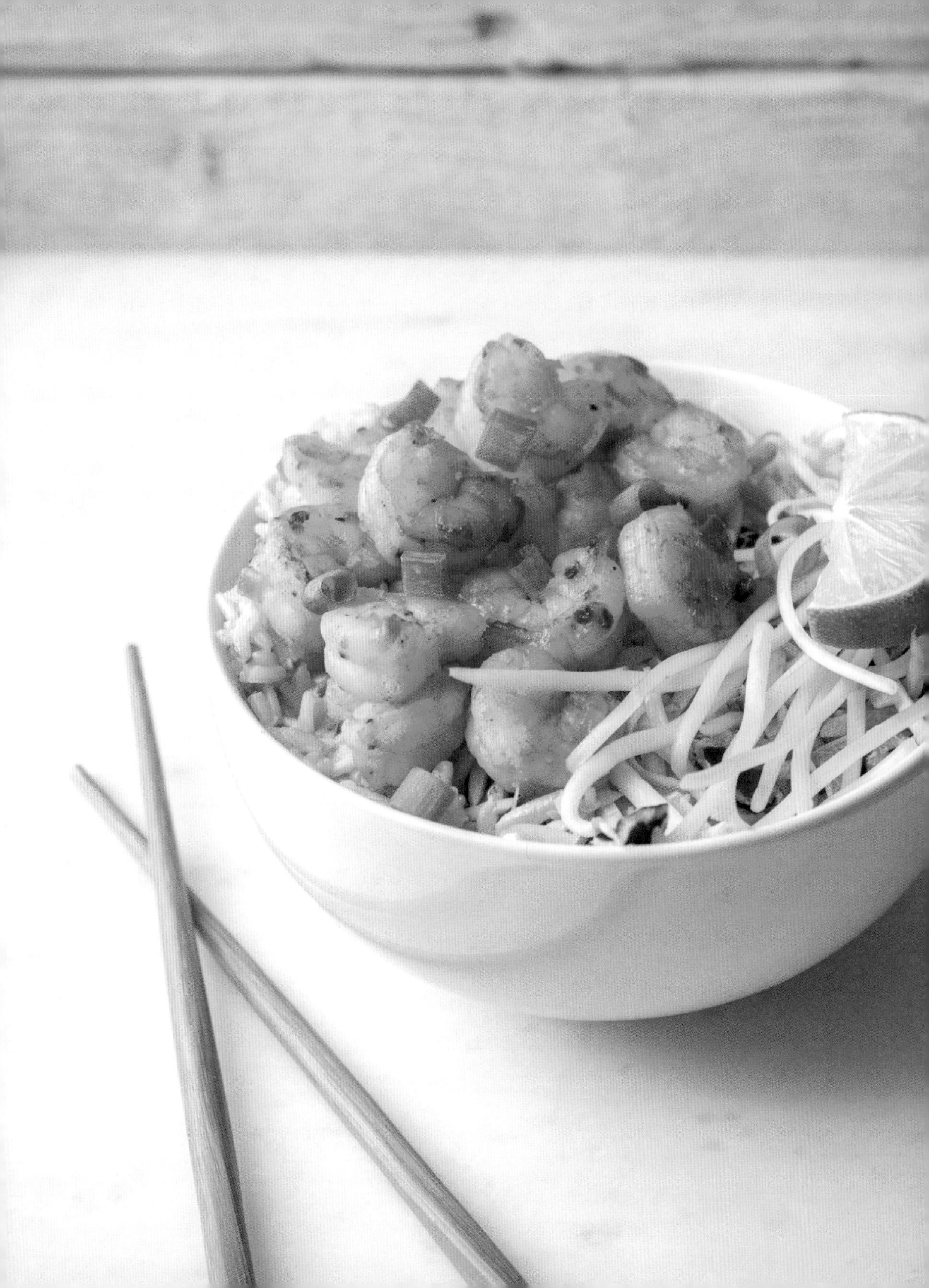

SWEET POTATO TURKEY BOATS

SERVES 4

TIME: 45 TO 60 MINUTES

The slightly sweet, slightly spicy combination of the sweet potato and seasoned turkey is a crowd pleaser. Drizzle it with Homemade Ranch Dressing (page 211) for even more flavor.

SWEET POTATO BOATS

2 large sweet potatoes
1 tablespoon olive oil
Sea salt and black pepper

SEASONED TURKEY

1 tablespoon olive oil (not extra-virgin) or coconut oil
1½ pounds ground turkey or 12 ounces crumbled tempeh
1 tablespoon chili powder
1 tablespoon tomato paste
1 teaspoon ground cumin
1 teaspoon paprika
1 teaspoon sea salt
½ teaspoon black pepper
¼ cup water
Homemade Ranch Dressing (page 211)
Chopped cilantro, for garnish

1. Preheat the oven to 375°F. Poke each sweet potato with a fork a few times throughout and then slice them down the middle lengthwise. Brush each top with oil and then bake for 35 to 40 minutes or until the middle is soft.

2. Meanwhile, add oil to a large pan over medium-high heat, then add the turkey. Break up the meat as it cooks. Add chili powder, tomato paste, cumin, paprika, salt, and pepper to the turkey and mix thoroughly. Add the water and stir until the sauce thickens. Add more water if necessary.

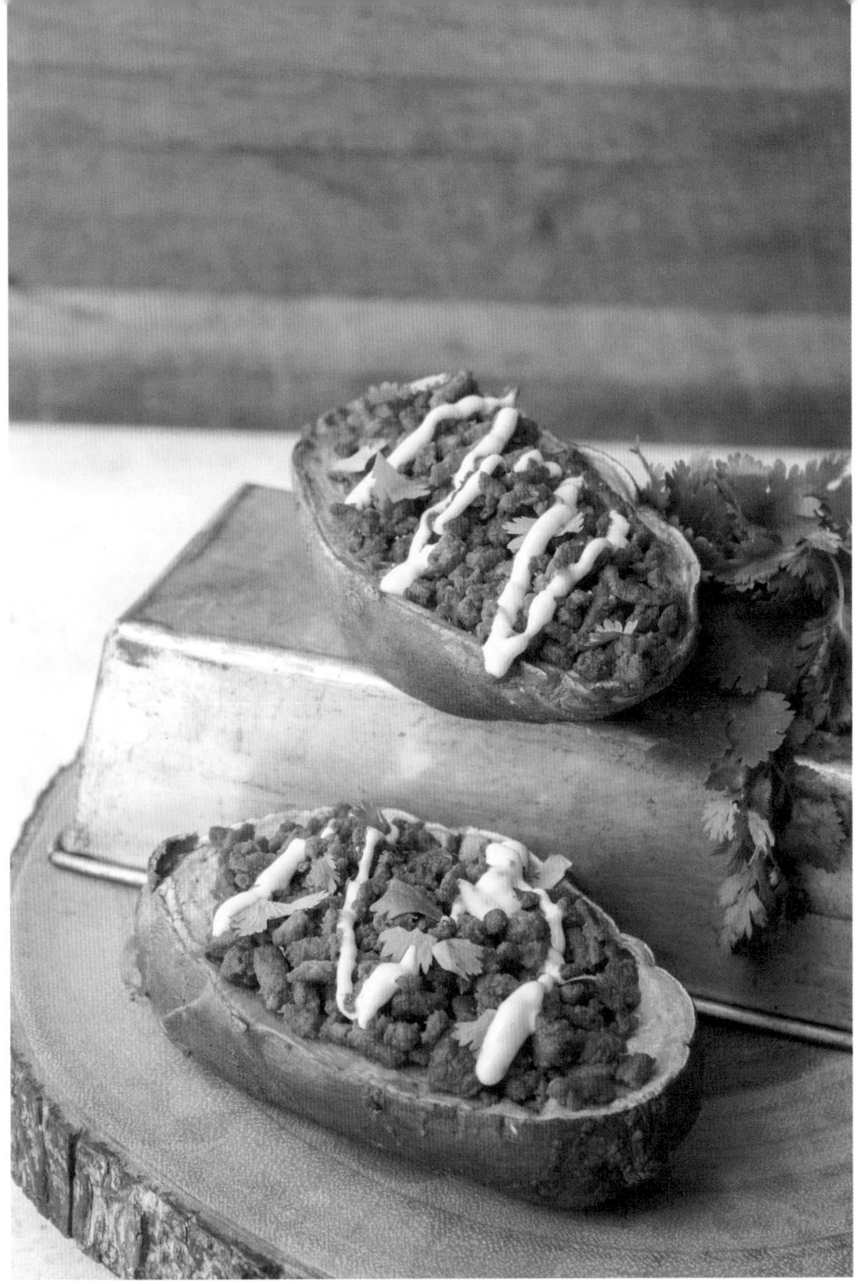

3. Scoop out the center of each sweet potato and save for another recipe. Fill each boat with ground turkey and pack it down. Drizzle them with ranch dressing and sprinkle with cilantro.

Note: Use the leftover sweet potato from this recipe for the Sweet Potato Falafel Bowl, page 234.

SWEET POTATO FALAFEL BOWL

SERVES 4

TIME: 30 MINUTES

Crunchy on the outside and soft on the inside, these sweet potato falafels are so simple to create that you will want to make a large batch for the entire week. Eat them on their own or on top of a bowl with brown rice and spinach. For grain-free and plant-based variations, see the recipe notes.

SWEET POTATO FALAFEL

1 cup cooked mashed sweet potato
1 cup cooked brown rice
¼ cup sliced almonds
1 egg
½ cup whole wheat flour
1 teaspoon sea salt
1 tablespoon plus 1 teaspoon olive oil or coconut oil, divided

BOWLS

1 cup white or brown sliced mushrooms
¼ cup Homemade Ranch Dressing (page 211)
1 tablespoon sriracha
1 cup spinach or artisan lettuce
2 cups cooked brown rice
Black sesame seeds

1. In a food processor, pulse the sweet potato, rice, and almonds together. Add the egg and pulse again. Pour the mixture into a bowl and stir in the flour and salt. Using your hands, shape the mixture into balls, about an inch in diameter. Flatten them slightly.

2. Heat a large skillet over medium-high heat. Add 1 tablespoon of the oil. Add the falafel patties and cook until one side is golden-brown, about 3 minutes. Flip the patties and cook until the other side is golden brown, about 2 minutes. Remove them from the pan and place them on a plate to cool.

CONTINUED

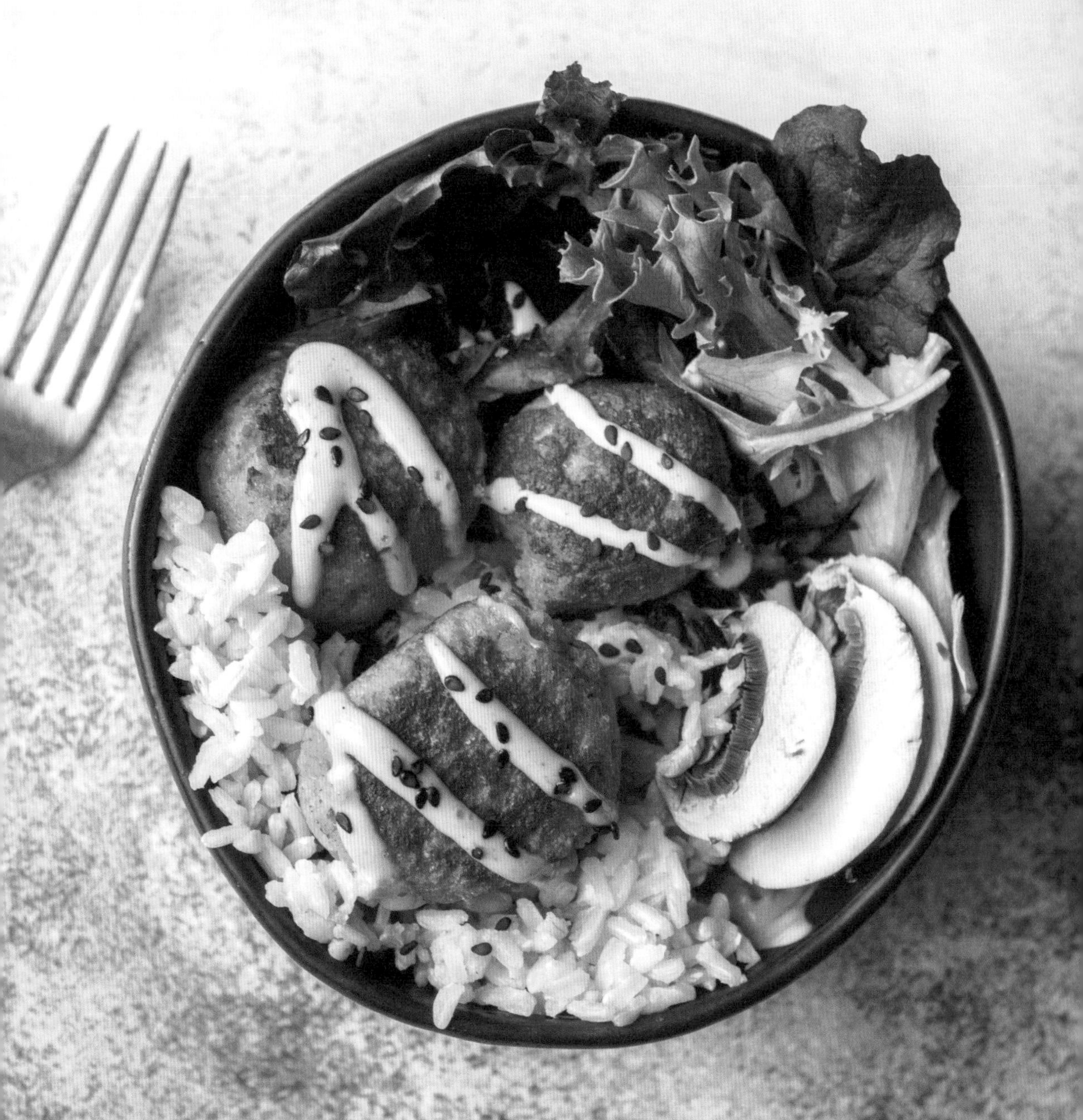

3. Add the remaining oil to the pan. Add the mushroom slices in a single layer. Let them cook without stirring until one side is golden brown, about 5 minutes. Flip the mushrooms and cook the other side about 3 minutes. Remove from the heat.

4. In a small bowl, stir together the Homemade Ranch Dressing and sriracha and set aside.

5. Construct the bowls by adding spinach and brown rice to the bottom, and topping with the mushrooms, falafel, sriracha-ranch mixture, and sesame seeds.

Grain-free variation: For the falafel, replace the brown rice with chopped-up chickpeas and replace the whole wheat flour with chickpea flour. In the salads, omit the brown rice or replace it with chopped raw or lightly steamed broccoli.

Plant-based variation: Use 2 ounces of silken tofu in place of the egg.

TURKEY MEATBALLS WITH TZATZIKI

SERVES 4

TIME: 30 MINUTES

Try this fresh, full-flavor Mediterranean-style dinner. It features a tasty sauce—and no pita bread is required (although you could add a whole-grain pita bread to get your resistant starch). For a plant-based variation, see the recipe note.

TURKEY MEATBALLS

1½ pounds ground turkey
1 egg, beaten
1 garlic clove, minced
1 teaspoon onion powder
1 teaspoon parsley
1 teaspoon sea salt
½ teaspoon black pepper
1 tablespoon olive oil (not extra-virgin) or coconut or grapeseed oil

TO SERVE

1 cucumber
½ cup cherry tomatoes
Tzatziki (recipe follows)
1 teaspoon lemon pepper
Chopped dill, for garnish
½ lemon, sliced

1. Make the meatballs: In a medium bowl, combine all of the meatball ingredients except the oil, and mix well with your hands. Wash your hands, then leaving them wet, form small balls and place them on a plate.

2. In a medium saucepan, heat the oil over medium heat. Add meatballs and move them around until they are brown on all sides and cooked through (about 10 minutes). Remove them from the pan and set them on a plate covered with a paper towel.

CONTINUED

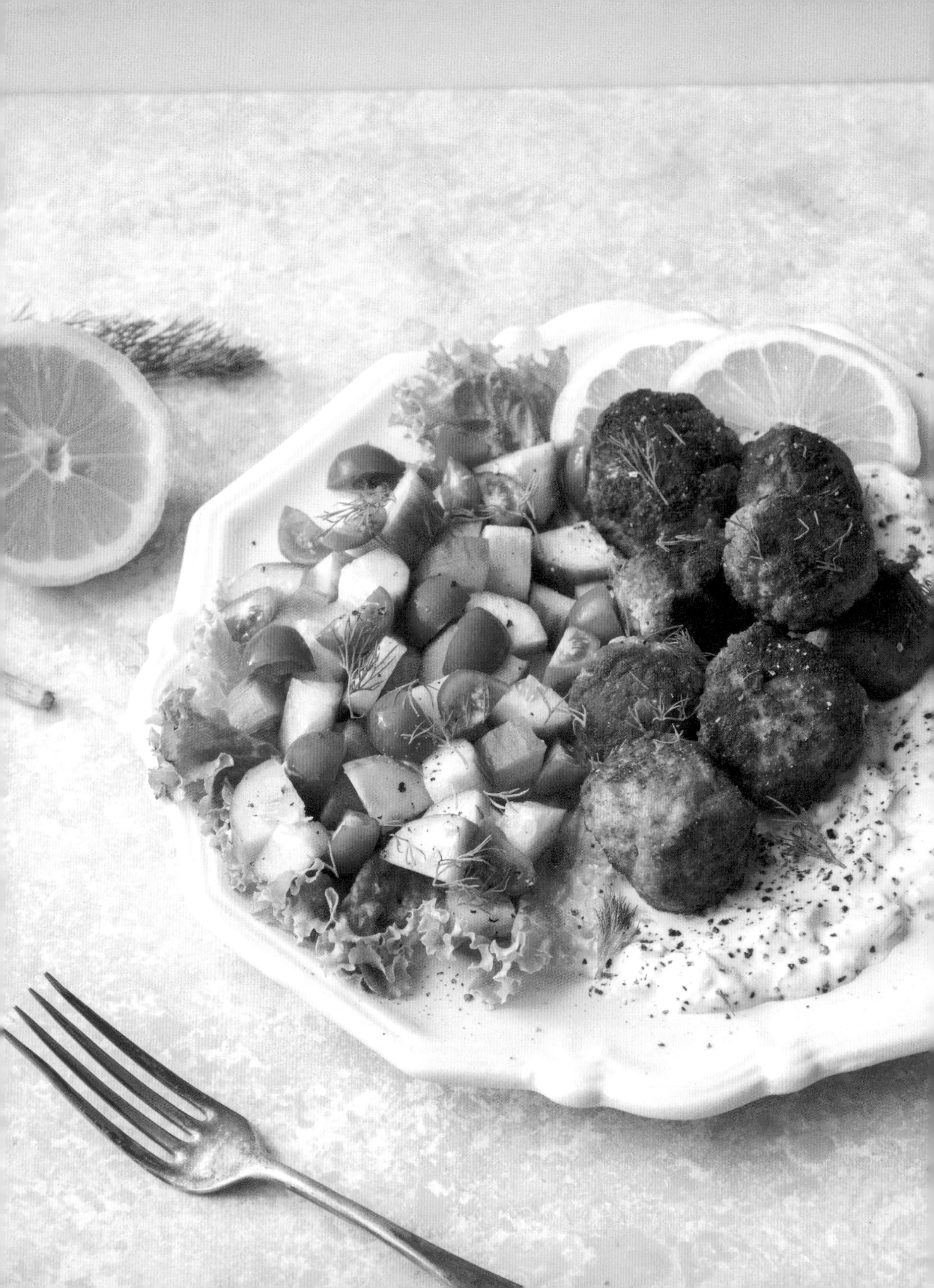

3. To assemble the dish, chop the cucumber and the tomatoes. Divide the meatballs and the vegetable mixture between four plates. Drizzle the tzatziki sauce over each plate or serve it on the side. Top everything with lemon pepper, dill, and sliced lemons.

TZATZIKI

MAKES ABOUT 1 CUP

TIME: 5 MINUTES PLUS CHILLING TIME

1 cucumber
6 ounces plain, unsweetened nonfat or low-fat dairy or plant-based Greek yogurt
2 tablespoons lemon juice
1 garlic clove, minced
1 tablespoon chopped fresh dill
1 teaspoon sea salt

Using a cheese grater, grate cucumber into shreds and strain the excess liquid. Combine all tzatziki ingredients in a small bowl, then cover and refrigerate until ready to use.

Plant-based variation: In place of turkey meatballs, rinse and drain one 15-ounce can of kidney beans. Mash them up so no whole beans remain. Prepare them as you would the turkey meatballs, but substitute ¼ cup hummus for the egg and add 1 tablespoon tomato paste and 1 teaspoon olive oil to the mixture.

THAI BUTTERNUT SQUASH SOUP

SERVES 4

TIME: 35 MINUTES

The creamy texture of butternut squash combined with the sweet coconut milk base makes a one-of-a-kind soup that you will want to keep in your dinner rotation. Not only does it taste amazing, it also gives the body vitamins A, C, and E, which help promote healthy hair and skin. And of course it's an excellent prebiotic source, so it's good food for your microbiome.

1 tablespoon coconut oil
½ yellow onion, diced
1 tablespoon Thai red curry paste
1 butternut squash, peeled with seeds removed and cut into cubes
2 cups vegetable stock or broth
One 13.5-ounce can coconut milk
1 teaspoon sea salt
Maca powder (optional)
4 tablespoons unsweetened coconut cream, or scoop the solid coconut cream from the top of the can of coconut milk used in the soup
Crushed peanuts for garnish
Chopped cilantro for garnish
1 lime, sliced

1. In a large pot, heat oil over medium heat. Add onions and cook until translucent and soft, about 5 minutes. Add curry paste and stir well. Add cubed butternut squash to the pot and then add vegetable stock, coconut milk, and salt. Cover and simmer for 15 to 20 minutes or until the squash is cooked through.

2. Using an immersion blender, blend the butternut squash into soup to create a creamy texture. Stir in the maca powder, if using. Ladle the soup into the bowls. Top each bowl of soup with 1 tablespoon coconut cream, then garnish with peanuts and cilantro. Serve with lime slices.

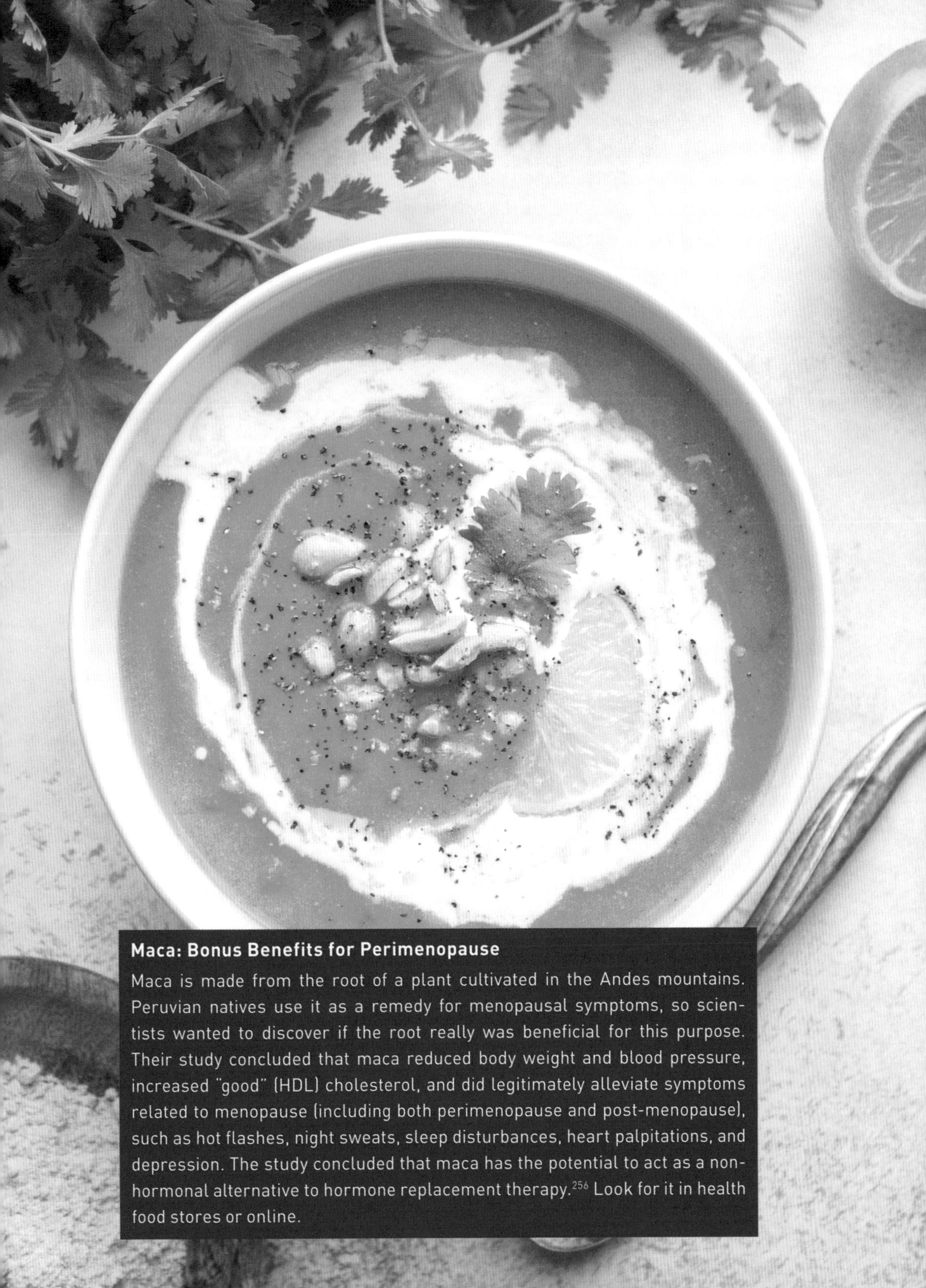

Maca: Bonus Benefits for Perimenopause

Maca is made from the root of a plant cultivated in the Andes mountains. Peruvian natives use it as a remedy for menopausal symptoms, so scientists wanted to discover if the root really was beneficial for this purpose. Their study concluded that maca reduced body weight and blood pressure, increased "good" (HDL) cholesterol, and did legitimately alleviate symptoms related to menopause (including both perimenopause and post-menopause), such as hot flashes, night sweats, sleep disturbances, heart palpitations, and depression. The study concluded that maca has the potential to act as a nonhormonal alternative to hormone replacement therapy.[256] Look for it in health food stores or online.

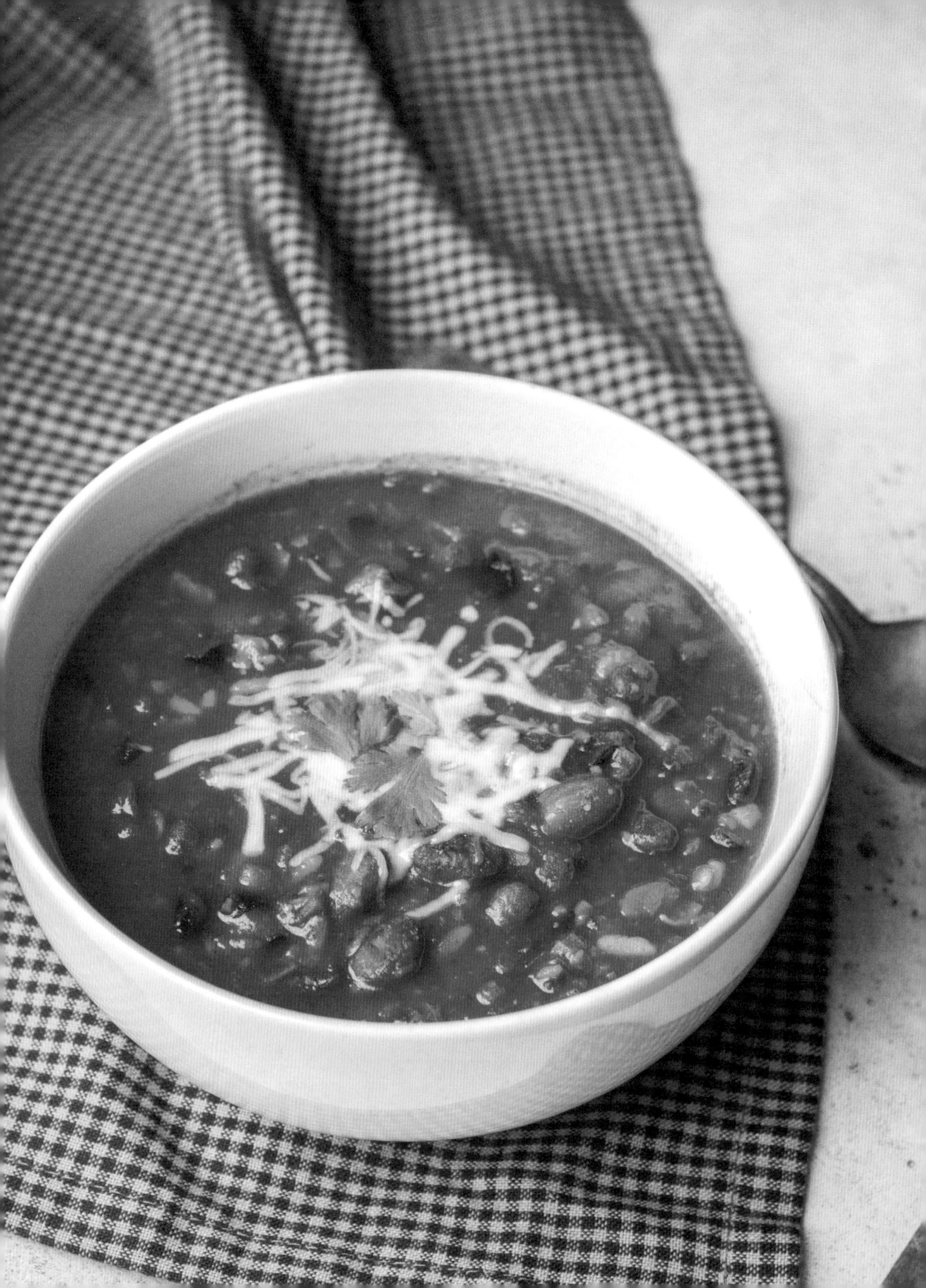

VEGETABLE CHILI WITH BROWN RICE

SERVES 4

TIME: 35 MINUTES

Chili is a dinnertime staple. This veggie version has plenty of prebiotic-rich brown rice, beans, and peppers. It keeps well, freezes well, and it's also delicious over a baked potato or sweet potato. You could even use it to top sweet potato fries, for an upgraded version of chili fries.

3 tablespoons olive oil (not extra-virgin) or grapeseed oil
1 large onion, chopped
4 large garlic cloves, minced
Three 14.5-ounce cans diced tomatoes in juice
One 4-ounce can diced mild green chilies
3 tablespoons chili powder
1 tablespoon ground cumin
1 tablespoon dried oregano
One 15-ounce can kidney beans, drained
One 15-ounce can black beans, drained
2 green bell peppers, chopped into small pieces
1 cup brown rice, cooked (or 1 cup cubed sweet potatoes or butternut squash, baked or boiled until tender)
1 teaspoon sea salt
½ teaspoon black pepper
Low-fat mozzarella cheese or vegan Parmesan for garnish
Chopped cilantro, for garnish

Heat oil in a large pot then add onion and garlic. Cook for 5 minutes. Add tomatoes, green chilies, chili powder, cumin, and oregano. Cook on medium heat for 10 minutes. Reduce heat to low and add the beans and bell peppers. Cook for about 10 more minutes, stirring occasionally. Stir in brown rice and add salt and pepper. Top with cheese and cilantro.

WHOLE WHEAT PASTA WITH ZUCCHINI AND BROCCOLINI

SERVES 4

TIME: 25 MINUTES

Adding green vegetables to pasta adds nutritional value as well as flavor. Get creative with the vegetables you have available—you can swap out any green vegetables for the zucchini and broccolini.

1 pound 100% whole wheat farfalle pasta (or use gluten-free or grain-free pasta)
2 tablespoons olive oil (not extra-virgin) or grapeseed oil
2 garlic cloves, minced
1 zucchini, chopped
2 bunches broccolini, chopped
1 teaspoon sea salt
¼ cup low-fat Parmesan cheese or vegan Parmesan (optional)

1. Boil a large pot of water and cook the pasta until it's *al dente*, about 11 minutes. Drain and set aside.

2. In a medium skillet, add 1 tablespoon of the olive oil and the garlic, sautéing until fragrant, about 5 minutes. Add zucchini and broccolini and cook until soft, about 8 minutes.

3. Mix the vegetables with pasta then add the remaining olive oil and salt. Toss to coat. Top with optional Parmesan cheese.

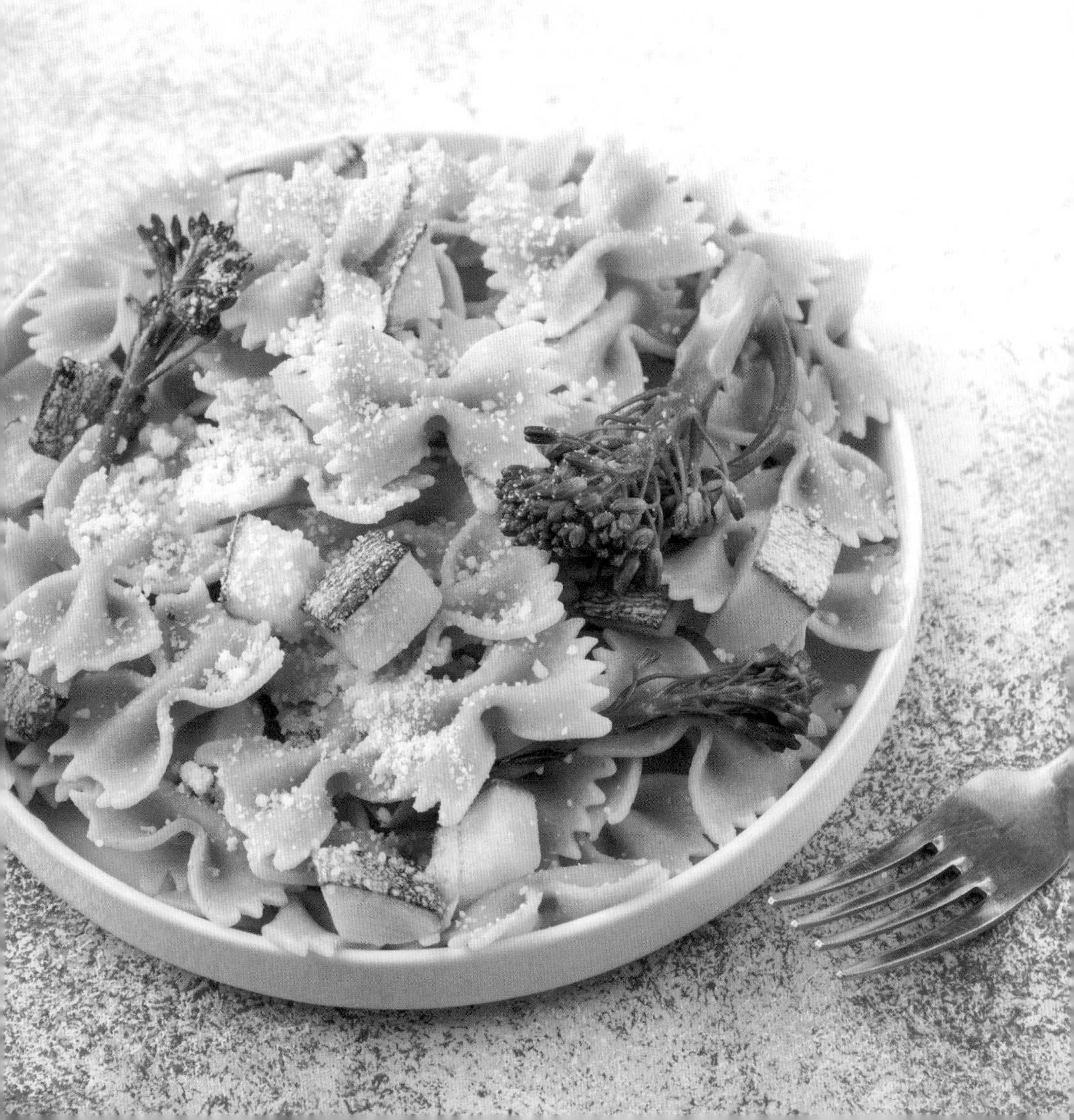

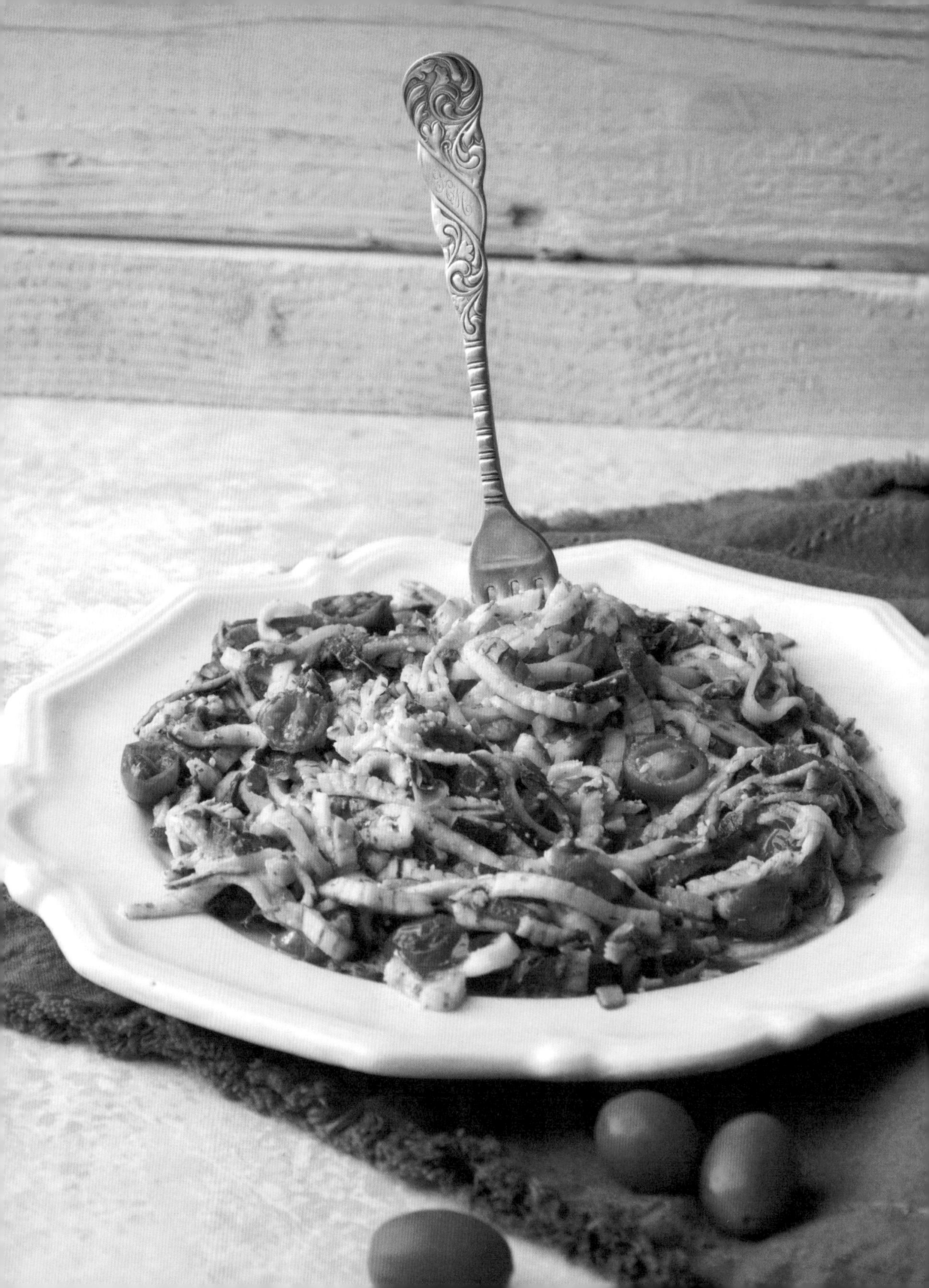

ZUCCHINI "PASTA" WITH CHERRY TOMATOES

SERVES 4

TIME: 25 MINUTES

This filling entrée uses only a handful of ingredients and takes less than a half hour to prepare. It's low in fat and carbs and high in prebiotic fiber. Serve it alongside a soup or salad to make it even more filling. For a plant-based option, see the recipe note.

5 large zucchini
3 teaspoons sea salt
1 tablespoon olive oil (not extra-virgin) or grapeseed oil
1 cup cherry tomatoes, cut in half
½ cup Homemade Pesto (page 250)
¼ cup low-fat or nonfat shredded mozzarella or grated Parmesan cheese (or plant-based cheese such as vegan Parmesan)

1. Make zucchini into noodles using a vegetable spiralizer or food processor. Put the "pasta" into a colander to drain excess liquid. Season with salt.

2. In a medium skillet over medium heat, warm the olive oil. Add the cherry tomatoes and pesto. Add the noodles to the pan and toss to coat. Cook until everything is warm. Serve on a platter or divide between four plates, and sprinkle with the cheese.

Plant-based variation: As an alternative to cheese, warm up ¼ cup of peanut butter or sesame butter (tahini) with 1 tablespoon water to make a sauce. Drizzle it over the "pasta" before serving.

ZUCCHINI AND CORN PIZZA

SERVES 4

TIME: 25 MINUTES

Using whole wheat naan bread, you can create your very own one-of-a-kind vegetable pizza with corn and zucchini. Don't feel limited by these vegetables—use whatever you have or what you can get fresh from your garden.

1 batch Homemade Pesto (recipe follows)
4 pieces whole wheat naan bread (or pita bread or whole-grain tortillas; or gluten-free or grain-free substitute)
1 zucchini, thinly sliced
½ cup fresh or defrosted corn
¼ red onion, thinly sliced
¼ cup nonfat or low-fat shredded dairy or plant-based mozzarella cheese (optional)
1 teaspoon Italian seasoning

1. Preheat the oven to 350°F.

2. Spread the Homemade Pesto on each piece of naan. Top with the sliced zucchini, corn, and red onion. Sprinkle with the cheese and seasoning.

3. Put the pizzas on a baking sheet or pizza stone and bake for 15 to 20 minutes or until the cheese is melted and the bread is slightly crispy.

CONTINUED

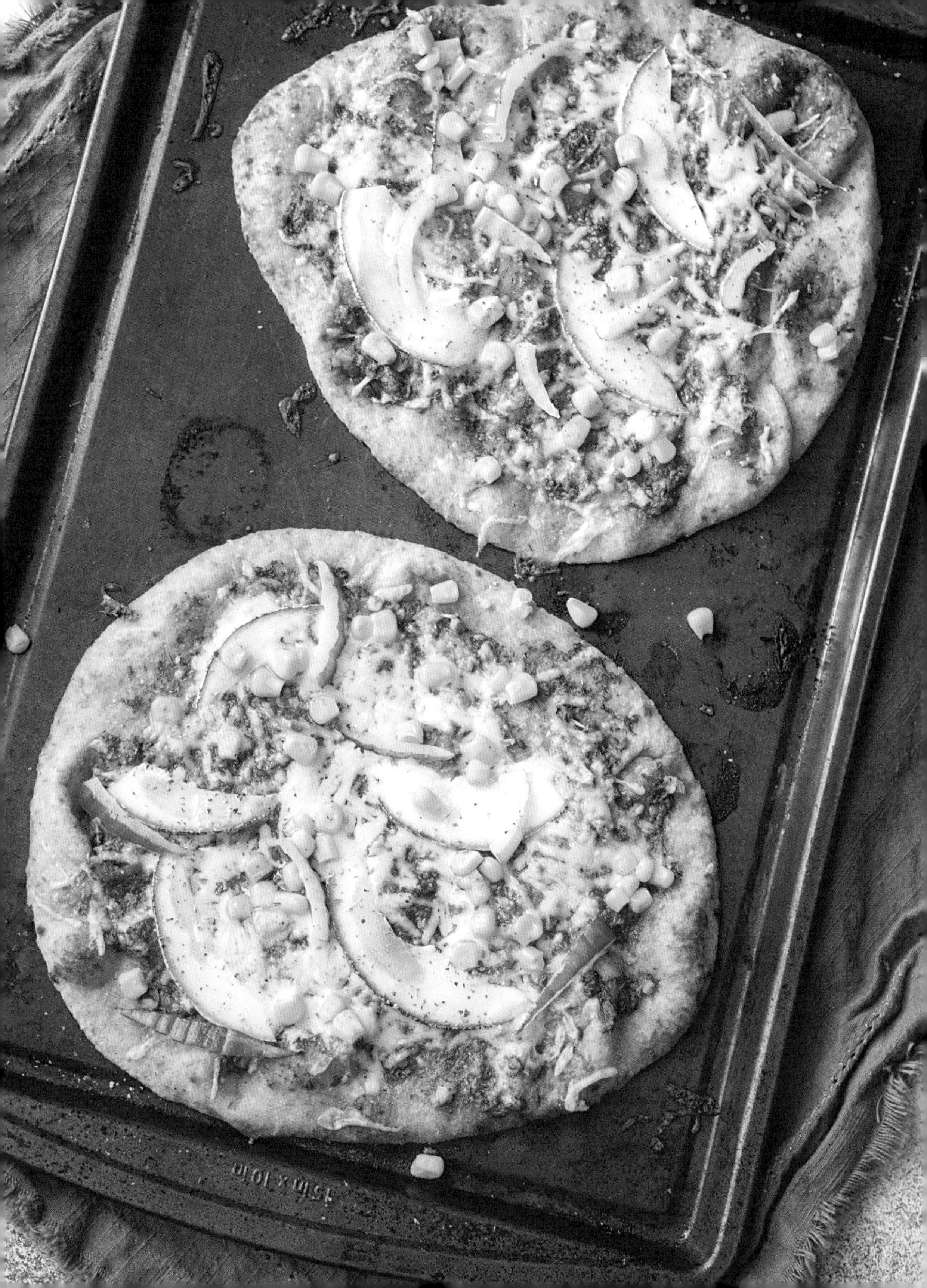

HOMEMADE PESTO

MAKES ABOUT ½ CUP

TIME: 5 MINUTES

You could pay a lot for gourmet pesto in a fancy store, or you could make your own in 5 minutes using fresh ingredients and no preservatives. This is a great recipe for summer when fresh basil is at its peak.

¼ cup tightly packed fresh basil leaves
¼ cup pine nuts or walnuts
1 tablespoon low-fat or nonfat Parmesan cheese
  or vegan Parmesan (optional)
1 teaspoon extra-virgin olive oil

In a blender or food processor, combine basil, pine nuts, optional Parmesan, and olive oil. Blend into a smooth pesto.

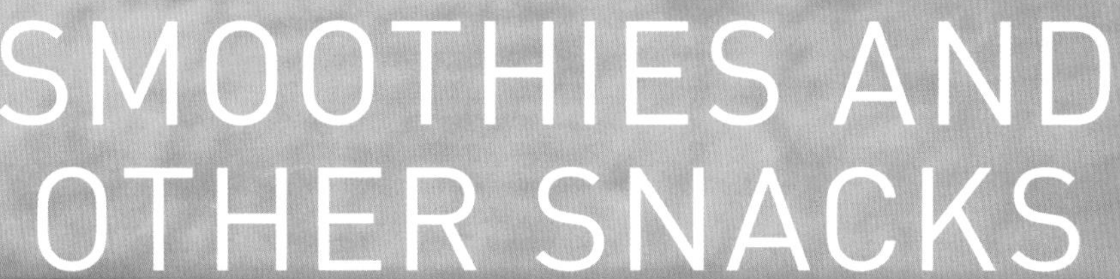
SMOOTHIES AND
OTHER SNACKS

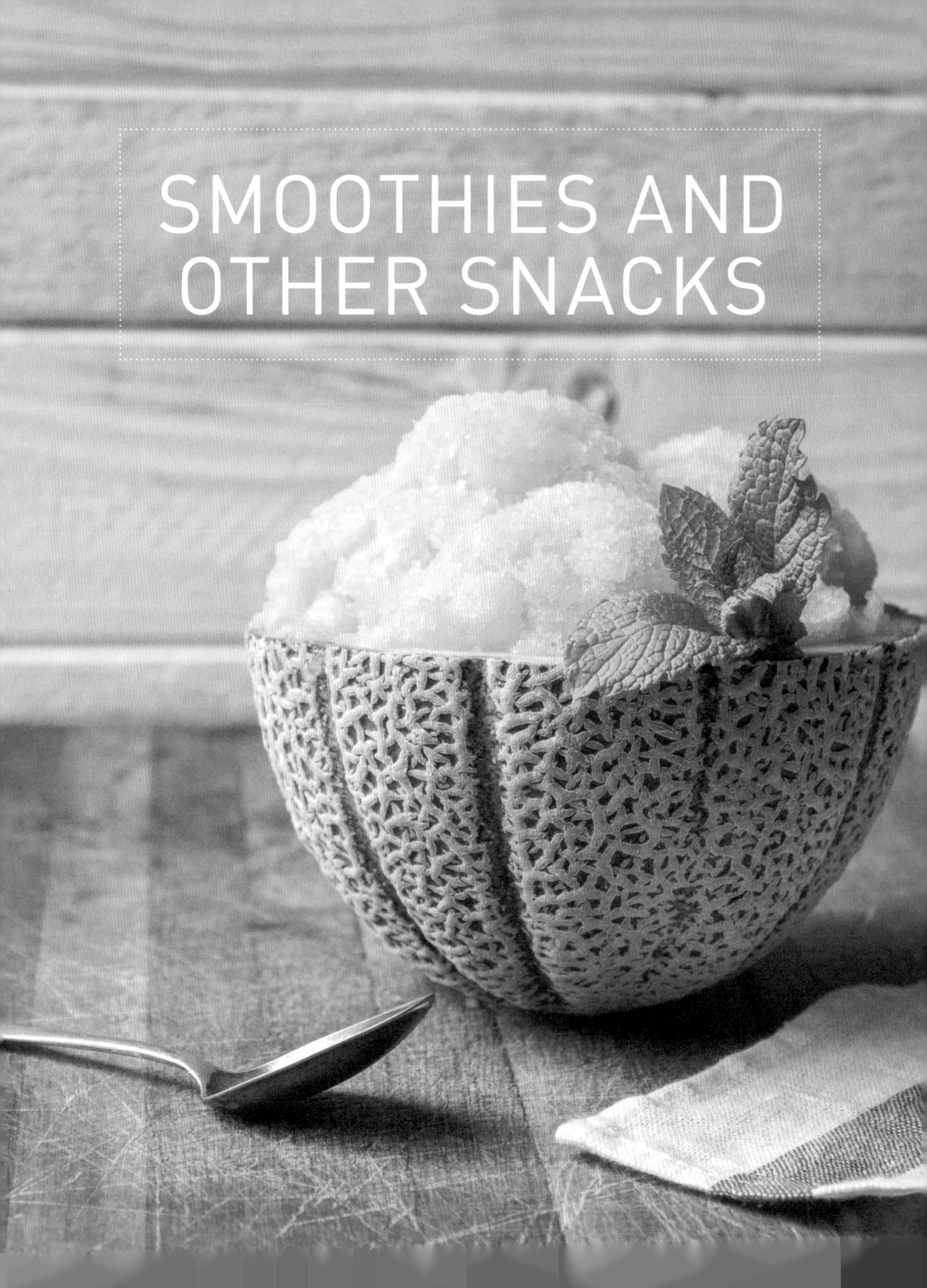

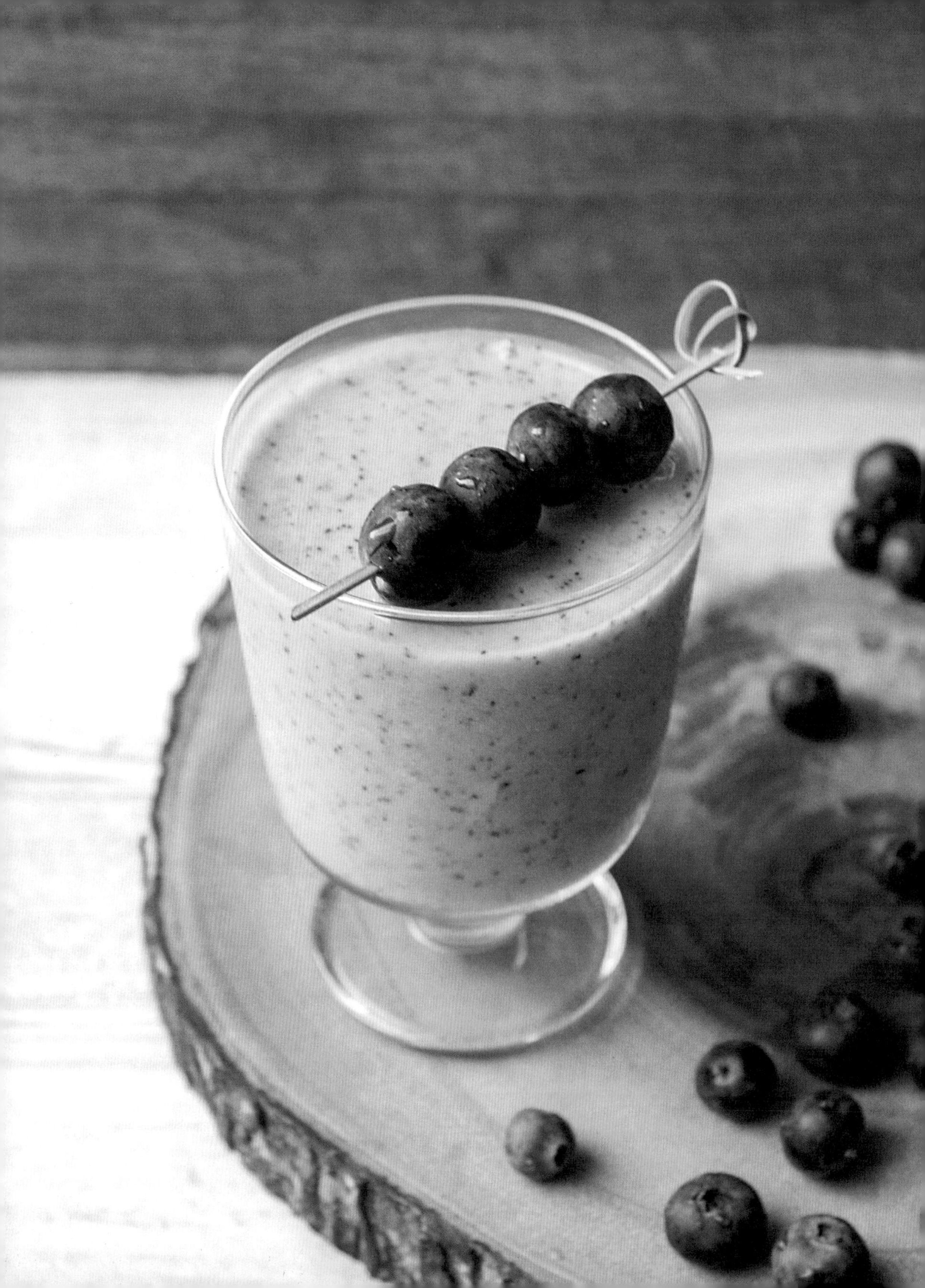

BLUEBERRY SMOOTHIE

SERVES 1

TIME: 5 MINUTES

Simple, classic smoothie recipes never go out of style especially when they are packed with antioxidants and potassium. This cold drink is naturally sweetened just enough to make a tasty vessel for all your protein or probiotic powders. If you use powders just add a serving's worth before blending.

1 frozen banana
½ pint blueberries
Honey or maple syrup to taste (optional, 1 tablespoon max)
1 cup any low-fat, nonfat, or unsweetened plant-based milk (such as Homemade Almond Milk, page 156)

Put all the ingredients in a blender jar and blend until smooth. Garnish with extra blueberries to make it fancy.

CANTALOUPE GINGER GRANITA

SERVES 1

TIME: 1 HOUR 10 MINUTES (MOSTLY FREEZING TIME)

Getting your daily intake of fruit never tasted so refreshing. Using cantaloupe as the base fruit, this granita recipe also works wonderfully with watermelon or honeydew. Just blend everything together with a simple honey syrup, freeze, and enjoy! This recipe makes one serving, but you can use a regular-sized cantaloupe and double the other ingredients to serve two.

½ cup water
Honey or maple syrup to taste (optional, 1 tablespoon max)
1 personal-size ripe cantaloupe (about 4 inches in diameter)
One 2-inch piece of ginger, peeled and minced

1. In a medium saucepan over medium heat, prepare a simple honey syrup: Whisk the water and honey together until the sweetener completely dissolves. Pour the mixture into a bowl and add a few ice cubes to cool it down. (If you aren't using sweetener, skip this step.)

2. Slice the cantaloupe in half and scoop out the seeds and pulp. Cut off the skin (or scoop out the fruit carefully if you want to reserve half of the cantaloupe for a bowl). Put the fruit in a food processor along with the (sweetened or not) water and ginger.

3. Pulse until the cantaloupe pieces are fully pureed. Pour the cantaloupe mixture into a rectangular baking dish (about 9-by-12 inches) and put it in the freezer. Freeze for one hour.

4. Using a fork, scrape the frozen fruit mixture to loosen it and make it spoonable. Spoon it into a bowl or into the scooped-out cantaloupe. Serve immediately.

GOLDEN MILK

SERVES 1

TIME: 5 MINUTES

This special recipe will help you get your weekly turmeric allowance. It makes a nice evening drink to settle the stomach as you prepare to get a good night's sleep. If the taste of turmeric is too strong for you, start with just a few dashes and then gradually work up to ½ teaspoon. You might also find you prefer the taste of the fresh turmeric root over the dried powder. You should be able to find turmeric root in well-stocked, health-oriented grocery stores and markets.

Note: Many people feel that this drink needs a sweetener. If you use a full tablespoon of honey or maple syrup in this drink, keep in mind that this is your total for the day.

1 cup nonfat or low-fat dairy or unsweetened soy, almond, or coconut milk (or use Homemade Almond Milk, page 156)
One 1-inch piece fresh turmeric root, peeled, or ½ teaspoon dried turmeric
1 dash cinnamon
1 dash dried ginger
1 dash black pepper
Honey or maple syrup to taste (optional, 1 tablespoon max)

Whisk all the ingredients together in a saucepan (you can also blend everything in a blender before heating). Turn the heat to medium and continue to stir the mixture as it heats. Just as it comes to a simmer, remove it from the heat (don't let it boil). If you used fresh turmeric root, remove it. Pour the golden milk into a mug and sip.

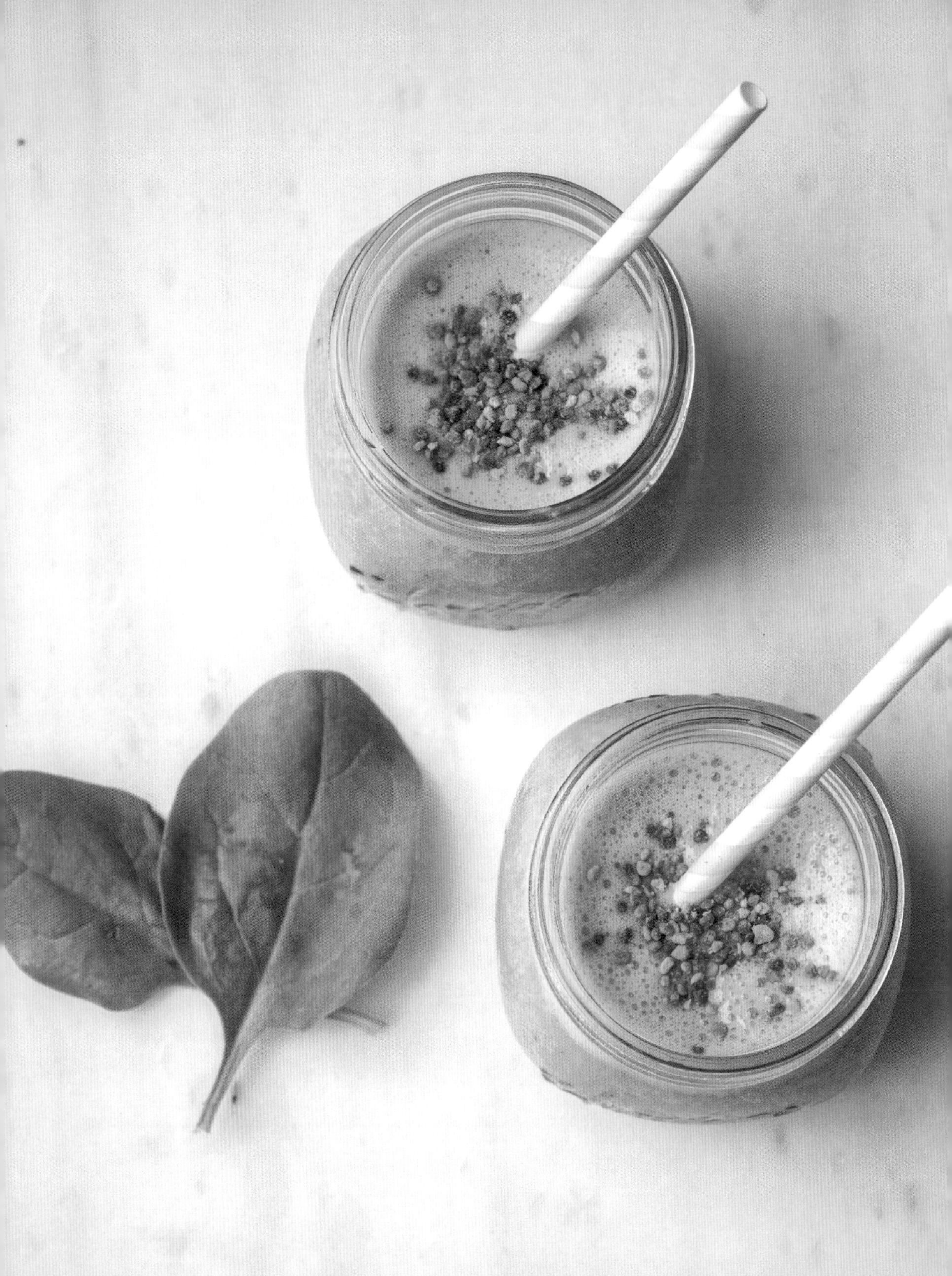

GREEN GODDESS SMOOTHIE

SERVES 1

TIME: 10 MINUTES

Here's a smoothie that will make you glow from the inside out. Filled with iron-rich spinach and banana along with gut-friendly chia seeds, this sweet green drink will start your day out right. The bee pollen is optional, but if you want to try it, you can find it in health food stores.

1 frozen banana
1 handful spinach or kale
Honey or maple syrup to taste (optional, 1 tablespoon max)
1 cup milk (nonfat, low-fat, or unsweetened plant milk such as Homemade Almond Milk, page 156)
2 tablespoons chia seeds
Bee pollen (optional)

In a blender, blend all ingredients together except the chia seeds and bee pollen. Pour into one large glass, or two small ones. Top with chia seeds (or mix them in) and a sprinkle of bee pollen, if desired.

The Microbiomes of . . . Bees?

Here's an interesting fact: All animals have their own microbiomes . . . even bees. A honeybee's microbiome is highly specialized to digest pollen, and research shows that a healthy bee microbiome is necessary for bee health and growth. Bees don't have as many microbes as we do, but like us, their microbiomes contain both bacteria and fungi. The most common fungus in the bee microbiome is *Saccharomyces*, but some foraging and queen bees contain many other types of fungus. Honey—that bee product so many humans enjoy—is also full of fungi, a product of honey-producing bees' microbiomes. Research also suggests that the recent severe decline in honeybee colonies may be related to dysbiosis in the honeybee microbiome, disrupting a bee's immune system and making it more susceptible to pathogens.[257]

TROPICAL MANGO SMOOTHIE

SERVES 1

TIME: 10 MINUTES

No need for a flight to the tropics when you have the flavors of banana and mango in this refreshing smoothie recipe. Blend these fruits with orange juice for some serious natural sweetness and an antioxidant boost.

1 frozen banana
½ cup plain, unsweetened nonfat or low-fat dairy yogurt or plant-based yogurt
1 mango, peeled with seed removed
¼ cup orange juice
¼ cup milk (nonfat, low-fat, or unsweetened plant milk such as Homemade Almond Milk, page 156)
Honey or maple syrup to taste (optional, 1 tablespoon max)
2 tablespoons chia seeds
Fresh mint, for garnish

In a blender, blend all ingredients except chia seeds and mint together and pour into one large glass or two small ones. Top with chia seeds (or mix them in) and mint.

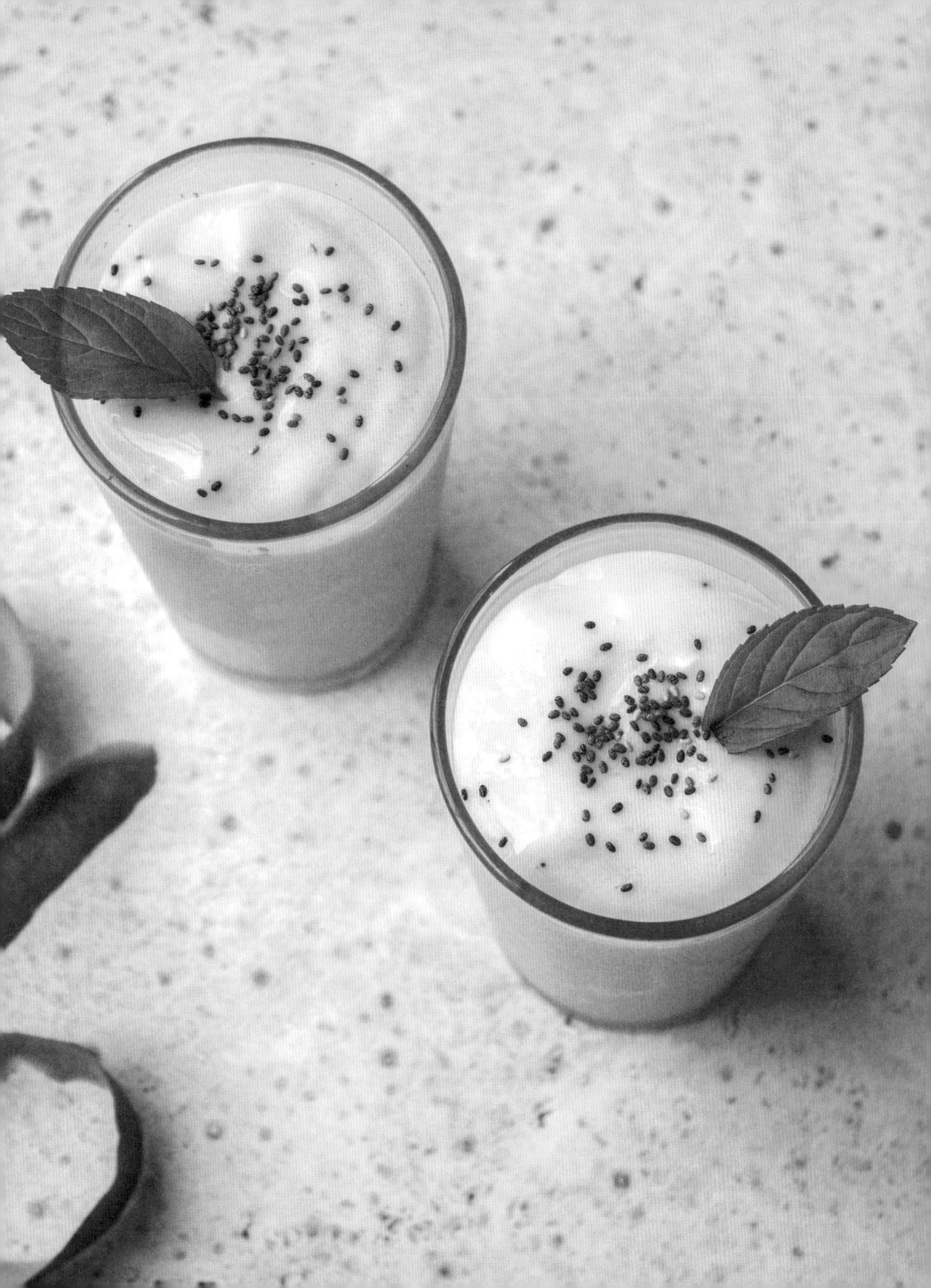

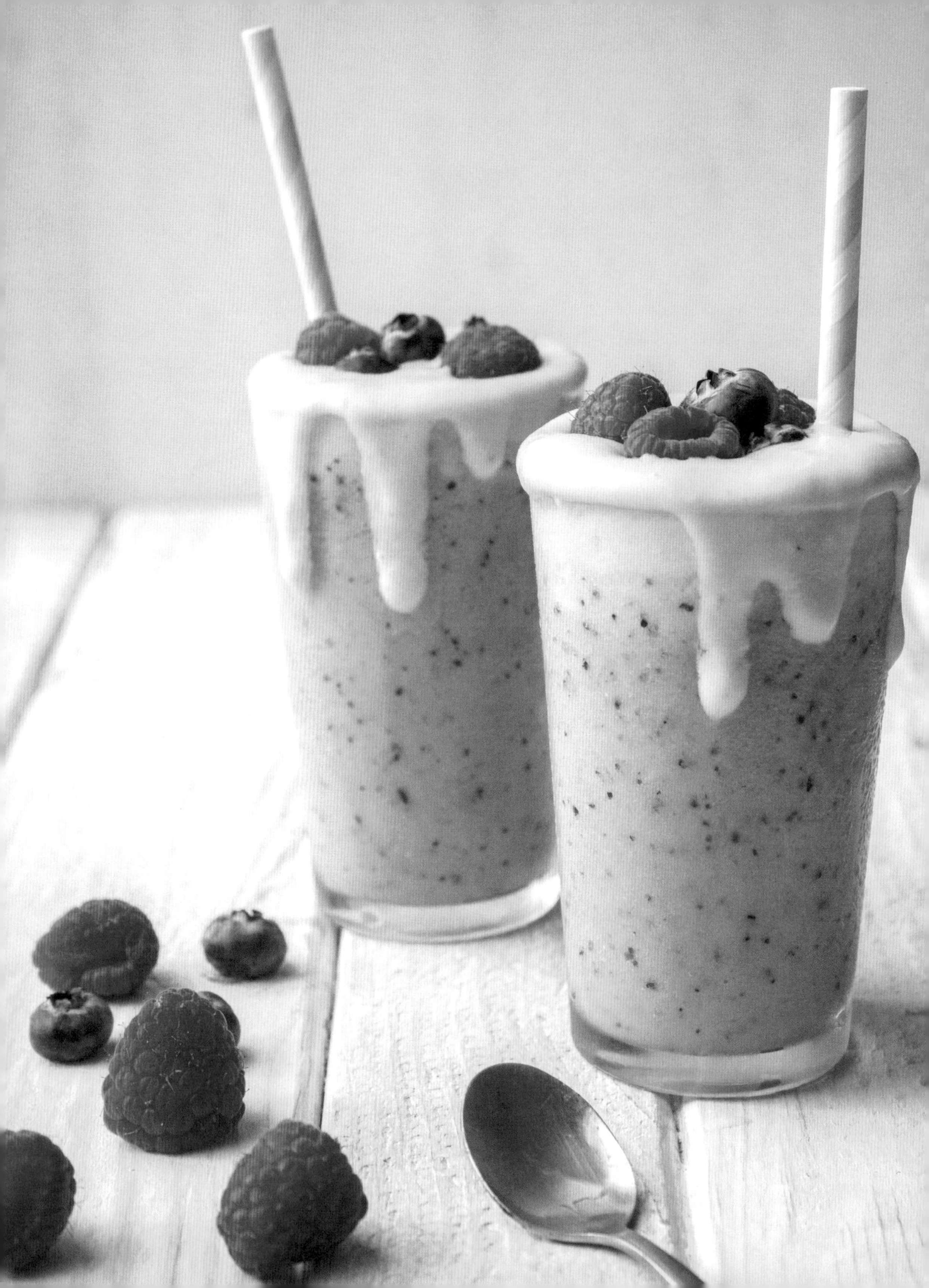

VERY BERRY SMOOTHIE

SERVES 1

TIME: 15 MINUTES

Layer your next smoothie with a fresh berry base and a naturally sweetened coconut whipped cream. It offers plenty of antioxidants, healthy fats, and electrolytes.

½ frozen banana
¼ cup blueberries
¼ cup raspberries
½ cup milk (nonfat, low-fat, or unsweetened plant milk such as Homemade Almond Milk, page 156)

WHIPPED COCONUT CREAM TOPPING
One 13-ounce can coconut milk
½ frozen banana
Honey or maple syrup to taste (optional, 1 tablespoon max)
Extra blueberries and raspberries, for topping

1. In a blender, pulse all ingredients for the smoothie portion. Pour into your glass.

2. Rinse out the blender. Scoop out just the fatty cream portion from the can of coconut milk. Reserve the liquid for another use. Put the coconut cream, banana, and optional sweetener in the blender. Blend until creamy.

3. Spoon the whipped cream on top of smoothie. Top with berries and enjoy.

BEET HUMMUS

SERVES 2

TIME: 15 MINUTES

Take ordinary hummus to a new level by adding bright red beets. Beets are naturally low in calories and help lower blood pressure—and they turn everything an attractive bright pink. Serve this dip with raw carrots and celery to stay full until your next meal. For regular hummus, leave out the beets.

2 small roasted beets (you can buy beets preroasted and vacuum sealed, for convenience)
One 15-ounce can chickpeas, rinsed and drained
1 tablespoon extra-virgin olive oil or coconut oil
2 tablespoons tahini (sesame "butter")
½ lemon, juiced
2 cloves garlic, roughly chopped
½ teaspoon sea salt
4 celery stalks, trimmed and cut into 4- to 6-inch pieces
2 to 3 carrots, trimmed and cut into sticks

1. Cut one slice out of a roasted beet and set it aside. In a food processor, combine the rest of the beets with chickpeas, oil, tahini, lemon juice, garlic, and salt. Puree. If it's too thick, add a teaspoon of water at a time until it is the consistency you like. It should be thick enough to scoop with a celery stalk.

2. Serve with raw carrots and celery and garnish with the extra slice of roasted beet.

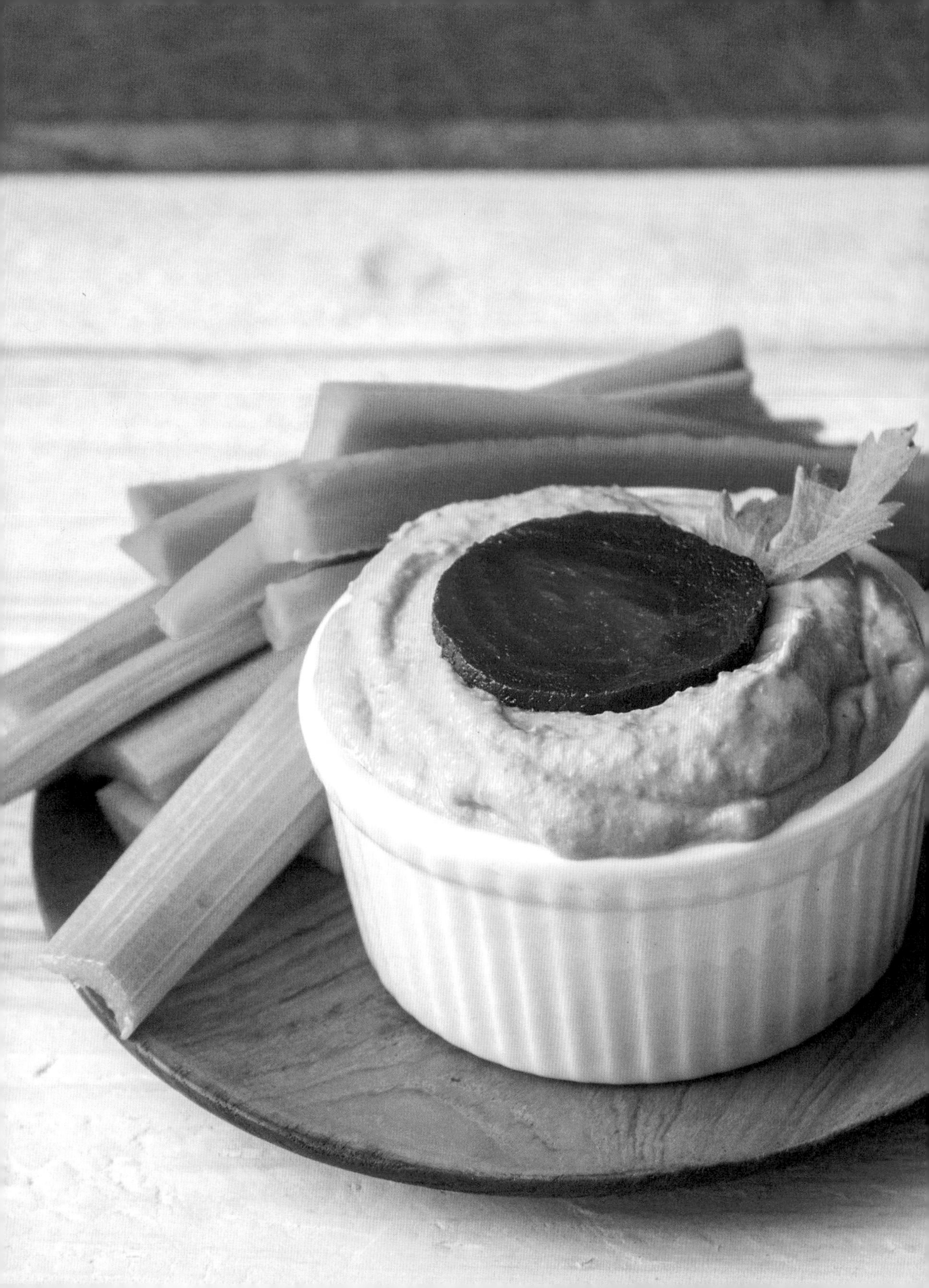

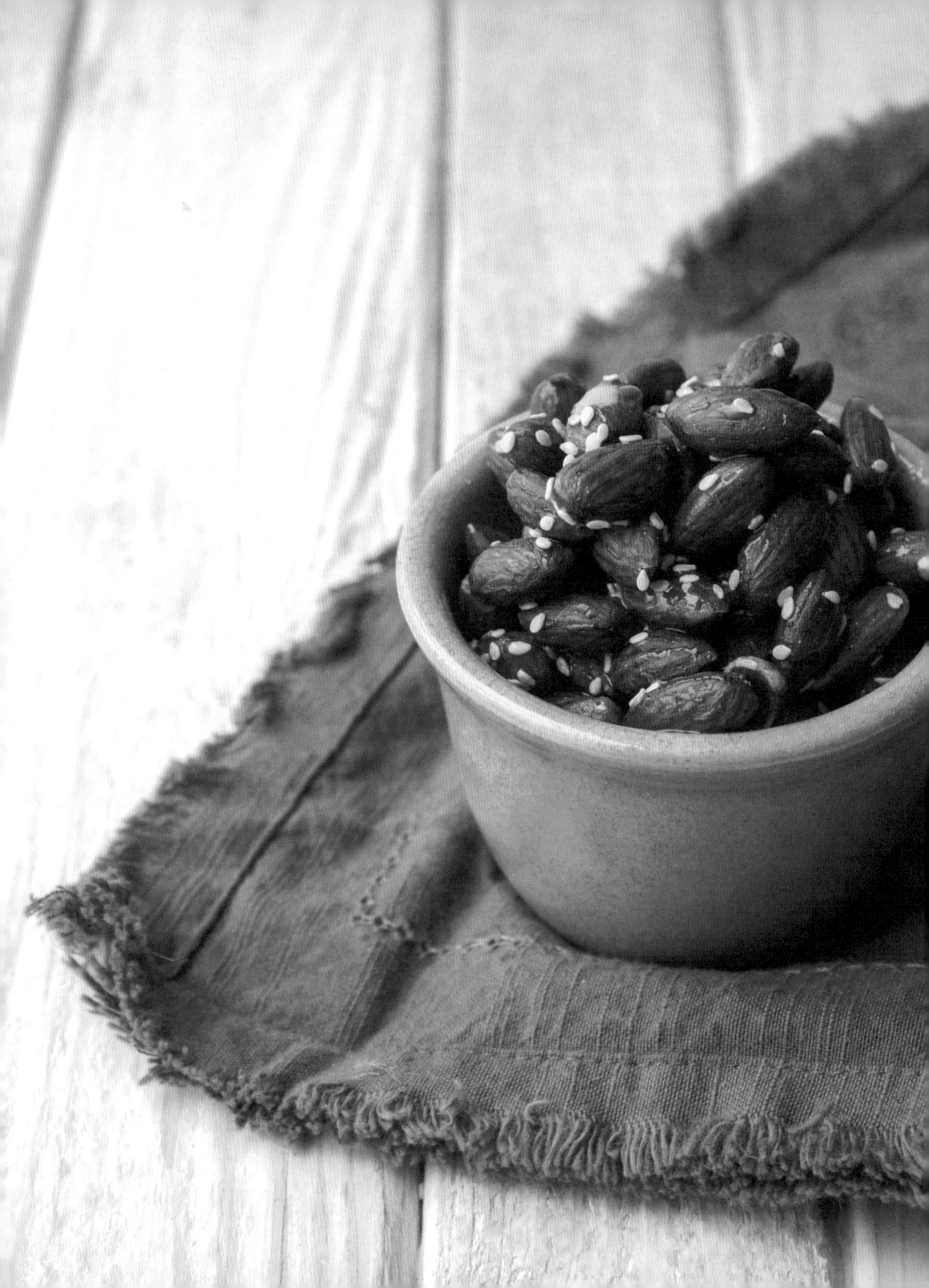

SESAME ALMONDS

SERVES 1

TIME: 15 MINUTES

In-between-meal snacks can be dangerous when they have hidden calories or loads of sugar. Avoid that conundrum with these tasty almonds. They are coated in honey and sprinkled with sesame seeds, and they offer magnesium, fiber, and plenty of vitamin E. This recipe makes one serving, but you can easily double, triple, or quadruple this recipe to feed more people. (Don't expect it to last long, but it can keep in an airtight container for 2 to 3 weeks.)

¼ cup whole raw almonds
1 tablespoon honey (this is your sweetener allowance for the day)
1 teaspoon sesame seeds
1 teaspoon water

Preheat oven to 350°F. Mix all ingredients together in a small saucepan over medium heat until well coated. Line a baking sheet with parchment paper. Pour the almond mixture onto the baking sheet and bake for 10 minutes. Cool slightly and serve warm.

ROASTED CURRIED CAULIFLOWER

SERVES 1

TIME: 15 MINUTES

Not only does cauliflower aid in digestion, it also helps your body detoxify. This makes cauliflower the perfect vegetable to grab when you're in between meals. Season it with yellow curry powder and a dash of salt, and you have a nutrient-rich snack you can feel good about.

2 cups cauliflower florets
1 tablespoon olive oil (not extra-virgin) or coconut oil
1 teaspoon curry powder
1 pinch sea salt

Preheat the oven to 425°F. Put all the ingredients in a sealable plastic bag and mix everything together until the cauliflower florets are well-coated. Spread the cauliflower onto a baking sheet and bake for 10 to 15 minutes, or until the edges start to brown. Serve warm.

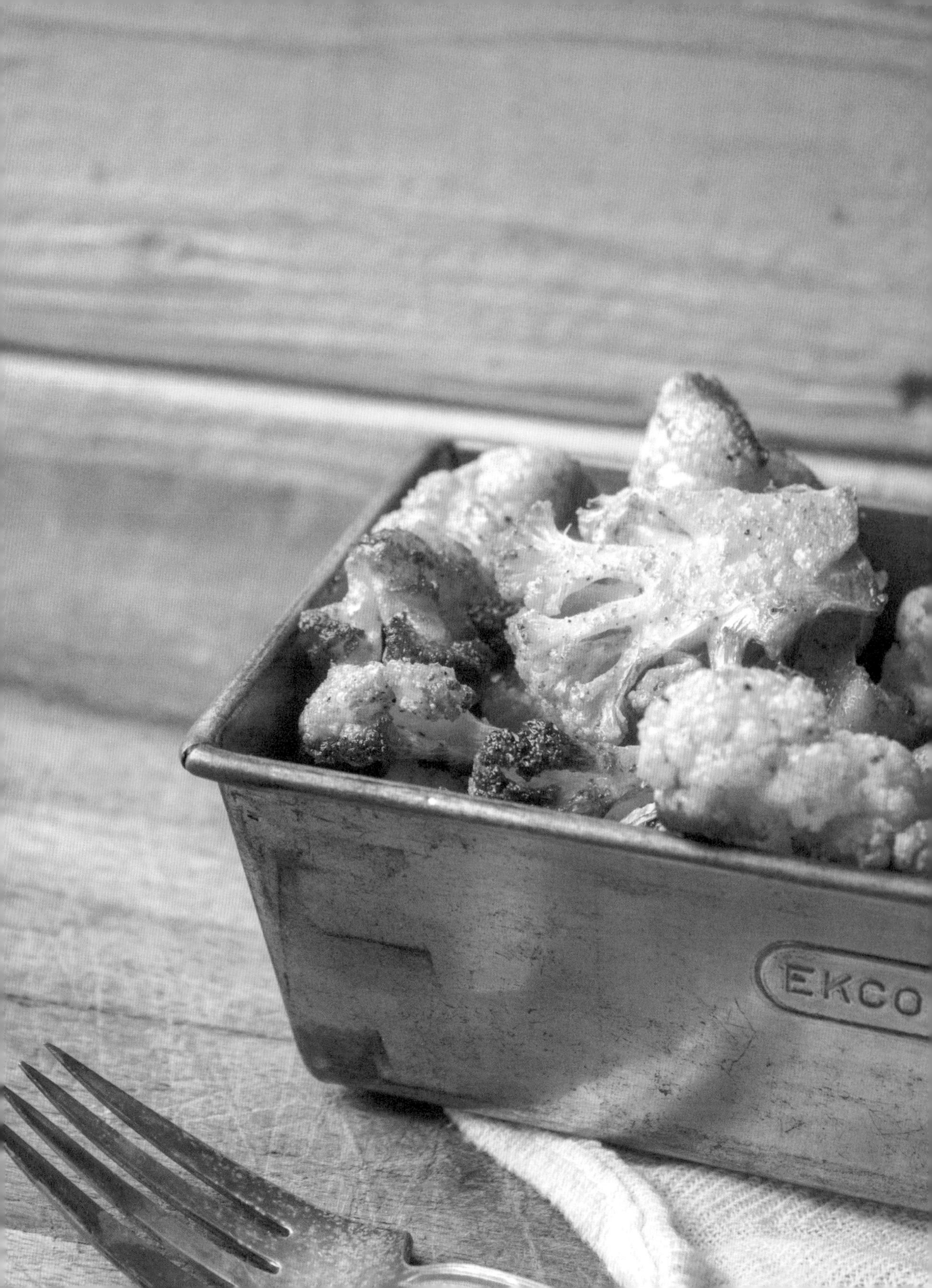
EKCO

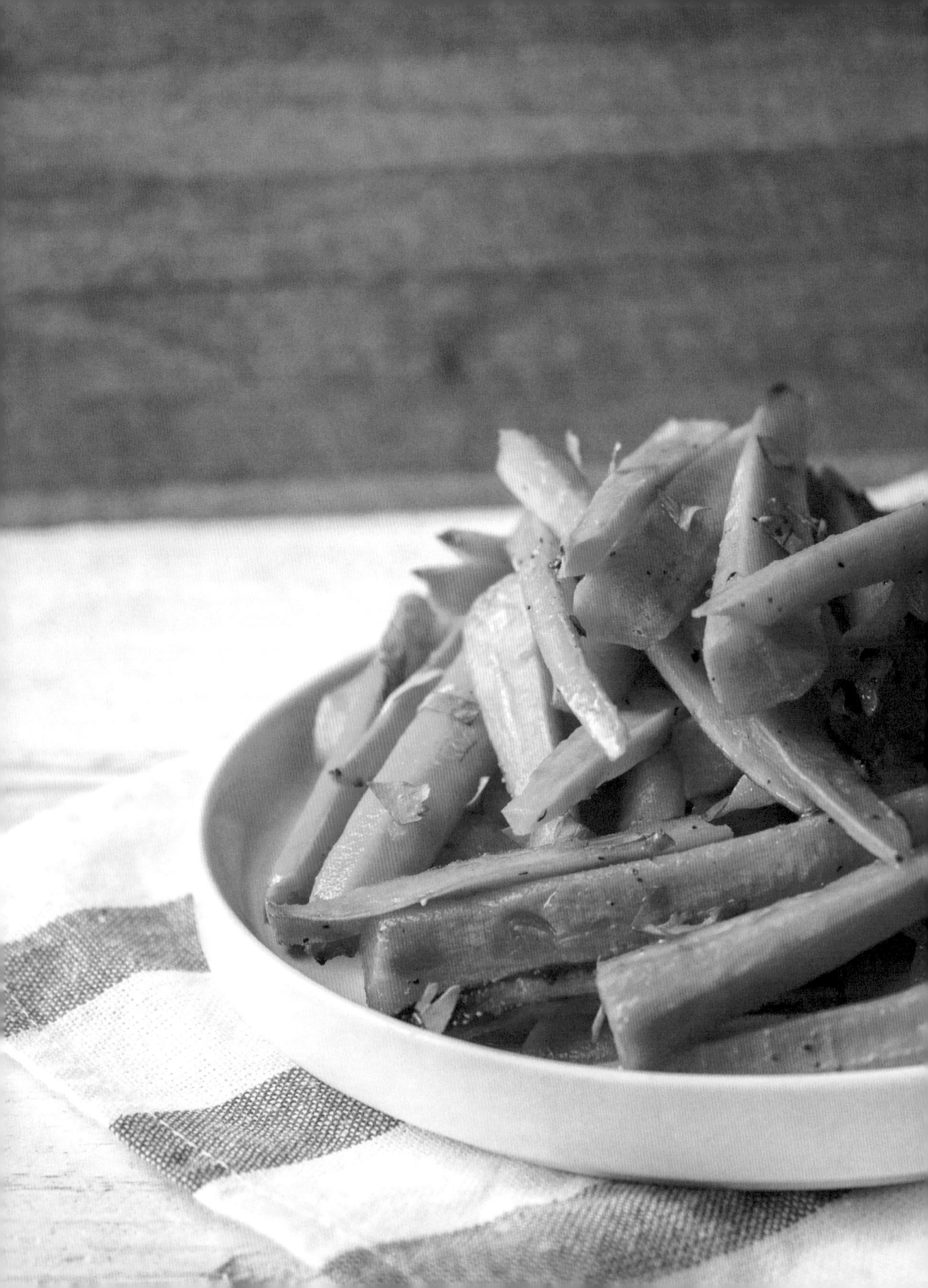

SEASONED ROASTED CARROTS

SERVES 1

TIME: 15 MINUTES

Whether you eat them raw or roasted, carrots make an optimal snack because they are loaded with vitamin A and beta-carotene.

1 tablespoon plus 1 teaspoon olive oil (not extra-virgin) or coconut oil
1 tablespoon apple cider vinegar
1 tablespoon minced cilantro leaves
1 teaspoon Dijon mustard
1 pinch each sea salt and black pepper
2 large or 3 medium carrots, trimmed, cut lengthwise into quarters, then sliced into 2-inch pieces

1. Preheat the oven to 475°F.

2. Make the vinaigrette by whisking together 1 tablespoon of the oil, vinegar, cilantro, mustard, salt, and pepper, or put it all in a jar with a lid and shake it.

3. Spread the carrots on a baking sheet and drizzle with one teaspoon of the oil. Bake for 10 to 15 minutes, or until they are soft. Put the warm carrots into a bowl and drizzle with the vinaigrette.

Note: Save any extra vinaigrette to put on a future salad or for dipping raw vegetables.

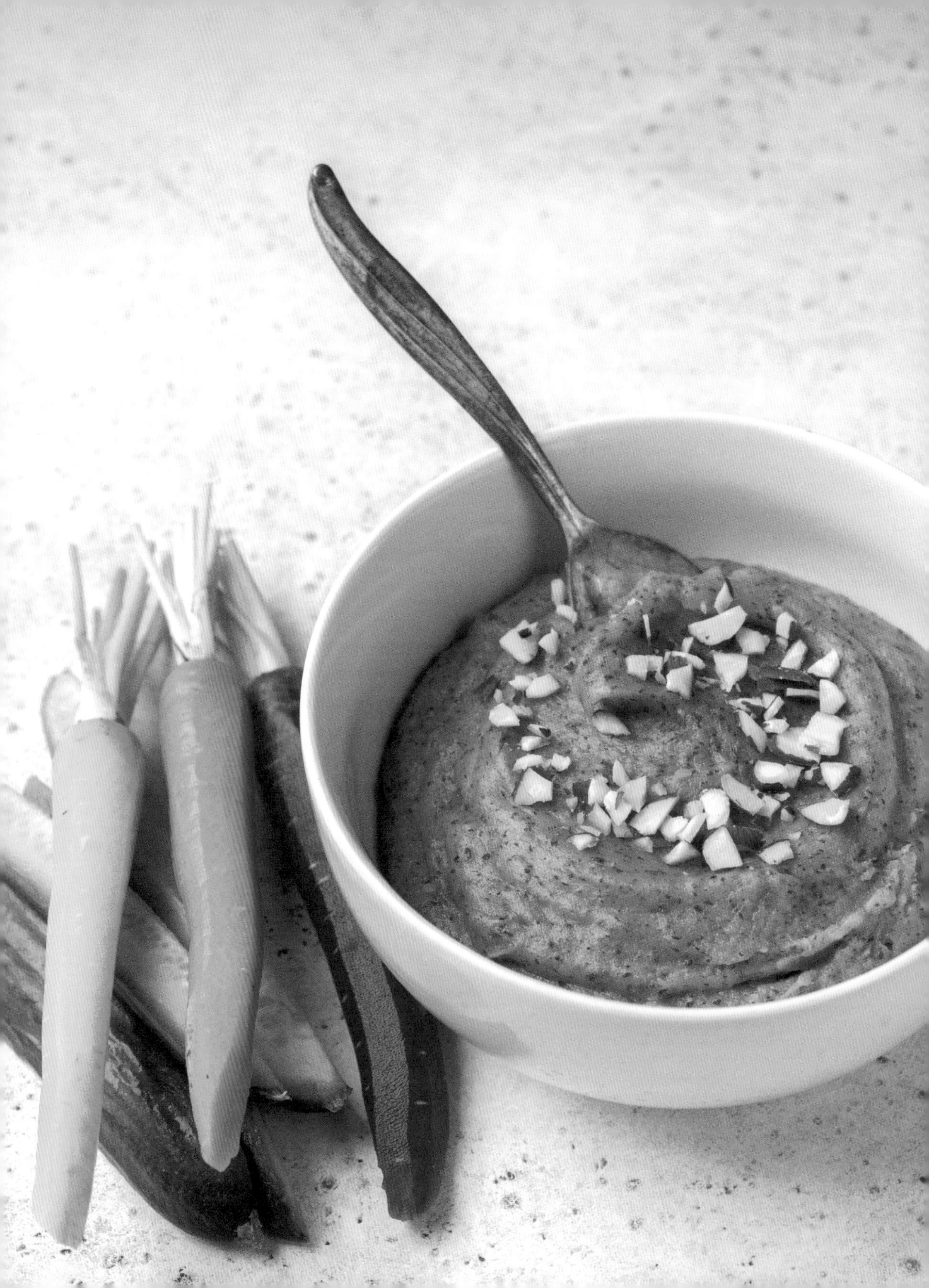

SPINACH MASHED POTATOES

SERVES 1

TIME: 20 MINUTES

Adding spinach to mashed potatoes is a genius idea because it adds loads of fiber and protein all while giving your dish a vibrant, beautiful color—yet it still tastes like mashed potatoes. Eat these potatoes as a side dish, or even as a snack. If you make this and immediately refrigerate it, you can eat it cold the next day and take advantage of its increased resistant starch content (see the Carley's Corner box that follows).

3 small gold potatoes, peeled and cut into cubes
1 cup fresh spinach
1 tablespoon milk (nonfat or low-fat dairy or plant-based)
1 tablespoon extra-virgin olive oil
1 teaspoon sea salt
1 tablespoon sliced almonds, for garnish

Boil water in a large saucepan. Add the potatoes and cook them until they are soft and easy to pierce with a fork, about 8 to 10 minutes, depending on the size of the potatoes.. Drain the potatoes and put them in a food processor. Add the spinach, milk, oil, and salt. Blend until creamy. Spoon the mixture into a bowl and top with almonds. Serve with vegetables for dipping or eat it with a spoon.

Carley's Corner: Oven-Roasted Smashed Potatoes

Resistant starch helps promote the growth of beneficial bacteria in the gut by providing nutrients for them to thrive. Resistant starch is named for being just that: *resistant* to digestion. It travels to the large intestine undigested, where gut bacteria can consume it, producing short-chain fatty acids (SCFAs).[258] Low SCFAs have been linked to dysfunction of the gut,[259] including irritable bowel syndrome (IBS) and even colon cancer.[260] Some of the foods with the highest levels of resistant starch are potatoes, legumes, oats, and banana flour. However, it is important that these foods are properly prepared in order to obtain the most resistant starch.

Potatoes, for instance, must be cooked and immediately cooled, which helps preserve the resistant starch. Legumes and rice are similar in that they must be soaked in water for at least 24 hours, then boiled and cooked according to the directions on the package. Not only is this going to boost the available resistant starch, but it will also help eliminate any anti-nutrients or protective barriers the legumes have, which can negatively impair digestion. While this may seem like a tedious extra step in preparing these foods, it takes minimal time and effort. What's more, you can make these foods in large quantities in advance and then freeze them so they are readily available when needed. If you have the time, why not go the extra mile?

Who knew potatoes were good for gut health? That is, if they are properly prepared. These potatoes are a tasty treat that is perfect for the entire family as an easy side dish at dinnertime. They are also a fun party appetizer!

SERVES 4 • TIME: 1 HOUR

Approximately 2 to 3 cups cubed potatoes (I like to use a combination of red and Dutch yellow baby potatoes)
4 tablespoons olive oil plus more for drizzling
2 to 3 tablespoons chopped fresh rosemary
2 teaspoons Himalayan sea salt

1. Preheat the oven to 350°F. Meanwhile, fill a large pot with water and bring it to a boil. Add the potatoes and boil for about 15 to 20 minutes or until softened. Immediately place in an ice bath (bowl of ice and cold water) or run under cool water until the potatoes are chilled.
2. Dry off the potatoes and place them in a mixing bowl. Add the oil, rosemary, and sea salt, mixing until the potatoes are well coated.
3. Transfer the potatoes to a baking sheet and gently press each one with the palm of your hand until it's "smashed." Drizzle the potatoes with a little extra oil, then roast them in the oven for 15 to 20 minutes or until golden and crisp.

FINAL THOUGHTS

We are at the end of our time together. This is where we part, and one of my great hopes for you is that this book has made a difference in your life. I hope you have learned some important things about your own health and have taken steps to improve your total gut balance, and by association your whole body and brain, for the better. I hope you have learned to eat, not just for enjoyment but also with the purpose of feeding your microbiome and optimizing your health. I also hope (and expect) that you are already seeing positive results, such as more energy, fewer uncomfortable symptoms, better digestion, better sleep, less pain, the loss of excess weight, and a happier state of mind. Life is a journey and we all have the opportunity to make the most of the lives we are given. May you go forward in great health with joy and a commitment to take care of your mind, your body, and the microbes within that are along for the ride.

APPENDIX: BIOHM HEALTH PROBIOTICS AND MICROBIOME TESTING

Throughout this book, I have talked a little bit about prebiotic and probiotic supplements, and also about getting your own microbiome tested. My company, BIOHM Health, manufactures these supplements and also does microbiome testing, but as I've said before, there is nothing in the Mycobiome Diet that requires the use of any of these products. However, for those who are interested in learning more, taking a good quality probiotic supplement, or getting their own microbiome tested, I'm including this information here.

PROBIOTICS

I truly believe that you can rebalance and maintain your microbiome through dietary and lifestyle changes alone. However, nutritional supplements can be a great *supplement* to your diet and lifestyle—they don't make up for poor dietary choices, but they can boost good choices.

In 2016, I discovered a particular need in this area. I published my research on a clinical trial my team and I conducted to examine the microbiomes of patients with Crohn's disease (CD). In that paper, we found that bacteria and fungi were working together in the gut to create biofilms (digestive plaque), to the great devastation of these patients. That paper got wide coverage around the world, and I had many people reach out to me, asking what they could do to control bacteria, fungi, and biofilms in their own guts. I thought about recommending probiotics, but when I looked at the probiotics available, I was surprised to see that no one had created a probiotic specifically designed to balance both the bacteria *and* the fungi in the gut. They had also failed to address the role of digestive biofilms.

When you need something and it doesn't exist, it makes sense to create it. That's exactly what we set out to do with the probiotic we now call BIOHM Probiotic. We recognized that it would be important to use and combine the right probiotic strains for maximum therapeutic value.

In designing a probiotic that would reduce intestinal dysbiosis, it was critical that we selected appropriate microbes that could target pathogenic bacterial and fungal strains while supporting beneficial ones. My team knew we wanted to include both bacteria *and* fungi, so we conducted research regarding the interactions between various bacterial strains, as well as the interactions between bacteria and fungi, to identify which probiotic strains (both bacterial and fungal) were best able to antagonize harmful microbes while also supporting beneficial ones. We concluded that there were four species that would do these jobs most effectively:

- *Bifidobacterium breve*
- *Saccharomyces boulardii*
- *Lactobacillus acidophilus*
- *Lactobacillus rhamnosus*

In addition to these probiotic strains, we also included a digestive enzyme called amylase, which is known to possess anti-biofilm activity. This, we believed, would be critical for enhancing anti-biofilm action.

The next step was to test BIOHM Probiotic[261] for safety and efficacy. We gave healthy volunteers BIOHM Probiotic over four weeks, taking stool samples before they began taking it and after they stopped taking it four weeks later. We sequenced the samples to create microbiome reports, and we compared their bacteriomes to the microbiomes of healthy subjects used in the Human Microbiome Project and to data captured from control subjects studied at Case Western Reserve University's Center for Medical Mycology.

Before the test, our subjects had low levels of beneficial *Ascomycota* and high levels of harmful *Zygomycota* fungi, as well as elevated *Candida* species, especially *Candida albicans*. Subjects also had elevated Firmicutes, which as you know from reading this book is associated with obesity, disordered sleep, and other health issues.

After four weeks on our probiotic, the subjects had normalized Firmicutes, *Ascomycota, Zygomycota,* and *Candida,* including *Candida albicans*—in particular, levels of *Candida* species were significantly lower. (And, anecdotally, many reported liking the probiotic and feeling better on it.) These findings suggest that the use of BIOHM Probiotic leads to both structural and functional changes in the gut bacteriome and gut mycobiome that could be supportive in resolving gut dysbiosis and benefiting microbiome balance.

This test confirmed that we had a probiotic that could control bad bacteria and fungi in the gut, while also breaking down digestive biofilms. No other probiotic has ever been proven to both balance bad bacteria and fungi, and also control digestive biofilms.

If you are interested in learning more about these products, please visit our BIOHM Probiotic website at BIOHMHealth.com. We also make a prebiotic supplement, to help provide optimal food for beneficial gut microbes, although you should be getting plenty of good microbiome food on the Mycobiome Diet.

MICROBIOME TESTING

As you know from reading this book, there are ways to make pretty good guesses about what species are likely to be out of balance in your own microbiome. However, some people want to know *for sure.* I know I did.

That is why, as another part of BIOHM Health, we decided to develop a microbiome testing kit, called the BIOHM Gut Report. Our test is sent directly to you through the mail. It includes a swab for you to provide a stool sample, simple instructions, and a self-addressed stamped envelope to mail your sample back to us. In addition to the sample collection kit, we include a lifestyle questionnaire. Once we receive your sample and questionnaire, we use state-of-the-art DNA technology and bioinformatics to analyze the bacteria and fungi present in your gut. We then compare your microbial profile with our in-house data, data from the Human Microbiome Project, and peer reviewed literature, to tell you whether your bacterial and fungal levels fall within normal ranges. To make it easy to understand your results, the report indicates which microbes live in your gut, and whether the levels of those nicrobes are in the high, low, or normal range. While we are not the only company with a microbiome test, a typical test is limited to the bacteria in your gut. Depending on the test, it may show you how your levels compare to levels normally found in the gut. You may also receive recommendations on how to actually use the results. However, many tests are limited to a general overview of the data, and don't really provide you with actionable recommendations.

Of course, I wanted to create a test that not only tested bacteria, but that also looked at the fungi in your gut—your mycobiome. My team also had a lot of ideas about how to make gut testing even easier and more effective. So that's what we did.

For example, your microbiome profile will reveal whether your gut contains enough good bacteria (for example *Bifidobacteria, Lactobacilli,* and the anti-inflammatory *Faecalibacterium*) and fungi (*Saccharomyces*), which are important for your gut health and consequently your overall health. You will also learn about the abundance of the bad microbes (such as *Escherichia coli* and *Clostridium difficile*). Even more, you are able to see if you have elevated levels of *Candida,* and if so, which species are the problem. In fact, if you are only interested in *Candida,* we have a test that only measures and gives you a full report on how much *Candida* you have, and what species, along with recommendations for reestablishing balance.

We also strive to make our test results easy to understand. Here's how I think about it. When people do an ancestry test and they get a result saying (for example), "You are 80% Irish," that's about all they wanted to know. That's useful, and just that information is useful to them because it answers the question, "What's my ancestry?" But with a microbiome test, if the result says, "You have high levels of *Bacteroides,*" that is essentially meaningless to the vast majority of people. What people really want to know when they do a microbiome test is, "Is my gut okay, or do I need to do something to improve it?"

So that's how we designed the BIOHM Gut Report's results. You will learn the exact types of organisms and their levels; you will also learn whether your microbiome balance is healthy or needs improvement. The report is designed like a credit report. We give you a Gut Score, or a score reflecting the health of your microbiome balance, with 1 being very bad, and 10 being very good.

We also give you actionable dietary, lifestyle, and supplement recommendations, so that it's easy to understand what you should be doing to optimize your gut. The recommendations are tailored to your specific microbiome and health profiles. You will gain insight into how to increase the levels of beneficial microbes that boost gut health while at the same time reduce the problematic ones. You will know which missing beneficial bacteria (like *Bifidobacterium* and *Lactobacillus*) your gut needs, whether you need fiber to support good bacteria and reduce bad ones (for example Proteobacteria), and which vitamin supplements you may need based on your current diet and lifestyle as well as your microbiome results. Finally, you will learn ways to optimize the digestion and absorption of nutrients to maintain the health of your gut lining and increase your gut immunity. We also have microbiome-trained nutritionists who are available for consults. Our nutritionist team has been trained how to interpret microbiome results, and every nutritionist has reviewed and interpreted thousands of test results. They are available for wellness consults and to answer any questions and to walk you through your results.

If you are interested in learning more, or having your own microbiome tested through our company, please visit our BIOHM Gut Report page at BIOHMHealth.com.

ADDITIONAL RESOURCES

Congratulations! My hope is that after engaging with *Total Gut Balance*, you are now well down the path to total gut optimization! For further help in putting your Mycobiome Diet into action, check out the following resources:

- Be sure to claim your *Total Gut Balance* Bonus Free Resources, where I've shared recipe videos, handy shopping guides, and video interviews with me and a number of my favorite microbiome experts: TotalGutBalanceBook.com/free-resources.
- For my latest insights on the microbiome, check out my personal site: DrMicrobiome.com.
- To dive deeper into optimizing your gut directly with my team and myself, be sure to check out my private 8-week coaching program: DrMicrobiome.com/coaching.
- For probiotics and gut testing designed to address both the bacteria and fungi in your gut, check out my company BIOHM: www.BIOHMHealth.com.
- Listen to my interviews with other leading experts as we discuss topics ranging from optimizing your child's microbiome to skincare regimens to balancing your skin's microbiome: *The Microbiome Report Podcast* on iTunes.
- Connect with me on social media:
  - Instagram: Instagram.com/Dr.Ghannoum
  - Facebook: Facebook.com/drmicrobiome
  - Twitter: Twitter.com/Dr_Microbiome

GLOSSARY

Abundance: A scientific term to describe the number of specific microbes. For example, "The Mycobiome Diet helps to decrease the abundance or level of *Candida* in the gastrointestinal tract."

Akkermansia muciniphila: A mucin-degrading bacterium commonly found in the human gut and often associated with obesity, diabetes, inflammation, and metabolic disorders.

Allergic airway diseases: Inflammatory diseases caused by allergens that negatively impact breathing, such as asthma and allergic rhinitis.

Amoeba, amaoebae (plural): Single-cell eukaryotic microorganisms.

Antibiosis: A biological interaction between two or more organisms (especially microorganisms) that is detrimental to at least one of them.

Archaea: Single-cell microorganisms that are not fungi, bacteria, or viruses. These organisms often inhabit and are able to survive in extreme environmental conditions.

Aspergillus: A genus of molds, including *Aspergillus fumigatus,* which is a common allergen that can cause sinus infections and life-threatening lung and blood infections.

Atherosclerosis: Hardening of the arteries.

Attention-Deficit/Hyperactivity Disorder (ADHD): A chronic disorder marked by problems paying attention, sustaining attention, focusing, hyperactivity, and concentrating.

Autochthonous: Resident, such as fungi that have colonized the human gut, living and reproducing there.

Bacteria: A type of single-celled microorganism common in many environments that often live on and within other life forms, with positive, neutral, or negative effects.

Bacteriophages: Viruses that only infect bacteria.

Bacteroides fragilis: A bacterium that is a normal part of the human microbiome but that could cause infection if it enters the bloodstream or tissue outside the GI tract.

Bacteroidetes: A phylum of bacteria that has colonized virtually all types of habitats on earth, including humans.

BFI: An acronym for bacterial-fungali interactions.

Bifidobacterium: A genus of beneficial bacteria found in the human microbiome that produce short-chain fatty acids (SCFAs), which lower inflammation.

Bilophila: A pro-inflammatory bacterium of the human microbiome.

Biofilms: A slimy film of exopolymeric material secreted by microorganisms that protect them from the external environment.

Candida: A common infectious fungus that includes many species. Some of the more common that can infect humans include *Candida albicans, Candida tropicalis, Candida glabrata, Candida parapsilosis, Candida krusei,* and *Candida auris.* Infection with any *Candida* species is called candidiasis.

Candidiasis: An infection caused by the fungus *Candida.*

CD: An acronym for Crohn's disease (this is also sometimes used as an acronym for celiac disease, but in this book, it is exclusively used to refer to Crohn's disease).

Clostridium: A genus of bacteria with many species that produce toxins.

Clostridium difficile (C. diff): A bacterium that causes diarrhea and more serious intestinal conditions such as colitis—in extreme cases, this infection can permanently damage health or even be fatal.

Colitis: A condition characterized by inflammation in large intestine (or colon) lining. There are several types, including ulcerative colitis, Crohn's colitis, and microscopic colitis.

Colon: The large intestine.

Commensal: Neutral in influence.

Diversity: When talking about the microbiome, diversity refers to the number of different species. In general, the more diverse, the more robust the microbiome. Microbiomes with low diversity tend to be more susceptible to dysbiosis.

Dysbiosis: An imbalance of microbes inside or on the body that has a negative impact, such as when pathogenic microbes like *Candida* become too numerous in the body and cause infections, crowding out more beneficial microbes that should outnumber and control them. To be dysbiotic is to have dysbiosis.

Dysmotility: A condition in which muscles of the digestive system become impaired causing impairment in digestive function.

Escherichia coli (E. coli): A species of bacteria commonly found in the lower intestine of warm-blooded organisms. Several strains are infectious and exposure may cause serious intestinal illness or even death.

Eurotiomycetes: Fungi that have been associated with obesity.

Exopolymer: A substance produced by a living organism that is secreted into the environment. An example of an exopolymer is biofilm material.

Faecalibacterium prausnitzii: A species of bacteria that produces short-chain fatty acids (SCFAs) and has anti-inflammatory effects.

Fiber: A type of indigestible carbohydrate that may be soluble or insoluble.

Firmicutes: A phylum of bacteria associated with gut health in moderate amounts.

Functional bowel disorders: Digestive disorders that have to do with problems in function, such as with the muscles that move food through the digestive tract, rather than with microbes or immunity.

Fungus: Any member of the group of eukaryotic organisms that includes microorganisms such as yeasts, mushrooms, molds, and dermatophytes.

Fusarium: A genus of molds.

Galactomyces geotrichum: A species of fungus associated with microbial balance and a healthy gut.

Genus: A principal taxonomic category that ranks above species and below family, and is denoted by a capitalized Latin name, such as *Candida.*

GERD: Gastroesophageal reflux disease, characterized by chronic acid reflux.

Gut-brain axis: The link between the central nervous system (the brain) and the enteric nervous system (nervous system tissue in the gastrointestinal tract), which allows the brain to influence gut function, and the gut to influence brain function.

Helicobacter pylori (H. pylori): a type of bacteria that causes infection in the stomach. Also the main cause of peptic ulcers and gastritis.

Histamine-2 blockers (H2 blockers): A medication that works to decrease the amount of acid produced by the stomach. Often used in the treatment of heartburn, acid reflux, and GERD.

Homeostasis: The dynamic state of steady stable internal conditions maintained by living things as a response to environmental conditions.

IBD: An acronym for inflammatory bowel disease, a condition characterized by chronic inflammation in the gastrointestinal tract, often related to immune system dysfunction.

IBS: An acronym for irritable bowel syndrome, a condition characterized by chronic gas, bloating, stomach pain, constipation, and/or diarrhea, probably caused by problems in the function of the gastrointestinal system. IBS is considered a functional bowel disorder.

Lactobacillus: A genus of bacteria found in the human microbiome and in some fermented foods.

Methanobrevibacter: A genus of archaea.

Microbes: A microorganism which may exist in its single-celled form or in as multiple cells.

Microbiome: The community of microbes living in the gut that includes bacteria, fungi, viruses, and archaea.

Mucor: Fungi more common in people of normal weight.

Mycobiome: The community of fungi living in different parts of our bodies including the gut.

NSAIDs: An acronym for nonsteroidal anti-inflammatory drugs. These include aspirin, ibuprofen, and naproxen.

Parasite: An organism that lives in or on an organism of another species (its host) and benefits by deriving nutrients at the other's expense.

Pathogenic: Causing disease. For example, the pathogenic fungus *Candida albicans* can cause infections in the human body.

Penicillium chrysogenum: The fungus, discovered in 1928, that is used to make the antibiotic medicine known as penicillin.

Phylum: A principal taxonomic category that ranks above class and below kingdom.

Pichia kluyveri: A species of yeast widely distributed in nature and commonly isolated from rotten fruit and the fleshy parts of plants.

PPIs: An acronym for proton pump inhibitors, which are a type of drug used to treat acid reflux and other digestion issues, including peptic ulcers.

Proteobacteria: A phylum of bacteria including a wide variety of pathogens such as *Escherichia, Salmonella, Vibrio, Helicobacter,* among others.

Protozoa: A phylum of single-celled microorganisms, including amoebas, flagellates, and many other forms.

Resistant starch: A kind of starch that humans cannot digest, but beneficial microbes can. This starch travels undigested to the large intestine, where microbes digest it, then release fermentation by-products that are generally beneficial to human health. Many plant foods contain resistant starches.

Roseburia: A genus of bacteria found in the human colon, and associated with weight loss and reduced glucose intolerance when abundant.

Ruminococcus: A genus of bacteria in the class of Clostridia. One or more species in this genus are found in significant numbers in the intestines of humans.

Saccharomyces: A genus of yeasts including the species *Saccharomyces cerevisiae,* which is brewer's yeast or baker's yeast used in brewing beer and baking bread. This genus also includes *Saccharomyces boulardii,* a yeast known to be beneficial in treating diarrhea related to traveling and antibiotic use.

SIBO: An acronym for small intestinal bacterial overgrowth, a condition in which bacteria that should reside in the colon grows up into the small intestine.

SIFO: An acronym for small intestinal fungal overgrowth, a condition in which fungi that should reside in the colon grow up into the small intestine.

Species: A principal taxonomic category that ranks below genus. A key characteristic is that they have the potential to interbreed.

Spore: A typically single-celled organism produced by plants, fungi, and some microorganisms that are capable of developing into a new individual plant, fungus, or microorganism.

Symbiosis (or symbiotic): A mutually beneficial relationship, such as the relationship between you and beneficial fungal species like *Saccharomyces boulardii.*

Syntrophism (or syntrophy): A specific type of symbiosis between two different microorganisms, in which they work together to perform a metabolic function neither can perform alone.

Tinea corporis: A fungal infection of the skin that typically forms ring shapes and is commonly known as ringworm.

Tinea cruris: A fungal infection of the groin and inner thighs, commonly known as jock itch.

Tinea pedis: A fungal infection of the foot, commonly known as athlete's foot.

Tinea versicolor: A fungal infection of the skin.

Transient: Passing through, such as bacteria from a probiotic that passes through the body and may have a temporary influence but does not colonize and reproduce in the body.

Virulence: How pathogenic or dangerous something is. For example, *Candida albicans* can become more virulent by changing shape so it can better penetrate tissue. This is called a virulence factor.

Virus: A microorganism that is smaller than a bacterium that invades living cells and cannot survive without using these cells to live and reproduce.

Visceral hypersensitivity: A term for internal pain, often associated with functional bowel disorders like irritable bowel syndrome.

Zygomycetes: A phylum of fungi mostly terrestrial in habitat, but in humans can be both pathogenic and potentially beneficial.

ACKNOWLEDGMENTS

To my children, Afif, Emma, and Adam—I love you and thank you so much for all your support!

To my dearest wife, Marie, from my PhD in 1976, to surviving a war, to living a life we only ever imagined in our dreams, you've believed in me always. I love you forever.

To Zach Schisgal, my literary agent, who had the foresight to reach out to me to start this project. Thank you for believing in the concept for the book!

To my dear friend and cowriter Eve Adamson, we did it! You took my vision and turned it into something that people can actually understand! I have written six scientific books, over 400 publications, and collaborated with many coauthors, and I must say I have never before had the pleasure of working with such a wonderful coauthor.

To my editors, Ann Treistman and Aurora Bell, and the whole Norton team, thank you for believing in me and seeing my vision for where this could go.

To Carley Smith, thank you for your help in so many ways!

I would also like to thank the volunteers who enrolled in the Mycobiome Diet test protocol. Your participation and feedback were invaluable in perfecting this diet and proving its effectiveness. Thank you!

To Rosie Hatch, thank you for your fabulous recipes and photography. I am in awe of your amazing talent.

To Dhru Purohit, thank you for your endless insights on what goes into making a book successful. Afif and I really appreciate your friendship and endless help.

To the BIOHM team, thank you for your constant encouragement. In particular, Marilyn Eisele, Ben Brucker, Aubrey Phelps, Mike Haritakis, Melanie Corrigan, Danielle Filip, and Chris Nader.

To my scientific colleagues, Nancy Isham, Chris Hager, Mauricio Retuerto, Iman Salem, Dan Winner, and Gurkan Bebek who allow me to be the best scientist I can be. It is a true pleasure to work with each of you.

This book could not have been created without my son Afif, who has always encouraged me in everything that I do. As we say to the kids, "We are fast, we are strong, we are very smart!"

Last but not least, thank you to all the people who contacted me from all over the world to share how my science has helped them improve their lives. That is truly what I live for.

NOTES

1. Eydokia K. Mitsou et al., "Adherence to the Mediterranean Diet is Associated with Gut Microbiota Pattern and Gastrointestinal Characteristics in an Adult Population," *British Journal of Nutrition* 117 (2017): 1645–55.
2. Nicholas P. Money, *The Triumph of the Fungi: A Rotten History* (Oxford: Oxford University Press, 2007), 107.
3. Maurizio Del Poeta, "Fungi Are Not All 'Fun-Guys' After All," *Frontiers in Microbiology* 1 (August 2010): 105, https://doi.org/10.3389/fmicb.2010.00105.
4. Karen R. Lips, "Witnessing Extinction in Real Time," *PLoS Biology* 16, no. 2 (February 2018): 1–5.
5. Arturo Casadevall, "Fungi and the Rise of Mammals," *PLoS Pathogens* 8, no. 8 (August 2012): 1–3.
6. Note that many previous articles drastically overestimated the number of microbiome cells in the human body, at a 10 to 1 ratio. This has since been disproven and we know the ratio is closer to 1:1. See Sunil Thomas et al., "The Host Microbiome Regulates and Maintains Human Health: A Primer for Non-Microbiologists," *Cancer Research* 77, no. 8 (April 2017): 1783–1812.
7. Najla El-Jurdi, Mahmoud A. Ghannoum, et al., "Microbiome: Its Impact Is Being Revealed!," *Current Clinical Microbiology Reports* 4, no. 2 (June 2017), 78–87.
8. All the items in the list following this footnote come from this article: Thomas et al., "The Host Microbiome."
9. Ibid.
10. Claire Maldarelli, "There Are Fungi Living inside Your Gut, and They're Probably Pretty Important," *Popular Science*, October 12, 2017, www.popsci.com/fungi-gut-microbiome-health.

11. M. Mar Rodríguez et al., "Obesity Changes the Human Gut Mycobiome," *Scientific Reports* 5 (October 2015): 21679, https://doi.org/10.1038/srep14600.
12. Ibid.
13. Benson J. Horowitz, Stanley W. Edelstein, and Leonard Lippmann, "Sugar Chromatography Studies in Recurrent *Candida* Vulvovaginitis," *Journal of Reproductive Medicine* 29, no. 7 (July 1984): 441–43, www.ncbi.nlm.nih.gov/pubmed/6481700.
14. Michael Gracey et al., "Isolation of *Candida* Species from the Gastrointestinal Tract of Malnourished Children," *American Journal of Clinical Nutrition* 27, no. 4 (1974): 345–49.
15. Qi Hui Sam, Matthew Wook Chang, and Louis Yi Ann Chai, "The Fungal Mycobiome and Its Interaction with Gut Bacteria in the Host," *International Journal of Molecular Sciences* 18, no. 2 (February 2017): 330.
16. Huacheng Tang et al., "*Galactomyces geotrichum* Isolated from Water Kefir: Interaction with Lactobacillus Kefir, *Italian Journal of Food Science* 28, no. 2 (January 2016): 287–97.
17. Pranab K. Mukherjee, Mahmoud A. Ghannoum, et al., "Oral Mycobiome Analysis of HIV-Infected Patients: Identification of *Pichia* as an Antagonist of Opportunistic Fungi, *PLOS Pathogens* 10, no. 3 (2014): e1003996.
18. Mitsou et al., "Adherence to the Mediterranean Diet."
19. A. F. Peery et al., "Burden of Gastrointestinal Disease in the United States: 2012 Update," *Gastroenterology* 143, no. 5 (November 2012): 1179–87.
20. S. F. Bloomfield, "Too Clean, or Not Too Clean: The Hygiene Hypothesis and Home Hygiene," *Clinical and Experimental Allergy* 36, no. 4 (April 2006): 402–25.
21. Andrew C. Dukowicz, Brian E. Lacy, and Gary M. Levine, "Small Intestinal Bacterial Overgrowth: A Comprehensive Review," *Gastroenterology & Hepatology* 3, no. 2 (February 2007): 112–22.
22. Askin Erdogan and Satish S. Rao, "Small Intestinal Fungal Overgrowth," *Current Gastroenterology Reports* 17, no. 4 (April 2015): 16, https://doi.org/10.1007/s11894-015-0436-2.
23. Ibid.
24. Carolyn Jacobs et al., "Dysmotility and Proton Pump Inhibitor Use Are Independent Risk Factors for Small Intestinal Bacterial and/or Fungal Overgrowth," *Alimentary Pharmacology and Therapeutics* 37, no. 11 (June 2013): 1103–111, https://doi.org/10.1111/apt.12304.
25. Carolyn Jacobs et al., "Investigation of Small Intestinal Fungal Overgrowth (SIFO) and/or Small Intestinal Bacterial Overgrowth (SIBO) in

Chronic, Unexplained Gastrointestinal Symptoms," *Gastroenterology* 140, no. 5, Supplement 1 (May 2011): S-810, https://doi.org/10.1016/S0016-5085(11)63354-4.

26. All of the risk factors in this list are discussed in Thomas et al., "The Host Microbiome."
27. Frederik Backhed et al., "Defining a Healthy Human Gut Microbiome: Current Concepts, Future Directions, and Clinical Applications," *Cell Host & Microbe* 12, no. 5 (November 2012): 611–20, https://doi.org/10.1016/j.chom.2012.10.012.
28. Xing Hua et al., "Allergy Associations with the Adult Fecal Microbiota: Analysis of the American Gut Project," *EBioMedicine* 3 (January 2016): 172–79, https://dx.doi.org/10.1016%2Fj.ebiom.2015.11.038.
29. Natasha Campbell-McBride, "Food Allergy: A Case Study," *Journal of Orthomolecular Medicine* 24, no. 1 (2009): 31–41.
30. Milena Sokolowska et al., "Microbiome and Asthma," *Asthma Research and Practice* 4, no. 1 (2018): 1, https://dx.doi.org/10.1186%2Fs40733-017-0037-y.
31. Svetlana N. Nedelskaya and Elena D. Kuznetsova, "State of Intestinal Microflora in Children with Atopic Dermatitis and Role of Probiotics in Its Correction," *АСТМА ТА АЛЕРГІЯ* 2 (2016): 1–6.
32. Natasha Campbell-McBride, "Gut and Psychology Syndrome," *Journal of Orthomolecular Medicine* 23, no. 2 (2008): 90–94.
33. Maria Klein-Laszlo, "Chronic Candidiasis—Pathogenesis, Symptoms, Diagnosis and Treatment," *Zbornik Matice srpske za prirodne nauke/Proc. Nat. Sci, Matica Srpska Novi Sad*, 16 (2009): 267–74.
34. Hakim Rahmoune and Nada Boutrid, "Migraine, Celiac Disease and Intestinal Microbiota," *Pediatric Neurology Briefs* 31, no. 2 (February 2017): 6, https://dx.doi.org/10.15844%2Fpedneurbriefs-31-2-3.
35. Erica White and Caroline Sherlock, "The Effect of Nutritional Therapy for Yeast Infection (Candidiasis) in Cases of Chronic Fatigue Syndrome," *Journal of Orthomolecular Medicine* 20, no. 3 (2005): 193–209.
36. You Lv et al., "The Relationship between Frequently Used Glucose-Lowering Agents and Gut Microbiota in Type 2 Diabetes Mellitus," *Journal of Diabetes Research* (2018): 1–10, https://doi.org/10.1155/2018/1890978.
37. Marjorie Mary Walker and Nicholas Talley, "Review Article: Bacteria and Pathogenesis of Disease in the Upper Gastrointestinal Tract—Beyond the Era of *Helicobacter pylori*," *Alimentary Pharmacology & Therapeutics* 39, no. 9 (February 2014): 767–79, http://dx.doi.org/10.1111/apt.12666.
38. Ibid.

39. Kimberley Lau et al., "Bridging the Gap between Gut Microbial Dysbiosis and Cardiovascular Diseases," *Nutrients* 9, no. 8 (August 2017): 859.
40. Maurits van den Nieuwboer et al., "The Administration of Probiotics and Synbiotics in Immune Compromised Adults: Is It Safe?," *Beneficial Microbes* 6, no. 1 (March 2015): 1–17, https://doi.org/10.3920/BM2014.0079; Sophie Viaud et al., "Harnessing the Intestinal Microbiome for Optimal Therapeutic Immunomodulation," *Cancer Research* 74, no. 16 (August 2014): 1–5, https://doi.org/10.1158/0008-5472.CAN-14-0987.
41. Christina Casén et al., "Deviations in Human Gut Microbiota: A Novel Diagnostic Test for Determining Dysbiosis in Patients with IBS or IBD," *Alimentary Pharmacology and Therapeutics* 42, no. 1 (July 2015): 71–83, https://doi.org/10.1111/apt.13236; Qasim Aziz et al., "Gut Microbiota and Gastrointestinal Health: Current Concepts and Future Directions," *Neurogastroenterology & Motility* 25, no. 1 (January 2013): 4–15, https://doi.org/10.1111/nmo.12046.
42. Ibid. Casén et al., "Deviations in Human Gut Microbiota." Anurag Agrawal et al., "Bloating and Distension in Irritable Bowel Syndrome: The Role of Gastrointestinal Transit," *The American Journal of Gastroenterology* 104, no. 8 (June 2009): 1998–2004, https://doi.org/10.1038/ajg.2009.251.
43. White and Sherlock, "The Effect of Nutritional Therapy for Yeast Infection," 193–209.
44. Aziz et al., "Gut Microbiota and Gastrointestinal Health."
45. Matam Vijay-Kumar et al., "Metabolic Syndrome and Altered Gut Microbiota in Mice Lacking Toll-Like Receptor 5," *Science* 328, no. 5975 (April 2010): 228–31, https://doi.org/10.1126/science.1179721.
46. Rahmoune and Boutrid, "Migraine, Celiac Disease and Intestinal Microbiota." Yu-Jie Dai et al., "Potential Beneficial Effects of Probiotics on Human Migraine Headache: A Literature Review," *Pain Physician* 20, no. 2 (February 2017): E251–E255.
47. Egle Cekanaviciute et al., "Gut Bacteria from Multiple Sclerosis Patients Modulate Human T Cells and Exacerbate Symptoms in Mouse Models," *PNAS* 114, no. 42 (October 2017): 1–6, https://doi.org/10.1073/pnas.1711235114.
48. Fernando Forato Anhê et al., "Gut Microbiota Dysbiosis in Obesity-Linked Metabolic Diseases and Prebiotic Potential of Polyphenol-Rich Extracts," *Current Obesity Reports* 4, no. 4 (December 2015): 389–400, https://doi.org/10.1007/s13679-015-0172-9.
49. Luis Vitetta, Matthew Bambling, and Hollie Alford, "The Gastrointesti-

nal Tract Microbiome, Probiotics, and Mood," *Inflammopharmacology* 22, no. 6 (December 2014): 333–9, https://doi.org/10.1007/s10787-014-0216-x; Campbell-McBride, "Gut and Psychology Syndrome." Eoin Sherwin et al., "May the Force Be with You: The Light and Dark Sides of the Microbiota-Gut-Brain Axis in Neuropsychiatry," *CNS Drugs* 30, no. 11 (November 2016): 1019–41, https://doi.org/10.1007/s40263-016-0370-3; Megan Clapp et al., "Gut Microbiota's Effect on Mental Health: The Gut-Brain Axis," *Clinics and Practice* 7, no. 4 (September 2017): 987, https://dx.doi.org/10.4081%2Fcp.2017.987.

50. Frederick T. Sutter, "Natural Therapies for Rheumatoid Arthritis and Other Chronic Inflammatory Conditions," *Applied Nutritional Science Reports* (August 2000); Kulveer Mankia and Paul Emery, "Preclinical Rheumatoid Arthritis: Progress Towards Prevention," *Arthritis & Rheumatology* 68, no. 4 (April 2016): 779–88, https://doi.org/10.1002/art.39603.
51. Jacobs et al., "Dysmotility and Proton Pump Inhibitor Use."
52. Arancha Hevia et al., "Intestinal Dysbiosis Associated with Systemic Lupus Erythematosus," *American Society for Microbiology* 5, no. 5 (September/October 2014): 1–10.
53. Vitetta, Bambling, and Alford, "The Gastrointestinal Tract Microbiome, Probiotics, and Mood." Campbell-McBride, "Gut and Psychology Syndrome"; Sherwin et al., "May the Force Be with You," 1019-41; Clapp et al., "Gut Microbiota's Effect on Mental Health," 987.
54. Ibid. Casén et al., "Deviations in Human Gut Microbiota." Agrawal et al., "Bloating and Distension in Irritable Bowel Syndrome," 1998–2004; Campbell-McBride, "Food Allergy," 31–41. Aziz et al., "Gut Microbiota and Gastrointestinal Health.
55. Rahmoune and Boutrid, "Migraine, Celiac Disease and Intestinal Microbiota." Dai et al., "Potential Beneficial Effects of Probiotics," E251–E255.
56. Nedelskaya and Kuznetsova, "State of Intestinal Microflora in Children"; Maria Klein-László, "Chronic Candidiasis—Pathogenesis, Symptoms, Diagnosis and Treatment," *Matica Srpska Journal of Natural Sciences* 116 (2009): 267–74; Campbell-McBride, "Food Allergy: A Case Study," 31–41.
57. Campbell-McBride, "Gut and Psychology Syndrome." Sherwin et al., "May the Force Be with You," 1019–41.
58. Walker and Talley, "Review Article: Bacteria and Pathogenesis of Disease."
59. Vijay-Kumar et al., "Metabolic Syndrome and Altered Gut Microbiota," 228–31.
60. James M. Baker, Layla Al-Nakkash, and Melissa M. Herbst-Kralovetz,

"Estrogen-Gut Microbiome Axis: Physiological and Clinical Implications," *Maturitas* 103 (Sept 2017): 45–53, https://doi.org/10.1016/j.maturitas.2017.06.025.

61. Brian Mowll and Razi Berry, *The Sugar Free Summer Program Manual,* http://thenatpath.com/wp-content/uploads/SFS-Program-Manual.pdf; Baker, Al-Nakkash, and Herbst-Kralovetz, "Estrogen-Gut Microbiome Axis," 45–53; Anhê et al., "Gut Microbiota Dysbiosis," 389–400; Vijay-Kumar et al., "Metabolic Syndrome and Altered Gut Microbiota," 228–31; Lv et al., "The Relationship between Frequently Used Glucose-Lowering Agents and Gut Microbiota," 1–10.
62. Luis Vitetta et al., "The Gastrointestinal Microbiome and Musculoskeletal Diseases: A Beneficial Role for Probiotics and Prebiotics," *Pathogens* 2, no. 4 (December 2013): 606–26, https://dx.doi.org/10.3390%2Fpathogens2040606; Sutter, "Natural Therapies for Rheumatoid Arthritis." Mankia and Emery, "Preclinical Rheumatoid Arthritis," 779–88.
63. White and Sherlock, "The Effect of Nutritional Therapy for Yeast Infection," 193–209; Lv et al., "The Relationship between Frequently Used Glucose-Lowering Agents and Gut Microbiota," 1–10.
64. Whitney P. Bowe and Alan C. Logan, "Acne Vulgaris, Probiotics and the Gut-Brain-Skin Axis—Back to the Future?," *Gut Pathology* 3, no. 1 (2011): 1–11, https://dx.doi.org/10.1186%2F1757-4749-3-1.
65. Vitetta, Bambling, and Alford, "The Gastrointestinal Tract Microbiome, Probiotics, and Mood," 333–39; Campbell-McBride, "Gut and Psychology Syndrome"; Sherwin et al., "May the Force Be with You," 1019–41; Clapp et al., "Gut Microbiota's Effect on Mental Health," 987.
66. Hua et al., "Allergy Associations with the Adult Fecal Microbiota," 172–79.
67. Baker, Al-Nakkash, and Herbst-Kralovetz, "Estrogen-Gut Microbiome Axis," 45–53. Anhê et al., "Gut Microbiota Dysbiosis," 389–400; Vijay-Kumar et al., "Metabolic Syndrome and Altered Gut Microbiota," 228–31; Lv et al., "The Relationship between Frequently Used Glucose-Lowering Agents and Gut Microbiota," 1–10.
68. Jacobs et al., "Dysmotility and Proton Pump Inhibitor Use."
69. This reference applies to all remaining bullets in this list: Lisa Maier et al., "Extensive Impact of Non-Antibiotic Drugs on Human Gut Bacteria," *Nature* 555 (March 2018): 623–28, https://doi.org/10.1038/nature25979.
70. Lisa Maier, et al., "Extensive Impact of Non-Antibiotic Drugs on Human Gut Bacteria," *Nature* 555, no. 7698 (March 2018):623-8, doi:10.1038/nature25979.

71. Anna-Carin Lundell et al., "High Proportion of CD5+ B Cells in Infants Predicts Development of Allergic Disease," *The Journal of Immunology* 193, no. 2 (July 2014): 510–18, https://doi.org/10.4049/jimmunol.1302990.
72. Meghan B. Azad et al., "Infant Gut Microbiota and the Hygiene Hypothesis of Allergic Disease: Impact of Household Pets and Siblings on Microbiota Composition and Diversity," *Allergy, Asthma, & Clinical Immunology* 9, no. 1 (2013): 15, https://doi.org/10.1186/1710-1492-9-15.
73. Sujata Gupta, "Microbiome: Puppy Power," *Nature* 543 (March 2017): S48-S49, www.nature.com/articles/543S48a#ref3.
74. Tove Fall et al., "Early Exposure to Dogs and Farm Animals and the Risk of Childhood Asthma," *JAMA Pediatrics* 169, no. 11 (November 2015): e153219, https://doi.org/10.1001/jamapediatrics.2015.3219.
75. Michael A. Conlon and Anthony R. Bird, "The Impact of Diet and Lifestyle on Gut Microbiota and Human Health," *Nutrients* 7, no. 1 (January 2015): 17–44.
76. Siobhan F. Clarke et al., "Exercise and Associated Dietary Extremes Impact on Gut Microbial Diversity," *Gut* 63, no. 12 (December 2014): 1913–20, https://doi.org/10.1136/gutjnl-2013-306541.
77. Rachel Allen, "5 Ways Spending Time in Nature Benefits Your Health (and Your Gut)," *Hyperbiotics*, www.hyperbiotics.com/blogs/recent-articles/5-ways-spending-time-in-nature-benefits-your-health-and-your-gut.
78. Michael A. Pfaller, et al., "National Surveillance of Nosocomial Blood Stream Infection Due to Species of *Candida* Other than *Candida albicans*: Frequency of Occurrence and Antifungal Susceptibility in the SCOPE Program," *Diagnostic Microbiology and Infectious Disease* 30, iss. 2 (February 1998): 121-129.
79. Rachna Singh and Arunaloke Chakrabarti, "Invasive Candidiasis in the Southeast-Asian Region," in *Candida albicans: Cellular and Molecular Biology*, 2nd ed., ed. Rajendra Prasad (Switzerland: Springer, 2017), 27.
80. Philippe Eggimann, Jorge Garbino, and Didier Pittet, "Epidemiology of Candida Species Infections in Critically Ill Non-Immunosuppressed Patients," *The Lancet Infectious Diseases* 3, no. 11 (November 2003): 685–702, https://doi.org/10.1016/S1473-3099(03)00801-6.
81. Ibid.
82. Ray Hachem, et al., "The Changing Epidemiology of Invasive Candidiasis Candida Glabrata and Candida Krusei as the Leading Causes of Candidemia in Hematologic Malignancy," American Cancer Society, doi 10.1002/cncr.23466 published online, *Wiley InterScience* (April 2008), www

.interscience.wiley.com; David W. Warnock, et al.,"Trends in the Epidemiology of Invasive Fungal Infections," *Journal of Medical Mycology* 48 (2007): 1-12; M. Bassetti et al., "Incidence of Candidaemia and Rlationship with Fuconazole Use in an Intensive Care Unit," *Journal of Antimicrobial Chemotherapy* 64 (2009): 625–9, doi:10.1093/jac/dkp251.

83. Ibid.
84. Gautier Hoarau, Mahmoud A. Ghannoum, et al., "Bacteriome and Mycobiome Interactions Underscore Microbial Dysbiosis in Familial Crohn's Disease," *mBio* 7, no. 5 (September 2016): e01250-16, https://doi.org/10.1128/mBio.01250-16.
85. Ibid.
86. Ibid.
87. Eggimann, Garbino, and Pittet, "Epidemiology of Candida Species Infections," 685–702.
88. Christina T. Piedrahita, Jennifer L. Cadnum, Annette L. Jencson, Aaron A. Shaikh, Mahmoud A. Ghannoum, Curtis J. Donskey. "Environmental Surfaces in Healthcare Facilities are a Potential Source for Transmission of Candida auris and Other Candida Species," *Infection Control & Hospital Epidemiology* (2017): 1-3.
89. Snigdha Vallabhaneni et al., "Investigation of the First Seven Reported Cases of Candida auris, a Globally Emerging Invasive, Multidrug-Resistant Fungus—United States, May 2013–August 2016," *American Journal of Transplantation* 17, no. 1 (January 2017): 65, https://doi.org/10.1111/ajt.14121.
90. William Crook, "The Effects of Candida on Mental Health," Safe Harbor, accessed September 13, 2018, www.alternativementalhealth.com/the-effects-of-candida-on-mental-health-by-william-crook-m-d.
91. Emily Larkin, Mahmoud Ghannoum, et al., "The Emerging Pathogen *Candida auris*: Growth Phenotype, Virulence Factors, Activity of Antifungals, and Effect of SCY-078, a Novel Glucan Synthesis Inhibitor, on Growth Morphology and Biofilm Formation," *Antimicrobial Agents and Chemotherapy* 61, no. 5 (April 2017): e02396-16, https://doi.org/10.1128/AAC.02396-16; Christopher L. Hager, Mahmoud A. Ghannoum, et al., "*In Vitro* and *In Vivo* Evaluation of the Antifungal Activity of APX001A/APX001 against *Candida auris*," *Antimicrobial Agents and Chemotherapy* 62, no. 3 (February 2018): e02319-17, https://doi.org/10.1128/AAC.02319-17; Christopher L. Hager, Mahmoud A. Ghannoum, et al., "Evaluation of the Efficacy of Rezafungin, a Novel Echinocandin, in the Treatment of Disseminated *Candida auris* Infection Using an Immunocompromised Mouse

Model," *Journal of Antimicrobial Chemotherapy* 73, no. 8 (August 2018): 2085–88, https://doi.org/10.1093/jac/dky153. Emily Larkin, Mahmoud Ghannoum, et al., "Evaluation of the *In Vitro* and *In Vivo* Antifungal Activity of APX001A/APX001 Against *Candida auris*," *Open Forum Infectious Diseases* 4, suppl. 1 (Fall 2017): S471–S472, https://doi.org/10.1093/ofid/ofx163.1206.

92. Dwayne C. Savage and Rene J. Dubos, "Localization of Indigenous Yeast in the Murine Stomach," *Journal of Bacteriology* 94, no. 6 (December 1967): 1811–16, www.ncbi.nlm.nih.gov/pmc/articles/PMC276909; Dwayne C. Savage, "Microbial Interference between Indigenous Yeast and Lactobacilli in the Rodent Stomach," *Journal of Bacteriology* 98, no. 3 (June 1969): 1278–83, www.ncbi.nlm.nih.gov/pmc/articles/PMC315325; Jose J. Limon, Joseph H. Skalski, and David M. Underhill, "Commensal Fungi in Health and Disease," *Cell Host & Microbe* 22, no. 2 (August 2017): 156–65, https://doi.org/10.1016/j.chom.2017.07.002.

93. Michael J. Kennedy and Paul A. Volz, "Ecology of *Candida albicans* Gut Colonization: Inhibition of *Candida* Adhesion, Colonization, and Dissemination from the Gastrointestinal Tract by Bacterial Antagonism," *Infection and Immunity* 49, no. 3 (September 1985): 654–63; Michael J. Kennedy and Paul A. Volz, "Effect of Various Antibiotics on Gastrointestinal Colonization and Dissemination by *Candida albicans*," *Sabouraudia* 23, no. 4 (August 1985): 265–73.

94. Katie L. Mason et al., "*Candida albicans* and Bacterial Microbiota Interactions in the Cecum during Recolonization Following Broad-Spectrum Antibiotic Therapy," *Infection and Immunity* 80, no. 10 (October 2012): 3371–80, https://doi.org/10.1128/IAI.00449-12.

95. Mason et al., "*Candida albicans* and Bacterial Microbiota Interactions in the Cecum," 3371–80; Paul B. Helstrom and Edward Balish, "Effect of Oral Tetracycline, the Microbial Flora, and the Athymic State on Gastrointestinal Colonization and Infection of BALB/c Mice with *Candida albicans*," *Infection and Immunity* 23, no. 3 (March 1979): 764–74.

96. Mahmoud A. Ghannoum and Samir S. Radwan, *Candida Adherence to Epithelial Cells* (Boca Raton, FL:, 1990); Mahmoud Ghannoum and S. Radwan, *Candida Adherence to Epithelial Cells* (Boca Raton, FL: CRC Press, 1990).

97. Eggimann, Garbino, and Pittet, "Epidemiology of Candida Species Infections," 685–702.

98. W. Krause, H. Matheis, and K. Wulf, "Fungaemia and Funguria After Oral Administration of *Candida albicans*," *Lancet* 1 (1969): 598–99.

99. Sergio B. Wey et al., "Risk Factors for Hospital-Acquired Candidemia: A Matched Case-Control Study," *Archives of Internal Medicine* 149, no. 10 (October 1989): 2349–53.

100. Victoria J. Fraser et al., "Candidemia in a Tertiary Care Hospital: Epidemiology, Risk Factors, and Predictors of Mortality," *Clinical Infectious Diseases* 15, no. 3 (September 1992): 414–21.

101. Eliane Haron et al., "Primary Candida Pneumonia. Experience at a Large Cancer Center and Review of the Literature," *Medicine* 72, no. 3 (May 1993): 137–42.

102. Eggimann, Garbino, and Pittet, "Epidemiology of Candida Species Infections," 685–702.

103. Didier Pittet et al., "Candida Colonization and Subsequent Infections in Critically Ill Surgical Patients," *Annals of Surgery* 220, no. 6 (December 1994): 751–58.

104. Ibid.

105. Richard R. Watkins, Mahmoud A. Ghannoum, et al., "Admission to the Intensive Care Unit is Associated with Changes in the Oral Mycobiome," *Journal of Intensive Care Medicine* 32, no. 4 (May 2017): 1–5, https://doi.org/10.1177/0885066615627757.

106. Christy A. Varughese, Niyati H. Vakil, and Kristy M. Phillips, "Antibiotic-Associated Diarrhea: A Refresher on Causes and Possible Prevention with Probiotics—Continuing Education Article," *Journal of Pharmacy Practice* 26, no. 5 (October 2015): 476–82, https://doi.org/10.1177/0897190013499523.

107. Stephen J. Ott et al., "Fungi and Inflammatory Bowel Diseases: Alterations of Composition and Diversity," *Scandinavian Journal of Gastroenterology* 43, no. 7 (2008): 831–41, https://doi.org/10.1080/00365520801935434.

108. Malgorzata Zwolinska-Wcislo et al., "Effect of Candida Colonization on Human Ulcerative Colitis and the Healing of Inflammatory Changes of the Colon in the Experimental Model of Colitis Ulcerosa," *Journal of Physiology and Pharmacology* 60, no. 1 (March 2009): 107–18.

109. Hoarau, Ghannoum, et al., "Bacteriome and Mycobiome Interactions," e01250-16.

110. Stephen J. Middleton, A. Coley, and John O. Hunter, "The Role of Faecal Candida albicans in the Pathogenesis of Food-Intolerant Irritable Bowel Syndrome," *Postgraduate Medical Journal* 68, no. 800 (June 1992): 453–54.

111. Heiko Santelmann and John McLaren Howard, "Yeast Metabolic Products, Yeast Antigens and Yeasts as Possible Triggers for Irritable Bowel

Syndrome," *European Journal of Gastroenterology and Hepatology* 17, no. 1 (January 2005): 21–26, www.ncbi.nlm.nih.gov/pubmed/15647635.

112. Maria N. Gamaletsou et al., "*Candida* Arthritis: Analysis of 112 Pediatric and Adult Cases," *Open Forum Infectious Diseases* 3, no. 1 (December 2015): https://dx.doi.org/10.1093%2Fofid%2Fofv207.
113. Middleton, Coley, and Hunter, "The Role of Faecal Candida albicans."
114. Mairi C. Noverr et al., "Role of Antibiotics and Fungal Microbiota in Driving Pulmonary Allergic Responses," *Infection and Immunity* 72, no. 9 (September 2004): 4996–5003, https://dx.doi.org/10.1128%2FIAI.72.9.4996-5003.2004.
115. Carol A. Kumamoto, "Inflammation and Gastrointestinal *Candida* Colonization," *Current Opinion in Microbiology* 14, no. 4 (August 2011): 386–91, https://dx.doi.org/10.1016%2Fj.mib.2011.07.015.
116. Candida infections in human beings: spectrum of diseases (adapted from Eggimann, Garbino, and Pittet, "Epidemiology of Candida Species Infections," 685–702).
117. Mahmoud A. Ghannoum et al., "A Large-Scale North American Study of Fungal Isolates from Nails: The Frequency of Onychomycosis, Fungal Distribution, and Antifungal Susceptibility Patterns," *Journal of the American Academy of Dermatology* 43, no. 4 (October 2000): 641–48, https://doi.org/10.1067/mjd.2000.107754.
118. Pascale Frey-Klett et al., "Bacterial-Fungal Interactions: Hyphens between Agricultural, Clinical, Environmental, and Food Microbiologists," *Microbiology and Molecular Biology Reviews* 75, no. 4 (December 2011): 583–609, https://doi.org/10.1128/MMBR.00020-11.
119. Matthew L. Wheeler et al., "Immunological Consequences of Intestinal Fungal Dysbiosis," *Cell Host & Microbe* 19, no. 6 (June 2016): 865–73, https://doi.org/10.1016/j.chom.2016.05.003.
120. Louis Yi Ann Chai et al., "Fungal Strategies for Overcoming Host Innate Immune Response," *Medical Mycology* 47, no. 3 (May 2009): 227–36, https://doi.org/10.1080/13693780802209082.
121. Duncan McNicol Kuhn, Mahmoud A. Ghannoum, et al., "Comparison of Biofilms Formed by *Candida albicans* and *Candida parapsilosis* on Bioprosthetic Surfaces," *Infection and Immunity* 70, no. 2 (February 2002): 878–88.
122. Mahmoud A. Ghannoum et al., "The Role of Echinocandins in *Candida* Biofilm-Related Vascular Catheter infections: *In Vitro* ad *In Vivo* Model Systems," *Clinical Infectious Diseases* 1, no. 61, suppl. 6 (December 2015): S618-21, https://doi.org/10.1093/cid/civ815.

123. Hoarau, Ghannoum et al., "Bacteriome and Mycobiome Interactions," e01250-16.
124. Johnson et al., "Metabolism Links Bacterial Biofilms and Colon Carcinogenesis," 891–97.
125. Cynthia L. Sears and Wendy S. Garrett, "Microbes, Microbiota, and Colon Cancer," *Cell Host & Microbe* 15, no. 3 (March 2014): 317–28, https://dx.doi.org/10.1016%2Fj.chom.2014.02.007.
126. Hollie M. Probert and Glenn R. Gibson, "Bacterial Biofilms in the Human Gastrointestinal Tract," *Current Issues in Intestinal Microbiology* 3, no. 2 (September 2002): 23–27; Pratik Shah and Edwin Swiatlo, "A Multifaceted Role for Polyamines in Bacterial Pathogens," *Molecular Microbiology* 68, no.1 (April 2008): 4–16, https://doi.org/10.1111/j.1365-2958.2008.06126.x.
127. Christine M. Dejea et al., "Microbiota Organization Is a Distinct Feature of Proximal Colorectal Cancers," *Proceedings of the National Academy of Science of the United States of America* 111, no. 51 (December 2014): 18321–26, https://doi.org/10.1073/pnas.1406199111.
128. C.L. Hager, M.A. Ghannoum, et al., "Effects of a novel probiotic combination on pathogenic bacterial-fungal polymicrobial biofilms," *mBio* 10 (2019): e00338-19, https://doi.org/10.1128/mBio.00338-19.
129. G. Hoarau, M.A. Ghannoum, et al., "Bacteriome and mycobiome interactions underscore microbial dysbiosis in familial Crohn's disease," *mBio* 7 (2016): e01250-16, https://doi.org/10.1128/mBio.01250-16.
130. Gary D. Wu et al., "Linking Long-Term Dietary Patterns with Gut Microbial Enterotypes," *Science* 334, no. 6052 (October 2011): 105–8, https://dx.doi.org/10.1126%2Fscience.1208344.
131. David et al., "Diet Rapidly and Reproducibly Alters the Human Gut Microbiome."
132. Ibid.
133. Jeremiah J. Faith et al., "The Long-Term Stability of the Human Gut Microbiota," *Science* 341, no. 6141 (July 2013): 6141, https://doi.org/10.1126/science.1237439.
134. Abigail R. Basson, Minh Lam, and Fabio Cominelli, "Complementary and Alternative Medicine Strategies for Therapeutic Gut Microbiota Modulation in Inflammatory Bowel Disease and their Next-Generation Approaches," *Gastroenterology Clinics of North America* 46, no. 4 (December 2017): 689–729, https://doi.org/10.1016/j.gtc.2017.08.002.
135. Ibid. (for above two references).

136. Basson, Lam, and Cominelli, "Complementary and Alternative Medicine Strategies."
137. Robert Caesar et al., "Crosstalk between Gut Microbiota and Dietary Lipids Aggravates WAT Inflammation through TLR Signaling," *Cell Metabolism* 22, no. 4 (October 2015): 658–68, https://doi.org/10.1016/j.cmet.2015.07.026.
138. Jotham Suez et al., "Artificial Sweeteners Induce Glucose Intolerance by Altering the Gut Microbiota," *Nature* 514, no. 7521 (October 2014): 181–86, https://doi.org/10.1038/nature13793.
139. Alexander Rodriguez-Palacios, Mahmoud A. Ghannoum, et al., "The Artificial Sweetener Splenda Promotes Gut Proteobacteria, Dysbiosis, and Myeloperoxidase Reactivity in Crohn's Disease–Like Ileitis," *Inflammatory Bowel Diseases* 24, no.5 (April 2018): 1005–20, https://doi.org/10.1093/ibd/izy060.
140. Allison Webster, "Gut Check: Sugars and the Gut Microbiome," Food Insight, International Food Information Council Foundation, July 6, 2018, www.foodinsight.org/gut-check-sugars-and-the-gut-microbiome.
141. Victoria Brown, Jessica A. Sexton, and Mark Johnston, "A Glucose Sensor in *Candida albicans*," *Eukaryotic Cell* 5, no. 10 (October 2006): 1726–37, https://doi.org/10.1128/EC.00186-06.
142. Singh et al., "Influence of Diet on the Gut Microbiome."
143. Connie M. Weaver et al., "Galactooligosaccharides Improve Mineral Absorption and Bone Properties in Growing Rats through Gut Fermentation," *Journal of Agricultural and Food Chemistry* 59, no. 12 (Jun 2011): 6501–10, https://doi.org/10.1021/jf2009777. Steven A. Jakeman et al., "Soluble Corn Fiber Increases Bone Calcium Retention in Postmenopausal Women in a Dose-Dependent Manner: A Randomized Crossover Trial," *The American Journal of Clinical Nutrition* 104, no. 3 (September 2016): 837–43, https://doi.org/10.3945/ajcn.116.132761.
144. Multiple studies: Zeinab Faghfoori et al., "Effects of an Oral Supplementation of Germinated Barley Foodstuff on Serum Tumour Necrosis Factor-Alpha, Interleukin-6 and -8 in Patients with Ulcerative Colitis," *Annals of Clinical Biochemistry* 48, pt. 3 (May 2011): 233–37, https://doi.org/10.1258/acb.2010.010093; Hiroyuki Hanai et al., "Germinated Barley Foodstuff Prolongs Remission in Patients with Ulcerative Colitis," *International Journal of Molecular Medicine* 13, no. 5 (May 2004): 643–37; Osamu Kanauchi et al., "Effect of Germinated Barley Foodstuff Administration on Mineral Utilization in Rodents," *Journal of Gastroenterology* 35, no. 3 (2000): 188–94; Keiichi Mitsuyama et al., "Treatment of Ulcerative Colitis with Germinated

Barley Foodstuff Feeding: A Pilot Study," *Alimentary Pharmacology and Therapeutics* 12, no. 12 (1998): 1225–30.

145. Singh et al., "Influence of Diet on the Gut Microbiome."
146. Roy Fuller and Glenn R. Gibson, "Probiotics and Prebiotics: Microflora Management for Improved Gut Health," *Clinical Microbiology and Infection* 4, no. 9 (September 1998): 477–80, https://doi.org/10.1111/j.1469-0691.1998.tb00401.x.
147. This reference applies to all compounds listed as biofilm inhibitors: Chieu Anh Kim Ta and John Thor Arnason, "Mini Review of Phytochemicals and Plant Taxa with Activity as Microbial Biofilm and Quorum Sensing Inhibitor," *Molecules* 21, no. 1 (December 2015): E29, https://doi.org/10.3390/molecules21010029.
148. Dae-Bang Seo et al., "Fermented Green Tea Extract Alleviates Obesity and Related Complications and Alters Gut Microbiota Composition in Diet-Induced Obese Mice," *Journal of Medicinal Food* 18, no. 5 (May 2015): 549–56, https://doi.org/10.1089/jmf.2014.3265.
149. Ibid.
150. Namrita Lall, ed., *Medicinal Plants for Holistic Health and Well-Being* (London: Academic Press, 2018), as referenced on "Ajoene," ScienceDirect, www.sciencedirect.com/topics/medicine-and-dentistry/ajoene.
151. Mahmoud A. Ghannoum, "Studies on the Anticandidal Mode of Action of Allium sativum (Garlic)," *Journal of General Microbiology* 134, no. 11 (November 1988): 2917–24, https://doi.org/10.1099/00221287-134-11-2917.
152. Soheil Zorofchian Moghadamtousi et al., "A Review on Antibacterial, Antiviral, and Antifungal Activity of Curcumin," *BioMed Research International* (2014): http://doi.org/10.1155/2014/186864.
153. Fernando Forato Anhê et al., "A Polyphenol-Rich Cranberry Extract Protects from Diet-Induced Obesity, Insulin Resistance and Intestinal Inflammation in Association with Increased Akkermansia spp. Population in the Gut Microbiota of Mice," *Gut* 64, no. 6 (July 2014): 872–83, https://doi.org/10.1136/gutjnl-2014-307142.
154. Anhê et al., "A Polyphenol-Rich Cranberry Extract Protects from Diet-Induced Obesity," 872–83.
155. Anna Lewinska et al., "Ursolic Acid-Mediated Changes in Glycolytic Pathway Promote Cytotoxic Autophagy and Apoptosis in Phenotypically Different Breast Cancer Cells," *Apoptosis* 22, no. 6 (June 2017): 800–15, https://doi.org/10.1007/s10495-017-1353-7.

156. "Vanillin," Phenol-Explorer, http://phenol-explorer.eu/contents/polyphenol/724.
157. Haigiu Huang et al., "Soy and Gut Microbiota: Interaction and Implication for Human Health," *Journal of Agricultural and Food Chemistry* 64, no. 46 (November 2016): 8695–8709, https://doi.org/10.1021/acs.jafc.6b03725.
158. Thomas Bjarnsholt et al., "Antibiofilm Properties of Acetic Acid," *Advances in Wound Care* 4, no. 7 (July 2015): 363–72, https://doi.org/10.1089/wound.2014.0554.
159. Maria Ukhanova et al., "Effects of Almond and Pistachio Consumption on Gut Microbiota Composition in a Randomized Cross-Over Human Feeding Study," *British Journal of Nutrition* 11, no. 12 (June 2014): 2145–52, https://doi.org/10.1017/S0007114514000385.
160. Lauri O. Byerley et al., "Changes in the Gut Microbial Communities Following Addition of Walnuts to the Diet," *The Journal of Nutritional Biochemistry* 48 (October 2017): 94–102, https://doi.org/10.1016/j.jnutbio.2017.07.001.
161. Charlotte Bamberger et al., "A Walnut-Enriched Diet Affects Gut Microbiome in Healthy Caucasian Subjects: A Randomized, Controlled Trial," *Nutrients* 10, no. 2 (February 2018): 244, https://doi.org/10.3390/nu10020244.
162. Muthukumaran Jayachandran, Jianbo Xiao, and Baojun Xu, "A Critical Review on Health Promoting Benefits of Edible Mushrooms Through Gut Microbiota," *International Journal of Molecular Sciences* 18, no. 9 (September 2017): 1934, https://doi.org/10.3390/ijms18091934.
163. Case Western Reserve University, "High Fat Diet Reduces Gut Bacteria, Crohn's Disease Symptoms," ScienceDaily, June 22, 2017, www.sciencedaily.com/releases/2017/06/170622121911.htm.
164. Sabri Ahmed Rial et al., "Gut Microbiota and Metabolic Health: The Potential Beneficial Effects of a Medium Chain Triglyceride Diet in Obese Individuals," *Nutrients* 8, no. 5 (May 2016): 281, https://dx.doi.org/10.3390%2Fnu8050281.
165. Jose C. Clemente et al., "The Microbiome of Uncontacted Amerindians," *Science Advances* 1, no. 3 (April 2015): https://doi.org/10.1126/sciadv.1500183.
166. Erica Sonnenburg, "You May Be on a Paleo Diet, but Is Your Microbiome?," *Psychology Today*, June 22, 2015, www.psychologytoday.com/us/blog/the-good-gut/201506/you-may-be-paleo-diet-is-your-microbiome.
167. Francesca De Filippis et al., "High-Level Adherence to a Mediterranean Diet Beneficially Impacts the Gut Microbiota and Associated Metabolome,"

Gut 65, no. 11 (November 2016): 1812–21, https://doi.org/10.1136/gutjnl-2015-309957.

168. Evdokia K. Mitsou et al., "Adherence to the Mediterranean Diet Is Associated with the Gut Microbiota Pattern and Gastrointestinal Characteristics in an Adult Population," *British Journal of Nutrition* 117, no. 12 (June 2017): 1645–55, https://doi.org/10.1017/S0007114517001593.
169. Aurélie Cotillard et al., "Dietary Intervention Impact on Gut Microbial Gene Richness," *Nature* 502, no. 7472 (August 2013): 585, https://doi.org/10.1038/nature12480.
170. Basson, Lam, and Cominelli, "Complementary and Alternative Medicine Strategies."
171. Emma P. Halmos et al., "Diets That Differ in Their FODMAP content Alter the Colonic Luminal Microenvironment," *Gut* 64, no. 1 (January 2015): 93–100, https://doi.org/10.1136/gutjnl-2014-307264; T. J. Sloan et al., "A low FODMAP diet is associated with changes in the microbiota and reduction in breath hydrogen but not colonic volume in healthy subjects," *PLoS ONE* 13, no. 7 (2018): e0201410, https://doi.org/10.1371/journal.pone.0201410; Sofia Reddel, Lorenza Putignani, Federica Del Chierico, "The Impact of Low-FODMAPs, Gluten-Free, and Ketogenic Diets on Gut Microbiota Modulation in Pathological Conditions, *Nutrients* 11, no. 2 (2019): 373.
172. Erica D. Sonnenburg and Justin L. Sonnenburg, "Starving Our Microbial Self: The Deleterious Consequences of a Diet Deficient in Microbiota-Accessible Carbohydrates," *Cell Metabolism* 4, no. 20 (November 2014): 779–86, https://doi.org/10.1016/j.cmet.2014.07.003.
173. Femke Lutgendorff, Louis M.A. Akkermans, and Johan D. Söderholm, "The Role of Microbiota and Probiotics in Stress-Induced Gastro-Intestinal Damage," *Current Molecular Medicine* 8, no. 4 (June 2008): 282–98, https://doi.org/10.2174/156652408784533779.
174. American Psychological Association, "Stress in America: The State of Our Nation," news release, November 1, 2017, www.apa.org/news/press/releases/stress/2017/state-nation.pdf.
175. Jeffrey D. Galley and Michael T. Bailey, "Impact of Stressor Exposure on the Interplay between Commensal Microbiota and Host Inflammation," *Gut Microbes* 5, no. 3 (May/June 2014): 390–96, https://doi.org/10.4161/gmic.28683.
176. Basson, Lam, and Cominelli, "Complementary and Alternative Medicine Strategies."

177. Jacob M. Allen et al., "Exercise Alters Gut Microbiota Composition and Function in Lean and Obese Humans," *Medicine and Science in Sports and Exercise* 50, no. 4 (April 2018): 747–57, https://doi.org/10.1249/MSS.0000000000001495.
178. Jane L. Benjamin et al., "Smokers with Active Crohn's Disease Have a Clinically Relevant Dysbiosis of the Gastrointestinal Microbiota," *Inflammatory Bowel Diseases* 18, no. 6 (June 2012): 1092–1100, https://doi.org/10.1002/ibd.21864.
179. Christoph A. Thaiss et al., "Transkingdom Control of Microbiota Diurnal Oscillations Promotes Metabolic Homeostasis," *Cell* 159, no. 3 (October 2014): 514–29, https://doi.org/10.1016/j.cell.2014.09.048.
180. Robin M. Voigt et al., "Circadian Disorganization Alters Intestinal Microbiota," *PLoS One* 9, no. 5 (May 2014): 397500, https://doi.org/10.1371/journal.pone.0097500.
181. Ghannoum, "Studies on the Anticandidal Mode of Action of Allium Sativum (Garlic)."
182. Lara Bull-Otterson et al., "Metagenomic Analyses of Alcohol Induced Pathogenic Alterations in the Intestinal Microbiome and the Effect of *Lactobacillus rhamnosus* GG Treatment," *PLoS One* 8, no. 1 (January 2013): e53028, https://doi.org/10.1371/journal.pone.0053028. Ece A. Mutlu et al., "Colonic Microbiome Is Altered in Alcoholism," *American Journal of Physiology: Gastrointestinal and Liver Physiology* 302, no. 9 (May 2012): G966-G978, https://doi.org/10.1152/ajpgi.00380.2011.
183. C. Carvalho et al., "Organic and Conventional Coffee Arabic L.: A Comparative Study of the Chemical Composition and Physiological, Biochemical, and Toxicological Effects in Wistar Rats," *Plant Foods for Human Nutrition* 66, no. 2 (June 2011): 114–21.
184. Kimberly F. Allred et al., "Trigonelline is a Novel Phytoestrogen in Coffee Beans," *The Journal of Nutrition* 139, no. 10 (October 2009): 1833–38.
185. M. Messina, "Soy Foods, Isoflavones, and the Health of Postmenopausal Women," *American Journal of Clinical Nutrition* 100 Supplement 1 (July 2014): 423S-30S.
186. D. N. Butteiger et al., "Soy Protein Compared with Milk Protein in a Western Diet Increases Gut Microbial Diversity and Reduces Serum Lipids in Golden Syrian Hamsters," *The Journal of Nutrition*, published online March 2, 2016, www.ncbi.nlm.nih.gov/pubmed/26936141.
187. Inés Martinez et al., "Gut Microbiome Composition Is Linked to Whole Grain-Induced Immunological Improvements," *The International Society*

for Microbial Ecology Journal 7, no. 2 (February 2013): 269–80, https://dx.doi.org/10.1038%2Fismej.2012.104.

188. Phillip J. Brantley, Valerie H. Myers, and Heli J. Roy, "Environmental and Lifestyle Influences on Obesity," *The Journal of the Louisiana State Medical Society* 157, no. 1 (January 2005): S19-27, www.ncbi.nlm.nih.gov/pubmed/15751906.
189. Evangelia Legaki and Maria Gazouli, "Influence of Environmental Factors in the Development of Inflammatory Bowel Diseases," *World Journal of Gastrointestinal Pharmacology and Therapeutics* 7, no. 1 (February 2016): 112–25, https://doi.org/10.4292/wjgpt.v7.i1.112.
190. Curtiss B Cook, Kay E. Wellik, and Margaret Fowke, "Geoenvironmental Diabetology," *Journal of Diabetes Science and Technology* 5, no.4 (July 2011): 834–42, https://doi.org/10.1177/193229681100500402.
191. Balazs I. Bodai and Phillip Tuso, "Breast Cancer Survivorship: A Comprehensive Review of Long-Term Medical Issues and Lifestyle Recommendations," *The Permanente Journal* 19, no. 2 (Spring 2015): 48–79, https://dx.doi.org/10.7812%2FTPP%2F14-241.
192. Timothy E. O'Toole, Daniel J. Conklin, and Aruni Bhatnagar, "Environmental Risk Factors for Heart Disease," *Reviews on Environmental Health* 23, no. 3 (July-September 2008): 167–202, www.ncbi.nlm.nih.gov/pubmed/19119685.
193. Myles S. Faith and Tanja V. E. Kral, "Social Environmental and Genetic Influences on Obesity and Obesity-Promoting Behaviors: Fostering Research Integration," in *Genes, Behavior, and the Social Environment: Moving Beyond the Nature/Nurture Debate* (Washington, DC: National Academies Press, 2006), www.ncbi.nlm.nih.gov/books/NBK19935
194. Mark A. Hyman, Dean Ornish, and Michael Roizen, "Lifestyle Medicine: Treating the Causes of Disease," *Alternative Therapies* 15, no. 6 (November/December 2009): 12–14, https://drhyman.com/downloads/Lifestyle-Medicine.pdf.
195. Suleen S. Ho et al., "Effects of Chronic Exercise Training on Inflammatory Markers in Australian Overweight and Obese Individuals in a Randomized Controlled Trial," *Inflammation* 36, no. 3 (June 2013): 625–32, https://doi.org/10.1007/s10753-012-9584-9; Paul V. Tisi et al., "Exercise Training for Intermittent Claudication: Does It Adversely Affect Biochemical Markers of the Exercise-Induced Inflammatory Response?," *European Journal of Vascular and Endovascular Surgery* 14, no. 5 (1997): 344–50.
196. Stefano Balducci et al., "Anti-Inflammatory Effect of Exercise Training in

Subjects with Type 2 Diabetes and the Metabolic Syndrome Is Dependent on Exercise Modalities and Independent of Weight Loss," *Nutrition, Metabolism, and Cardiovascular Diseases* 20, no. 8 (October 2010): 608–17, https://doi.org/10.1016/j.numecd.2009.04.015.

197. BeiBei Luo et al., "The Effects of Moderate Exercise on Chronic Stress-Induced Intestinal Barrier Dysfunction and Antimicrobial Defense," *Brain, Bebavior, and Immunity* 39 (July 2014): 99–106, https://doi.org/10.1016/j.bbi.2013.11.013.

198. Mohyyodin Qamar and Alan E. A. Read, "Effects of Exercise on Mesenteric Blood Flow in Man," *Gut* 28, no. 5 (May 1987): 583–87.

199. Wojtek J. Chodzko-Zajko et al., "American College of Sports Medicine Position Stand: Exercise and Physical Activity for Older Adults," *Medicine and Science in Sports and Exercise* 41, no. 7 (July 2009): 1510–30, https://doi.org/10.1249/MSS.0b013e3181a0c95c.

200. "National Sleep Foundation Recommends New Sleep Times," National Sleep Foundation, February 2, 2015, www.sleepfoundation.org/press-release/national-sleep-foundation-recommends-new-sleep-times.

201. Valeriy A. Poroyko et al., "Chronic Sleep Disruption Alters Gut Microbiota, Induces Systemic and Adipose Tissue Inflammation and Insulin Resistance in Mice," *Scientific Reports* 6 (October 2016): 35405, https://doi.org/10.1038/srep35405.

202. Jonathan Halpern et al., "Yoga for Improving Sleep Quality and Quality of Life for Older Adults," *Alternative Therapies in Health and Medicine* 20, no. 3 (May-June 2014): 37–46, www.ncbi.nlm.nih.gov/pubmed/24755569.

203. Ziv Savin et al., "Smoking and the Intestinal Microbiome," *Archives of Microbiology* 200, no. 5 (July 2018): 677–84, https://doi.org/10.1007/s00203-018-1506-2.

204. Hans K. Biesalski, "Nutrition Meets the Microbiome: Micronutrients and the Microbiota," in "Nutrition and the Microbiome," ed. Karin Moelling, special issue, *Annals of the New York Academy of Sciences* 1372, no. 1 (May 2016): 53–64, https://doi.org/10.1111/nyas.13145.

205. Andrew L. Kau et al., "Human Nutrition, the Gut Microbiome, and Immune System: Envisioning the Future," *Nature* 474, no. 7351 (June 2011): 327–36, https://dx.doi.org/10.1038%2Fnature10213.

206. Sanil Rege and James Graham, "The Simplified Guide to the Gut-Brain Axis—How the Gut and The Brain Talk to Each Other," Psych Scene Hub, June 27, 2017, psychscenehub.com/psychinsights/the-simplified-guide-to-the-gut-brain-axis.

207. Marilia Carabotti et al., "The Gut-Brain Axis: Interactions between Enteric Microbiota, Central and Enteric Nervous Systems," *Annals of Gastroenterology* 28, no. 2 (April–June 2015): 203–9, www.ncbi.nlm.nih.gov/pmc/articles/PMC4367209.
208. Ibid.
209. Sang H. Rhee, Charalabos Pothoulakis, and Emeran A. Mayer, "Principles and Clinical Implications of the Brain-Gut-Enteric Microbiota Axis," *Nature Reviews Gastroenterology & Hepatology* 6, no. 5 (May 2009): 306–14, https://doi.org/10.1038/nrgastro.2009.35.
210. Raphael Enaud et al., "The Mycobiome: A Neglected Component in the Microbiota-Gut-Brain Axis," *Microorganisms* 6, no. 1 (March 2018): 22, https://doi.org/10.3390/microorganisms6010022.
211. Ibid.
212. Chloe E. Huseyin et al., "Forgotten Fungi—The Gut Mycobiome in Human Health and Disease," *FEMS Microbiol Reviews* 41, no. 4 (July 2017): 479–511, https://doi.org/10.1093/femsre/fuw047.
213. Rosa Krajmalnik-Brown et al., "Gut Bacteria in Children with Autism Spectrum Disorders: Challenges and Promise of Studying How a Complex Community Influences a Complex Disease," in "The Microbiome in Autism Spectrum Disorder," ed. Richard E. Frye and John Slattery, supplement, *Microbial Ecology in Health and Disease* 26, no. S1 (March 2015): 26914, https://doi.org/10.3402/mehd.v26.26914.
214. B. Rael Cahn et al., "Yoga, Meditation, and Mind-Body Health: Increased BDNF, Cortisol Awakening Response, and Altered Inflammatory Marker Expression After a 3-Month Yoga and Meditation Retreat," *Frontiers in Human Neuroscience* 11 (June 2017): 315, https://dx.doi.org/10.3389%2Ffnhum.2017.00315.
215. Jonathan Halpern et al., "Yoga for Improving Sleep Quality and Quality of Life for Older Adults," *Alternative Therapies in Health and Medicine* 20, no. 3 (2014): 37–46, www.ncbi.nlm.nih.gov/pubmed/24755569.
216. B. Real Cahn and John Polich, "Meditation States and Traits: EEG, ERP, and Neuroimaging Studies," *Psychology Bulletin* 132, no. 2 (March 2006): 180–211, https://doi.org/10.1037/0033-2909.132.2.180.
217. Ayman Mukerji Househam et al., "The Effects of Stress and Meditation on the Immune System, Human Microbiota, and Epigenetics," *Advances in Mind-Body Medicine* 31, no. 4 (Fall 2017).
218. Richard J. Davidson and Bruce S. McEwen, "Social Influences on Neuroplasticity: Stress and Interventions to Promote Well-Being," *Nature Neu-*

roscience 15, no. 2 (April 2012): 689–95, https://dx.doi.org/10.1038%2Fnn.3093; Katya Rubia, "The Neurobiology of Meditation and Its Clinical Effectiveness in Psychiatric Disorders," *Biological Psychology* 82, no. 1 (September 2009): 1–11, https://doi.org/10.1016/j.biopsycho.2009.04.003.

219. Individuals signed informed consent forms before sending their samples.
220. "Microbiome Analysis," *NIH Human Microbiome Project,* https://hmpdacc.org/hmp/micro_analysis/microbiome_analyses.php.
221. G. Rizzatti et al., "Proteobacteria: A Common Factor in Human Diseases," *BioMed Research International* 2017, Article ID 9351507 (November 2017): 7 pp. N. R. Shin, T. W. Whon, and J. W. Bae, "Proteobacteria: Microbial Signature of Dysbiosis in Gut Microbiota," *Trends in Biotechnology* 33, no. 9 (September 2015): 496–503.
222. M. Mar Rodríguez et al., "Obesity Changes the Human Gut Mycobiome."
223. Ming Cui, et al., "Circadian Rhythm Shapes the Gut Microbiota Affecting Host Radiosensitivity," *International Journal of Molecular Sciences,* 17, no. 11 (November 2016): 1786. Christoph A. Thaiss, et al., "Transkingdom Control of Microbiota Diurnal Oscillations Promotes Metabolic Homeostasis," *Cell* 159, no. 3 (October 2014): P514–29.
224. Ibid.
225. Ibid.
226. R. Jumpertz et al., "Energy-Balance Studies Reveal Associations Between Gut Microbes, Caloric Load, and Nutrient Absorption in Humans," *American Journal of Clinical Nutrition* 94, no. 1 (July 2011): 58–64.
227. American Dietetic Association, "Position of the American Dietetic Association: Food Fortification and Dietary Supplements," *Journal of the American Dietetic Association* 101 (2001): 115–25; Department of Agriculture, Department of Health and Human Services, "Nutrition and Your Health: Dietary Guidelines for Americans," 5th edition, Washington, D.C.: Government Printing Office, 2000.
228. BN Ames, "Micronutrient Deficiencies: A Major Cause of DNA Damage," *Annals of the New York Academy of Sciences* 889 (1999): 87–106.
229. Susanne Hempel, Sydne J. Newberry, Alicia R. Maher, "Probiotics for the Prevention and Treatment of Antibiotic-Associated Diarrhea," *JAMA* 307, no. 18 (2012): 1959–69.
230. Aeg Hovhannisyan et al., "Efficacy of Adaptogenic Supplements on Adapting to Stress: A Randomized, Controlled Trial," *Journal of Athletic Enhancement* 4, no. 4 (September 2016); Alexander Panossian, Georg Wikman, Punit Kaur, and Alexzander Asea, "Adaptogens Exert a Stress-Protective

Effect by Modulation of Expression of Molecular Chaperones," *Phytomedicine* 16, no. 6–7 (June 2009): 617–22; Alexander Panossian and George Wikman, "Effects of Adaptogens on the Central Nervous System and the Molecular Mechanisms Associated with Their Stress-Protective Activity," *Pharmaceuticals* 3, no. 1 (2010): 188–224.

231. Colin Hill et al., "Expert Consensus Document: The International Scientific Association for Probiotics and Prebiotics Consensus Statement on the Scope and Appropriate Use of the Term Probiotic," *Nature Reviews: Gastro Gastroenterology & Hepatology* 11, no. 8 (August 2014): 506–14.
232. Hovhannisyan et al., "Efficacy of Adaptogenic Supplements"; also Panossian, "Adaptogens Exert a Stress-Protective Effect"; and Panossian, "Effects of Adaptogens on the Central Nervous System."
233. Liyan Zhang, Nan Li, Ricardo Caicedo, and Josef Neu, "Alive and Dead *Lactobacillus rhamnosus* GG Decreases Tumor Necrosis Factor-Alpha-Induced Interleukin-8 Production in Caco-2 Cells," *The Journal of Nutrition* 135, no. 7 (July 2005): 1752–56; A. Oksaharju et al., "Probiotic *Lactobacillus rhamnosus* Downregulates FCER1 and HRH4 Expression in Human Mast Cells, *World Journal of Gastroenterology* 17, no. 6 (2011): 750–59.
234. Theodoros Kekesidis, Charalabos Pothoulakis, "Efficacy and Safety of the Probiotic *Saccharomyces boulardii* for the Prevention and Therapy of Gastrointestinal Disorders," *Therapeutic Advances in Gastroenterology* 5, no. 2 (March 2012): 111–25.
235. Jane Mea Natividad et al., "Differential Induction of Antimicrobial REGIII by the Intestinal Microbiota and *Bificobacterium breve* NCC2950," *Applied and Environmental Microbiology* 79, no. 24 (December 2013): 7745–54.
236. Conlon and Bird, "The Impact of Diet and Lifestyle on Gut Microbiota."
237. Thomas F. Hehemann et al., "Environmental and Gut Bacteroidetes: The Food Connection," *Frontiers in Microbiology* 2, no. 93 (May 2011).
238. J. Slavin, "Fiber and Prebiotics: Mechanisms and Health Benefits," *Nutrients* 5, no. 4 (April 2013): 1417–5.
239. Nikki Calabrese and Phyllis Cellini Braun, "The Effects of Tea Polyphenols on *Candida albicans*: Inhibition of Biofilm Formation and Proteasome Inactivation," *Canadian Journal of Microbiology* 55, no. 9 (September 2009): 1033–39.
240. Liyan Zhang, Nan Li, Ricardo Caicedo, and Josef Neu, "Alive and Dead *Lactobacillus rhamnosus* GG Decreases Tumor Necrosis Factor-Alpha-Induced Interleukin-8 Production in Caco-2 Cells," *The Journal of Nutrition* 135, no. 7 (July 2005): 1752–56; A. Oksaharju et al., "Probiotic *Lactobacillus rham-*

nosus Downregulates FCER1 and HRH4 Expression in Human Mast Cells, *World Journal of Gastroenterology* 17, no. 6 (2011): 750–59.

241. Jane Mea Natividad et al., "Differential Induction of Antimicrobial REGIII by the Intestinal Microbiota and *Bificobacterium breve* NCC2950, *Applied and Environmental Microbiology* 79, no. 24 (December 2013): 7745–54.
242. Theodoros Kekesidis and Charalabos Pothoulakis, "Efficacy and Safety of the Probiotic *Saccharomyces boulardii* for the Prevention and Therapy of Gastrointestinal Disorders," *Therapeutic Advances in Gastroenterology* 5, no. 2 (March 2012): 111–25.
243. C. Kumamoto, "Inflammation and Gastrointestinal *Candida* Colonization," *Current Opinions in Microbiology* 14, no. 4 (August 2011): 386–91.
244. Kadur Ramamurthy Raveendra et al., "An Extract of Glycyrrhiza glabra (GutGard) Alleviates Symptoms of Functional Dyspepsia: A Randomized, Double-Blind, Placebo-Controlled Study," *Evidence-Based Complementary and Alternative Medicine* 2012, Article ID 216970, 9 pp.
245. A. Deters et al., "Aqueous Extracts and Polysaccharides from Marshmallow Roots (althea officinalis L.): Cellular Internalisation and Stimulation of Cell Physiology of Human Epthithelial Cells in vitro," *Journal of Ethnopharmacology* 127, no. 1 (January 2010): 62–9.
246. W. W. Wang et al., "Amino Acids and Gut Function," *Amino Acids* 37, no. 1 (May 2009): 105–10.
247. E. Cario et al., "Effects of Exogenous Zinc Supplementation on Intestinal Epithelial Repair *in vitro*," *European Journal of Clinical Investigation* 30, no. 5 (May 2000): 419–28.
248. F.S.W. McCullough, Christine Northrop-Clewes, and David I. Thurnham, "The Effect of Vitamin A on Epithelial Integrity," *Proceedings of The Nutrition Society* 58, no. 2 (June 1999): 289–93.
249. A. W. Zhang et al., "The Relation Between Gastric Vitamin C Concentrations, Mucosal Histology, and CagA Seropositivity in the Human Stomach," *gut* 43 (1998): 322–26.
250. Katherine Harmon Courage, "Why Is Dark Chocolate Good for You? Thank Your Microbes," *Scientific American*, March 19, 2014, www.scientificamerican.com/article/why-is-dark-chocolate-good-for-you-thank-your-microbes.
251. Nabil Hayek, "Chocolate, Gut Microbiota, and Human Health," *Frontiers in Pharmacology* 4 (February 2013): 11.
252. Yi Zou et al., "Oregano Essential Oil Improves Intestinal Morphology and Expression of Tight Junction Proteins Associated with Modula-

tion of Selected Intestinal Bacteria and Immune Status in a Pig Model," *BioMed Research International* (2016): 5436738, https://dx.doi.org/10.1155%2F2016%2F5436738.

253. Victor Chedid et al., "Herbal Therapy Is Equivalent to Rifaximin for the Treatment of Small Intestinal Bacterial Overgrowth," *Global Advances in Health and Medicine* 3, no. 3 (May 2014): 16–24, https://dx.doi.org/10.7453%2Fgahmj.2014.019.

254. Penn State University, "Using Mushrooms as a Prebiotic May Help Improve Glucose Regulation," ScienceDaily, August 16, 2018, www.sciencedaily.com/releases/2018/08/180816105524.htm.

255. Muthukumaran Jayachandran, Jianbo Xiao, and Baoiun Xu, "A Critical Review on Health Promoting Benefits of Edible Mushrooms Through Gut Microbiota," *International Journal of Molecular Science* 18, no. 9 (September 2017): E1934, https://doi.org/10.3390/ijms18091934.

256. Henry Ostrowski Meissner et al., "Therapeutic Effects of Pre-Gelatinized Maca (Lepidium Peruvianum Chacon) Used as a Non-Hormonal Alternative to HRT in Perimenopausal Women—Clinical Pilot Study," *International Journal of Biomedical Science* 2, no. 2 (June 2006): 143–59, www.ncbi.nlm.nih.gov/pubmed/23674976.

257. Ji-Hyun Yun et al., "Social Status Shapes the Bacterial and Fungal Gut Communities of the Honey Bee," *Scientific Reports* 8 (January 2018): 2019, https://doi.org/10.1038/s41598-018-19860-7.

258. Michael J. Keenan et al., "Role of Resistant Starch in Improving Gut Health, Adiposity, and Insulin Resistance," Advances in Nutrition 6, no. 2 (March 2015): 192–205, https://doi.org/10.3945/an.114.007419.

259. Wolfgang Scheppach, "Effects of Short Chain Fatty Acids on Gut Morphology and Function," Gut 35, Supplement 1 (January 1994): S35–S38, www.ncbi.nlm.nih.gov/pmc/articles/PMC1378144.

260. Janine A. Higgins and Ian L. Brown, "Resistant Starch: A Promising Dietary Agent for the Prevention/Treatment of Inflammatory Bowel Disease and Bowel Cancer," Current Opinion in Gastroenterology 29, no. 2 (March 2013): 190–94.

261. K. Schrom, Mahmoud A. Ghannoum, et al., "Consumption of a Novel Probiotic Leads to Beneficial Structural Functional Changes in the Gut Bacteriome and Mycobiome of Human Volunteers," presented at ASM Microbes Meeting, Atlanta, Georgia, June 2018.

INDEX

Note: *Italicized* pages refer to diagrams, photos, or tables.

C

G

H

ABOUT THE AUTHOR

Dr. Mahmoud Ghannoum is a tenured professor and director of the Center for Medical Mycology at Case Western Reserve University and University Hospitals Cleveland Medical Center in Cleveland, Ohio. Educated in Lebanon, England, and the United States, he received his PhD in Microbial Physiology from University of Technology in England and an Executive MBA from the Weatherhead School of Management at Case Western Reserve University. He has spent his entire career studying medically important fungi and publishing extensively about their virulence factors, especially in microbial biofilms.

Over the past decade, Dr. Ghannoum recognized the role of the microbial community (both bacterial and fungal) in human health and published the first study describing the oral fungal community, coining the term "mycobiome." He described the bacterial microbiome (bacteriome) and the mycobiome in HIV-infected patients, and led the characterization of the interaction between bacteria and fungi as they relate to health and disease. In 2016, he published an opinion piece in *The Scientist* on the contribution of the mycobiome to human health and was consequently invited to speak at a number of meetings organized by the National Institutes of Health. He conducted a study characterizing the bacterial and fungal communities in Crohn's disease patients that resulted in the first model of microbiome dysbiosis that implicated cooperation between bacteria and fungi in biofilms. This work resulted in a publication that received national and international coverage.

Dr. Ghannoum is also a fellow of the Infectious Disease Society of America and past President of the Medical Mycological Society of the Americas (MMSA). He has received many distinguished awards for his research, and in 2013, he was selected as "Most Interesting Person" by *Cleveland Magazine*. In 2016, he received the Rohda Benham Award presented for his continuous outstanding and meritorious contributions to medical mycology from the Medical Mycological Society of the Americas and the Freedom to Discover Award from Bristol-Myers Squibb for his work on microbial biofilms. In 2017, he was inducted as a fellow of the American Academy of Microbiology. He continues to be a pioneer in the characterization of the human microbiome.

With over 400 peer-reviewed publications to his credit and six published books on antifungal therapy, microbial biofilms, *Candida* adherence, and related topics, Dr. Ghannoum continues to be a prominent leader in his field. The National Institutes of Health has continually funded his research since 1994, and he recently received a large NIH grant to study the mechanism(s) of bacterial/fungal interaction in intestinal inflammation, such as in colitis and Crohn's disease. He has also consulted for many international pharmaceutical and biotech companies, and cofounded multiple successful and profitable companies, including BIOHM Health, launched in 2016, that engineer products and services to address the critical role of the bacterial and fungal communities in digestive and overall health and wellness. BIOHM Health was just awarded the Science and Innovation Award by *Nutrition Business Journal*. He lives in Cleveland with his wife, children, and grandchildren.